Théodule Ribot

Heredity

A Psychological Study of its Phenomena, Laws, Causes and Consequences

Théodule Ribot

Heredity

A Psychological Study of its Phenomena, Laws, Causes and Consequences

ISBN/EAN: 9783337232153

Printed in Europe, USA, Canada, Australia, Japan

Cover: Foto ©Thomas Meinert / pixelio.de

More available books at **www.hansebooks.com**

HEREDITY:

A PSYCHOLOGICAL STUDY OF ITS PHENOMENA,
LAWS, CAUSES, AND CONSEQUENCES.

FROM THE FRENCH OF
TH. RIBOT,
AUTHOR OF "CONTEMPORARY ENGLISH PSYCHOLOGY."

NEW YORK:
D. APPLETON AND COMPANY,
1, 3, AND 5 BOND STREET.
1889.

CONTENTS.

INTRODUCTION.

PART FIRST.

THE FACTS.

CHAPTER III.

HEREDITY OF THE MEMORY.

CHAPTER IV.

HEREDITY OF THE IMAGINATION.

CHAPTER V.

HEREDITY OF THE INTELLECT.

CHAPTER VI.

HEREDITY OF THE SENTIMENTS AND THE PASSIONS.

CHAPTER VII.

HEREDITY OF THE WILL.

CHAPTER III.

ESSAYS IN STATISTICS.

CHAPTER IV.

EXCEPTIONS TO THE LAW OF HEREDITY.

PART THIRD.

THE CAUSES.

CHAPTER I.

GENERAL RELATIONS BETWEEN THE PHYSICAL AND THE MORAL.

HEREDITY.

———◆———

INTRODUCTION.

PHYSIOLOGICAL HEREDITY.

HEREDITY is that biological law by which all beings endowed with life tend to repeat themselves in their descendants: it is for the species what personal identity is for the individual. By it a groundwork remains unchanged amid incessant variation; by it Nature ever copies and imitates herself. Ideally considered, heredity would simply be the reproduction of like by like. But this conception is purely theoretical, for the phenomena of life do not lend themselves to such mathematical precision: the conditions of their occurrence grow more and more complex in proportion as we ascend from the vegetable world to the higher animals, and thence to man.

Man may be regarded either in his organism or in his dynamism: in the functions which constitute his physical life, or in the operations which constitute his mental life. Are both of these forms of life subject to the law of heredity? are they subject to it wholly, or only in part? and, in the latter case, to what extent are they so subject?

The physiological side of this question has been diligently studied, but not so its psychological side. We propose to supply this deficiency in the present work. But the hereditary transmission of mental faculties—considered in its phenomena, its laws, its consequences, and especially in its causes—is so closely connected with physiological heredity, that we are compelled to consider this latter subject at the outset. This we will do very briefly, referring the reader for fuller details to special treatises. It will suffice to show, by means of a few definite and well-ascertained facts, that heredity extends over all the elements and functions of the organism; to its external and internal structure, its maladies, its special characteristics, and its acquired modifications.

The first thing that attracts the attention, even of the unobservant, is the heredity of the external structure. This is a fact of everyday experience, and nothing is more common than to hear that such and such a child is the image of its father, mother, or grandparents. Hereditary influence may manifest itself in the limbs, the trunk, the head, even in the nails and the hair, but especially in the countenance, expression, or characteristic features. This is an observation made by the ancients; hence the Romans had their *Nasones, Labeones, Buccones, Capitones,* and other names, derived from hereditary peculiarities. According to Haller, the Bentivoglios had on their bodies a slightly prominent tumour, transmitted from father to son, which warned them of changes in the weather, and which grew larger whenever a moist wind was coming. The resemblance may be so close as to give rise to doubts concerning personal identity, or at once to betray parentage. Ten years before his death a singer at the opera, named Nourrit, appeared on the stage with one of his sons, who had inherited his physical constitution as well as his pleasing voice; and in a play with a plot like that of the *Menæchmi,* the extraordinary resemblance of the son to the father added a hundred-fold interest to the endless misunderstandings with which the play was filled.[1] These hereditary resemblances have sometimes led to the most unexpected and most romantic adventures, so that it is not surprising that Marryat has turned them to account in his novel, '*Japhet in Search of a Father.*'

It is still more singular that this resemblance between parents and children may undergo such metamorphoses as shall cause the child to resemble at one time the father, and at another the

---

[1] P. Lucas, *Traité Physiologique et Philosophique de l'Hérédité Naturelle,* vol. i. p. 195.

mother. Girou de Buzareingues, in his work *De la Génération*, containing some curious facts observed by him, tells us that he knew two brothers who in early life resembled their mother, while their sister resembled the father. These resemblances were such as to strike all who saw them. ' But now, ' says he, 'and ever since their youth, the two boys resemble the father, while the daughter has ceased to be like him.' This same author was led, in consequence of numerous observations, to believe that changes of this kind are more frequent and more thorough in the case of boys than in that of girls.

The system of intentional and conscious selection has been applied even to man. Frederick William I., the father of Frederick the Great, who was noted for his love of colossal men, dealt with his regiment of giants as stock-breeders deal with their cattle. He would not allow his guards to marry women of stature inferior to their own. Haller used to boast of his ' belonging to one of those races whose members, by reason of their imposing stature, seem born to rule other men.'

Heredity may be also traced in all that concerns the complexion of the skin, and the shape and size of the body. Thus, so truly is obesity the result of an organic predisposition, that it has often been known to make its appearance amid privations, and under all the disadvantages of hard labour and poverty.

Heredity influences the internal conformation no less than the external structure. Nothing is more undisputed than the heredity of the form, size, and anomalies of the osseous system ; and universal everyday experience proves the heredity of all the proportions of the cranium, thorax, pelvis, vertebral column, and the smallest bones of the skeleton. Even the heredity of excess or defect in the number of the vertebræ and the teeth has been ascertained. (Lucas.) The circulatory, digestive, and muscular systems obey the same laws which govern the transmission of the other internal systems of the organism. There are some families in which the heart and the size of the principal blood-vessels are naturally very large ; others in which they are comparatively small ; and others, again, which present identical faults of conformation. Lastly—and this is a point that more nearly concerns us— heredity regulates the proportions of the nervous system. It is evident in the general dimensions of the brain, the principal organ of that system; it is very often apparent in the size, and even in the form, of the cerebral convolutions. This fact was observed by Gall, who thereby accounted for the transmission of mental faculties. We need not here dwell upon this point, for we shall have frequent occasion to revert to it in the course of the present work.

Heredity of the internal elements occurs in the fluids of the organism, as well as in the solid parts : the blood is more abundant in some families than in others, and this superabundance transmits, or may transmit, to the members of such families, a pre-disposition to apoplexy, hemorrhage, and inflammation. Thus there exists in some families such a liability to hemorrhage that even the prick of a pin may cause in them a flow of blood that cannot be checked. The same may be said with regard to the bile and the lymph.

Nor is it merely, as might be supposed, the structure, whether internal or external, that is thus transmissible ; some quite peculiar characteristics of the mode of existence pass from parent to child. Heredity governs the subordinate no less than the domi-nant characteristics. Thus fecundity, length of life, and those purely personal characteristics which physicians call idiosyncrasies, are hereditarily transmitted. A few facts will confirm this.

There is no doubt of the influence of heredity on the repro-ductive power. Some families are noted for their fecundity, and this fecundity descends either through the father or through the mother.

A mother gave birth to twenty-four children, among them five girls, who in turn gave birth to forty-six children in all. The daughter of this woman's son, while still young, was brought to bed with her sixteenth child. (Girou.) The sons, daughters, and grand children of a couple who were the parents of nineteen children were nearly all gifted, says Lucas, with the same fecundity.

Several families belonging to the old French nobility possessed extraordinary powers of propagation. Anne de Montmorency (who when over seventy-five years of age was still able, at the battle of St. Denis, to break with his sword the teeth of the Scotch soldier who gave him his death-blow) was the father of twelve children. Three of his ancestors—Mathieu I., Mathieu II., and Mathieu III.—had altogether eighteen children, of whom fifteen were boys. The son and grandson of the great Condé reckoned nineteen children between them; and their great-grandfather, who was slain at Jarnac, had ten. The first four Guises had, in all, forty-three children, thirty of them boys. Achille de Harlay, father of the first President, had nine children; his father, ten; his great-grandfather, eighteen. In some families this fecundity has persisted for five or six generations.[1]

It is now generally understood that longevity depends far less on race, climate, profession, mode of life or food, than on hereditary transmission. If we consult special treatises on this subject, we find centenarians as well among blacks as among whites; in Russia and Scotland as in Italy and Spain; among those who take the greatest care of their health as among those who have led the hardest lives. A collier in Scotland prolonged his hard and dreary existence over one hundred and thirty-three years, and worked in the mines after he was eighty.

Similar facts are to be met with among prisoners, and even galley-slaves. 'The average of life,' says Dr. Lucas, 'plainly depends on locality, hygiene, and civilization; but individual longevity is entirely exempt from these conditions. Everything tends to show that long life is the result of an internal principle of vitality, which privileged individuals receive at their birth. It is so deeply imprinted in their nature as to make itself apparent in every part of their organization.' This kind of heredity has long been observed in England, where life-assurance companies require information as to the longevity of the ancestors of those who desire to effect an insurance.

There are, also, on the other hand, many families in which the hair turns grey in early youth, and in which the vigour of the physical and intellectual faculties fails prematurely. In others, early death is of such common occurrence that only a few individuals can escape it by great precaution. In the Turgot family the fifty-ninth year was rarely passed. The man who made that family

---

[1] Benoiston de Châteauneuf, *Mémoire sur la Durée des Familles Nobles en France.*

illustrious, when he saw that fatal term approaching, remarked—though he had then every appearance of health and strength—that it was time for him to put his affairs in order, and to finish the work he had then in hand, because in his family it was usual to die at that age. He died in fact at the age of fifty-three.

The immunity from contagious diseases, and especially from small-pox, with which some families are endowed, is a well-established fact.

Heredity may transmit muscular strength, and the various forms of motor energy. In ancient times there were families of athletes, and there have been families of prize-fighters. The recent researches of Galton as to wrestlers and oarsmen show that the victors generally belong to a small number of families among whom strength and skill are hereditary. As for motor energy, a point of special importance in horses, experience long ago taught breeders that speed on the turf—just like faulty action, or cribbiting—is transmitted. Among men there are families nearly all of whose members are possessed of exquisite dexterity and grace of movement. Heredity has oftentimes transmitted a talent for dancing, of which the celebrated Vestris family is an example.

It is the same with regard to the voice. Every animal possesses the voice peculiar to its kind; but even individual characteristics are transmitted; as, for instance, stammering, speaking through the nose, and lisping. There are many families of singers, and there are also families that have no ear at all for melody. Loquacity, too, is hereditary:—'Most of the children of talkative persons,' says Dr. Lucas, 'are chatterboxes from the cradle. Words—idealess, aimless, and unbridled—appear in them to be prompted by a sort of elastic spring over which they have no control. We once saw at a friend's house a servant-girl of irrepressible loquacity. She would talk to people, who could scarcely get in a word edgewise; she would talk to dumb beasts and to inanimate things; she would talk aloud to herself. She had to be sent away. " But," said she to her employer, "it is no fault of mine: it comes to me from my father; the same fault in him drove my mother distracted; and one of his brothers was like me."'

The heredity of anomalies of organization is a well-ascertained fact. One of the strangest and best known instances of this is the case of Edward Lambert, whose whole body, with the exception of the face, the palms of the hands and the soles of the feet, was covered with a sort of carapace of horny excrescences which rattled against each other. He was the father of six children, all of whom, from the age of six weeks, presented the same singularity. The only one of these who survived transmitted it to all his sons; and this transmission, going from male to male, was kept up during five generations.[1] Albinism, rickets, lameness, ectrodactylism and polydactylism, harelip—in fact, all deviations from the type, whether they be the result of an excess or of an arrest of organic development—are transmissible. These facts are of great interest, as showing that the individual type is subject to the law of heredity, no less than the specific type.

It is a disputed question whether we must conclude that deviations from the specific type, anomalies of all kinds—such as strabismus, myopia, atrophy and hypertrophy of members—remain fixed for ever, or that heredity in such cases is only of a restricted and temporary nature. These individual deviations from law are sometimes transmitted, sometimes not. Experience would appear to show that there is a tendency towards a return to the primitive type. Thus, in the Colburn family, which presented one of the most curious instances of sexdigitism—the members of this family had each a supernumerary finger and toe—the anomaly continued through four generations; but, says Burdach,[2] the normal was steadily gaining on the abnormal.

The ratio was—

1st generation, as 1 to 35
2nd   „   „ 1 „ 14
3rd   „   „ 1 „ 3¼

The return, therefore, to the normal type took place rapidly. This brings us to the important and difficult question of the heredity of acquired modifications. All of which we have spoken— the transmission of internal and external structure, of longevity, fecundity, and idiosyncrasies—is involved in the very nature of the being as virtually constituted by the act of generation, and belongs

[1] *Philosophical Transactions*, vol. xvii. and vol. xlix.
[2] *Physiologic*, vol. ii. p. 251.

to its essence; hence it is perfectly natural that all these qualities and modifications should be transmitted to its descendants. But man cannot, any more than other animals, live without contracting habits; without undergoing, under the influence of circumstances, or from an excess or deficiency in the exercise of each organ, modifications of all kinds, which remain fixed in him. Are these transmitted? Are they destined to perish with the individual, or do they become in his descendants a new, an acquired character? The brain, for example, like every other organ, is developed by exercise. If this increase, whether of size or of energy, is transmissible, some important consequences for the mental faculties must be the result; progress will then be determined, not only outwardly and traditionally, but inwardly and organically.

We will consider this question in the course of the work; for the present we consider only the physiological phenomena.

Habit is defined to be an acquired disposition. We ask if any purely individual habits are transmitted. Instances of this are cited. Girou de Buzareingues observes that he had known a man who had the habit, when in bed, of lying on his back and crossing the right leg over the left. One of his daughters had the same habit from birth; she constantly assumed that posture in the cradle, notwithstanding the resistance offered by the napkins. 'I know many girls,' says he, 'who resemble their fathers, and who have derived from them extraordinary habits, which cannot be attributed either to imitation or to training, and boys who have habits derived from their mothers.[1] But it is impossible to enter upon any details on this subject.' Darwin notes the following instance, which came under his own observation :—a boy had the singular habit, when pleased, of rapidly moving his fingers parallel to each other; and when much excited, of raising both hands, with the fingers still moving, to the sides of his face on a level with the eyes; this boy, when almost an old man, could still hardly resist this trick when much pleased, but, from its absurdity, concealed it. He had eight children. Of these, a girl, when pleased, at the age of four and a half years, moved her fingers in exactly

---

[1] *De la Génération*, 282.

the same way; and, what is still odder, when much excited she raised both her hands, with her fingers still moving, to the sides of her face, in exactly the same way as her father had done. Handwriting depends on several physical and mental habits, and we often see a great resemblance between the handwriting of a father and a son. Even those who have no great powers of observation must often have remarked this. 'Hofacker, in Germany, has remarked that handwriting is hereditary.' The same remark will apply to France; 'and it has even been asserted that English boys, when taught to write in France, naturally cling to their English manner of writing.'[1]

What is true of habits is also true of anomalies accidentally acquired,—that they are transmissible. Thus a man whose right hand had suffered an injury had one of his fingers badly set. He had several sons, each of whom had that same finger crooked. (Blumenbach.) Artificial deformities, too, are transmissible. Three tribes in Peru—the Aymaras, the Huancas, and the Chinchas—had each their own peculiar mode of deforming the heads of their children, and this deformity has since remained. The Esquimaux, says M. de Quatrefages, cut off the tails of the dogs they harness to their sledges; the pups are often born tailless.

Notwithstanding these facts, the transmission of acquired modifications appears to be very restricted, even when occurring in both of the parents. A deaf-mute married to a deaf-mute has children who can both hear and speak. The necessity of performing circumcision on Jews shows that an acquired modification, often repeated, is not therefore hereditary. Deviations from a type, after having subsisted for generations, return to the normal state; so that many naturalists hold it as a rule that accidental modifications are not perpetuated.

This is very different to the law formulated by Lamarck :—
'Whatever Nature has enabled individuals to gain or to lose, under the influence of circumstances to which their race has been long exposed, is preserved, by generation, for the new individuals

---

[1] Darwin, *Variation of Animals and Plants under Domestication*, vol. ii. p. 6. Edition. 1868.

which descend from them, provided the changes acquired are common to the two sexes, or to those which have produced new individuals.'[1]

Still, these two opposite opinions, both of which may be supported by facts, can be reconciled if we bear in mind that there are modifications which, by their very nature, are in antagonism with everything around them, and for which, in consequence, the conditions of existence grow more and more difficult; just as there are others which, when in conformity with everything around them, may become permanent by either natural or artificial selection : so that all things conspire to blot out the former class of modifications, and to perpetuate the latter. We shall meet this difficulty again, when treating of psychological heredity, and will there consider it more fully.

We have now to speak of the last form of heredity—that of disease. This seems to have been observed from the foundation of the art of medicine—in all times, in every land, and in every nation. Even the Greek physicians recognized hereditary diseases (νόσοι κληρονομίκαι). And yet in modern times the heredity of disease has given rise to all manner of debates among medical men. It would be beyond our subject, and beyond our power, to discuss this point. It is enough to say that the question appears to be substantially settled by the fact that the sturdiest opponents of morbid heredity admit, if not the heredity of disease itself, at least the heredity of a disposition to it. In Dr. Lucas's work on Heredity will be found facts of all kinds, sufficiently numerous and sufficiently clear to warrant a conclusion.

This hasty physiological sketch will show that the law of heredity influences every form of vital energy—a fact which is generally known and admitted. Is the same to be said with regard to the psychological aspect of the question? This we propose now to consider, and to begin with the study of the facts.

---

[1] In regard to the physiological side of this controversy, see the *Bulletins de la Société d'Anthropologie*, tome i. p. 339, and particularly p. 551, seq.; tome ii., *De l'Hérédité des Anomalies.*

PART FIRST.

THE FACTS.

Rassemblons des faits pour nous donner des idées.—Buffon.

CHAPTER I.

I.

WHEN we speak of instinct, our first difficulty is to define the term. Not to enumerate here all the various significations of the word as used in ordinary language, it is employed in at least three different senses even by naturalists and philosophers, whose language has to be more precise than that of other people. Sometimes instinct is intended to signify the automatic, almost mechanical, and probably unconscious action of animals, in pursuance of an object determined by their organization, and specific characters. Again, instinct is made synonymous with desire, inclination, propensity; as when we speak of good or evil instincts, a thievish or murderous instinct. Finally, we sometimes comprise under the term instinct all the psychological phenomena occurring in animals, and all forms of mental activity inferior to those of man. This latter signification of the word is plainly the result of our unwillingness to attribute intellect to brutes; and thus, contrary to all reason, we confound with blind and unconscious impulses the conscious acts which every animal performs under the guidance of its individual experience,[1] and which, consequently, are analogous to those which, in our own case, we call intelligent or intellectual acts.

Although, in our opinion, instinct and intelligence are one and the same, as we will try hereafter to show, and though the difference between them is one not of kind, but only of degree; still we will employ the word instinct here in its first signification only which alone we hold to be exact and in conformity with etymology. We must, for the sake of greater precision, begin with a good definition of this term; but, unfortunately, no such definition has yet

---

[1] For instance, the act performed by a dog carried far from his home, when from among a score of roads he selects the one which will bring him back.

been found. Still we may, with a contemporary German philosopher, define instinct to be 'an act conformed to an end, but without consciousness of that end;'[1] or we may say, with Darwin, that 'an action which we ourselves should require experience to enable us to perform, when performed by an animal, more especially by a very young one, without any experience, and when performed by many individuals in the same way without their knowing for what purpose it is performed, is usually said to be instinctive.'[2]

If, instead of defining instinct, we endeavour to determine its characteristics, not one of which perhaps is absolutely certain and unquestioned, we find a general agreement as to the following :

Instinct is innate, *i.e.* anterior to all individual experience. Whereas intelligence is developed slowly by accumulated experiences, instinct is perfect from the first. The duckling hatched by a hen makes straight for the water ; the squirrel, before it knows anything of winter, lays up a store of nuts. A bird hatched in a cage will, when given its freedom, build for itself a nest like that of its parents, out of the same materials, and of the same shape.

Intelligence gropes about, tries this way and that, misses its object, commits mistakes and corrects them : instinct advances with a mechanical certainty. Hence comes its unconscious character ; it knows nothing either of ends, or of the means of attaining them ; it implies no comparison, judgment, or choice. All seems directed by thought, without ever arriving at thought ; and if this phenomenon appear strange, it must be observed that analogous states occur in ourselves. All that we do from habit—walking, writing, or practising a mechanical art, for instance—all these, and many other very complex acts, are performed without consciousness.

Instinct appears stationary. It does not, like intelligence, seem to grow and decay, to gain and to lose. It does not improve. If it does not remain perfectly invariable, at least it varies only within very narrow limits ; and though this question has been warmly debated in our day, and is yet unsettled, we may yet say that in instinct immutability is the law, variation the exception.

---

[1] Hartmann, *Philosophie des Unbewussten*, p. 54. Berlin, 1869.
[2] Darwin, *Origin of Species*, p. 255. Fifth Edition, 1869.

Such are the admitted characters of instinct. Though none of them is out of the reach of minute criticism ; though none of them is absolutely true, still they are sufficiently exact to serve to distinguish instinct from all other psychological phenomena.

Instinct, so defined, is, beyond all question, transmissible, and subject to the law of heredity. The animal inherits the psychical dispositions, no less than the physiological constitutions of its parents. The naturalist takes account of the former characteristics, as well as of the latter. In his eyes it is as essential for the bee to extract the pollen of flowers, construct cells and in them deposit her honey, as for her to possess mandibles, six feet, and four wings. A worker-bee with the instincts of an ant would appear to him as strange a thing as a bee with wing-sheaths and eight feet. Every animal has two chief functions—one, nutrition, which preserves the individual; another, generation, which preserves the species. The latter transmits instincts together with physical forms—generation is moral as well as material. The beaver transmits to its young its anatomical and physiological characters as a rodent mammal, its constructive instincts, and architectural talent.

Thus we find at the outset a vast number of psychological facts —instinctive actions, strictly subject to the laws of hereditary transmission. It needs no long reflection to see how large is the domain of instinct : the Invertebrata seem to be completely restricted to this form of mental activity. In the sub-kingdom of the Vertebrata, the inferior classes, such as the Fishes, Batrachians, Reptiles, Birds, have oftentimes no other means save instinct, of supporting life, of attack, defence, and recognition of enemies. Finally, among Mammals, and even in Man, instinct gradually diminishes, but never entirely disappears. Its domain, therefore, is co-extensive with animal life ; and this vast domain is governed by the laws of heredity.

Since it is an evident fact, universally admitted, that heredity is the invariable rule of the transmission of instincts, we need not cite instances to confirm our position. The tenacity of instincts is so great, and their hereditary transmission so certain, that sometimes they are found to outlive for centuries the conditions of life to which they are adapted. ' We have reason to believe,' says Darwin.

2

'that aboriginal habits are long retained under domestication. Thus with the common ass we see signs of its original desert life in its strong dislike to cross the smallest stream of water, and in its pleasure in rolling in the dust. The same strong dislike to cross a stream is common to the camel, which has been domesticated from a very ancient period. Young pigs, though so tame, sometimes squat when frightened, and thus try to conceal themselves even in an open and bare place. Young turkeys, and occasionally even young fowls, when the hen gives the danger-cry, run away and try to hide themselves, like young partridges or pheasants, in order that their mother may take flight, of which she has lost the power. The musk-duck, in its native country, often perches and roosts on trees, and our domesticated musk-ducks, though sluggish birds, are fond of perching on the tops of barns, walls, etc. . . . . . We know that the dog, however well and regularly fed, often buries, like the fox, any superfluous food; we see him turning round and round on a carpet, as if to trample down grass to form a bed. . . . . In the delight with which lambs and kids crowd together and frisk on the smallest hillock, we see a vestige of their former alpine habits.'[1]

II.

Instead of dwelling unnecessarily on the heredity of natural and primitive instincts, it will be more instructive to inquire whether acquired instincts are transmissible. We have already said, when giving, according to F. Cuvier and Flourens, the characteristics generally attributed to instinctive acts, that none of them are absolutely true. Thus, instinct is not always invariable. The beaver changes, according to circumstances, the site and form of his house, and from being a builder becomes a miner. The bee can modify her plan of construction, and substitute for hexagonal cells pentagonal cavities. In the Island of Goree the swallows remain through the whole year, because the warmth of the climate enables them to find food at all seasons. In many species the mode of nest-building varies according to the nature of the soil, the locality, and the temperature of the country. Instinct is certainly not as pliant an instrument as intelligence; it cannot, like intelligence, adapt itself

---

[1] *Variation,* etc., vol. i. p. 180.

to all media, conform to all circumstances, or vary and modify its actions in a thousand ways ; yet it is capable of modification within certain limits, when subjected to strong and lasting influences.

Two causes chiefly produce these variations : external conditions and domestication. Climate, soil, food; the dangers which habitually surround the animal, and the impressions it receives, modify its organism and consequently its instincts. The action of man is still more powerful on the animal than that of Nature : by training, man fashions and bends it to his needs or his wishes. It is not for us to inquire here how these acquired or modified instincts are produced. We have only to ask whether they are hereditary. Experience answers in the affirmative ; many facts show that acquired instincts, as well as those which are natural, are transmitted by heredity. Such are the following :—.

G. Leroy observes that in districts where a sharp war is waged against the fox, the cubs, on first coming out of their earths, and before they can have acquired any experience, are more cautious, crafty, and suspicious than are old foxes in places where no attempt is made to trap them. This he explains by the hypothesis of a language among animals. F. Cuvier has furnished the solution of the enigma by referring the fact to the heredity of modifications which are acquired by instinct. There is no doubt that the instinct of fear is acquired in many wild animals, and transmitted to their descendants. Knight, who for sixty years devoted himself to systematic observation of this class of facts, says that during that time the habits of the English woodcock under-went great changes, and that its fear of man was considerably increased by its transmission through several generations. The same author discovered similar changes of habit, even in bees. Darwin has established the fact that animals living in desert islands gradually acquire a fear of man, in proportion as they become acquainted with our methods of destroying them. He says that in England large birds are much more shy than small ones, and this, no doubt, because they are much more persecuted by man. The proof that this is the reason of the difference is found in the fact that in uninhabited islands large birds are not any more timid than small ones.[1]

---

[1] *Origin of Species*, p. 260. Fifth Edition, 1869. Lucas, ii. 432.

When an animal is capable of education, that is, when its original instincts are capable of modification, it usually requires three or four generations to fix the results of training and to prevent a return to the instincts of the wild state. If we try to hatch the eggs of wild ducks under tame ducks, the ducklings will scarce have left the egg when they obey the instinct of their race, and take their flight. If they be prevented from flying away, and kept for repro- duction, it will be several generations before we have tame ducks. The same may be said of free, or wild herds of horses. Their colts are broken with great difficulty, and even after taming they are far less docile than horses born in a state of domestication. Nay, even the mongrel progeny of wild and domesticated horses, or of wild and domesticated reindeer, take three or four genera- tions before they entirely give up the shy habits of their natural state. On the other hand, colts bred of a well-broken sire and dam oftentimes come into the world with a marked aptitude for training; and some horse-trainers have even proposed to select brood stock exclusively from among horses that have been prac- tised in the circus.

Originally man had considerable trouble in taming the animals which are now domesticated; and his work would have been in vain had not heredity come to his aid. It may be said that after man has modified a wild animal to his will, there goes on in its progeny a silent conflict between two heredities, the one tending to fix the acquired modifications, and the other to preserve the primitive instincts. The latter often get the mastery, and only after several generations is training sure of victory. But we may see that in either case heredity always asserts its rights.

Among the higher animals, which are possessed not only of instinct but also of intelligence, nothing is more common than to see mental dispositions, which have evidently been acquired, so fixed by heredity that they are confounded with instinct, so spon- taneous and so automatic do they become. Young pointers have been known to point the first time they were taken out, sometimes even better than dogs that had been for a long time in training. The habit of saving life is hereditary in breeds that have been brought up to it, as is also the shepherd-dog's habit of moving around the flock and guarding it.

Knight has shown, experimentally, the truth of the proverb "a good hound is bred so." He took every care that when the pups were first taken into the field they should receive no guidance from older dogs. Yet the very first day one of the pups stood trembling with anxiety, having his eyes fixed and all his muscles strained at the partridges which their parents had been trained to point. A spaniel, belonging to a breed that had been trained to woodcock-shooting, knew perfectly well from the first how to act like an old dog, avoiding places where the soil was frozen, and where it was therefore useless to seek the game, as in such places there is no scent. Finally, a young polecat-terrier was thrown into a state of great excitement the first time he ever saw one of these animals, while a spaniel remained perfectly calm.

In South America, according to Roulin, dogs belonging to a breed that has long been trained to the dangerous chase of the peccary, when taken for the first time into the woods, know the tactics to adopt quite as well as the old dogs, and that without any instruction. Dogs of other races, and unacquainted with the tactics, are killed at once, no matter how strong they may be. The American greyhound, instead of leaping at the throat of the stag, attacks him by the belly and throws him over, as his ancestors had been trained to do in hunting down the Indians.

Thus, then, heredity transmits acquired modification no less than natural instincts. There is, however, an important difference to be noted : the heredity of instincts admits of no exceptions, while in that of modifications there are many. It is only when variations have been firmly rooted ; when, having become organic, they constitute a second nature, which supplants the first ; when, like instinct, they have assumed a mechanical character, that they can be transmitted. If we note these differences in passing, we shall find them lead us hereafter to important conclusions.

III.

WE have just shown, from indisputable facts, that heredity governs the transmission of instincts, whether acquired or primitive. It might seem that in this portion of our inquiry, which has to deal only with the facts, we ought to be content with that exposition of the case. But certain theories, put forth by distinguished writers in our own day, attribute to heredity so important a part in the formation of instincts, that they cannot be passed by in silence. Indeed, according to these theories, heredity is one of the essential factors of psychological development; and so mighty and supreme is its influence, that it not only preserves instincts, but also creates them. Hence we are obliged to study more closely the nature of instinct, and to abandon the domain of facts, in order to enter into that of causes, that is, of hypotheses. This is to be regretted, for it is no trifling thing to attempt cursorily a theory of instinct. To us it seems that there is not in the whole field of psychology a more intricate question than this; and Schelling did not at all exaggerate when he said,—'For the thinker there are no phenomena more important than the phenomena of animal instinct, nor is there any better criterion of true philosophy.'

We will restrict our brief inquiry into this subject to two questions—What is instinct? and, What is its origin?

To the first question we reply: Instinct is an unconscious mode of intelligence. To the second: It is possible that instincts are only habits fixed by heredity.

It cannot be denied that it is only within the past hundred years that instinct has been seriously studied. The present century especially has done much. In past times we find only confused views and ingenious paradoxes: but naturalists have now removed the question to its proper sphere, that of observation and experiment. But when we study instinct from the naturalist's standpoint, the first thing that strikes us is the perfect adaptation of organs to instinct. 'An animal's form corresponds perfectly with its habits; it desires only what it can attain by means of its organs, and its organs do not incite it to anything for which it has not a propensity. The mole, destined by its needs to live underground, has in its organs nothing that would lead it aside from that disposition. Although it can see, still its sight lacks precision, because its eyes are small, and surrounded by a close growth of hairs. Its fore-paws are altogether organized for burrowing, not for walking. The paw is so formed and so related to the fore-arm, that it can hardly be used for locomotion without delving. The sloth, which walks upon the outer edge of the feet with the toes doubled in, is extremely tardy of movement on level ground, a circumstance which gave rise to the erroneous idea that nature's treatment of the animal had been that of a stepmother. But this is not the case : the sloth is as perfect in its kind as all other animals ; its limbs are so arranged as to enable it to climb, and to live in trees. The spider's legs are so arranged and organized that it moves with difficulty over a plane surface : these organs are intended for use on a line or a thread, and the spider carries about the materials from which to spin such thread.[1] In general we might say : As is the organism, so are the instincts ; and *vice versâ.* Given the instincts of an animal, a good naturalist can infer its organization ; or, given its organization, he can infer its instincts.

This intimate correlation between the physiological and the mental constitution leads naturally to the conclusion that the instincts of an animal result from its organization. Each organ, even each tissue, has its special function to discharge, and this tendency to the discharge of functions constitutes the need or instinct; the same organ or the same tissue communicates to the being in which it exists this same need ; each additional organ or tissue adds a new need or instinct. Hence the instinct of an animal is the sum of the instincts of its various organs ; it is their necessary—their inevitable consequence, and it comes into play under influences to which the animal is unconsciously subject.

This explanation is simple enough, but may not be perfectly sound. It is certain that instinct depends on organization, but it is very questionable whether it results exclusively from it. This is a region where the phenomena are so complex that physiology is insufficient to explain them all, for here evidently occurs the mysterious transition from the purely organic to the mental life, by means of reflex action, which is principally physiological, and of instinct, which is principally psychological. This transition is insensible and incomprehensible, and serves well to show that any line of demarcation drawn between psychology and physiology is arbitrary, and that mental life is slowly and gradually disengaged from physical life, so that it is impossible to tell where or how it has its rise. Neither can mechanism—which seems to be the

---

[1] Müller, *Physiologie*, ii. 108.

ultimate, the irresolvable character of all vital phenomena—prove
sufficient to explain instinct.   For if mechanism explains the lower
forms of spiritual life, it must also explain the higher—the
difference is one only of degree and of complexity ; but then, also,
if mechanism does not explain the higher, neither can it explain
the lower.   It has been said that thought is only translated
motion, and that it is but the highest form of the universal
mechanism.   This theory is no doubt very alluring, inasmuch as
it enables us to bring under one law all the phenomena of the
universe, from simple impact up to the most complicated events of
social life and history.   But it is only an hypothesis, which is
rendered doubtful by the fact that we can perceive no equivalence
between thought and motion.   Each appears to us as an ultimate
fact, *sui generis*, and not reducible into the other.

   To these theoretic considerations we may add others drawn
from facts.   If organization is the cause of instincts, then, as it
varies, so must they.   But observation shows that this is not
the case.   Observation teaches us that the correlation between
instincts and organs is not absolute ; that we may have the same
organization with different instincts, and the same instincts with
different organizations.   Thus, the European beaver, which is
hardly to be distinguished from the American, burrows like the
mole, whereas the other builds houses.   All spiders have the same
apparatus for weaving their webs, and yet one spider weaves a
circular web, another weaves a web of irregular form; a third weaves
no web, but inhabits holes, simply making a door.   Birds have their
beaks and feet as their only instruments for nest building, yet how
great are the differences of the form, architecture, and position of
nests.

   Let it be granted for the moment that the opinion we are
discussing is correct, although in the present state of our knowledge
it is a mere hypothesis.   Science has accustomed us to revelations
so unexpected that it may be rash to say that the opinion is
untenable.   Assuming, then, that instinct is not the result of the
organization, we shall still have to study its nature; for this
hypothesis only enlightens us as to its cause.   It tells us whence it
comes, but not what it is.   The reduction of all physical phenomena
to motion does not bar the separate study of electricity, of sound,

heat, and light ; nor would the reduction of all psychical phenomena to motion bar the separate study of instinct, sensation, imagination, will, etc. In any case, therefore, the question remains, What is instinct ?

Instinct is an unconscious form of intelligence, determined by the organization.

We intend to give in another place (Part III. chap. i. § 2) a detailed exposition of unconscious psychological phenomena, and to insist upon a class of facts that have been somewhat overlooked, though they probably contain much instruction for us. For the present, we would merely observe that, besides the conscious action of the mind, there is also an unconscious action, with a far wider sphere ; that consciousness is an habitual, though not necessary, accompaniment of our mental life; that perhaps every one of these phenomena—instinct, sensation, perception, memory, etc.—is by turns conscious and unconscious. This consideration will probably aid us to throw light on the problem of instinct.

Suppose a highly civilized people, among whom the division of labour is carried to great lengths ; that it contains architects, poets, engineers, musicians, all incapable of any work save that which constitutes the specialty of each ; that the architect can only build houses, and only a certain kind of house ; the engineer only bridges, and such or such a kind of bridge ; that the poet can only make verses — let us suppose, further, that each of them works unconsciously. These acts will certainly be regarded as instinctive, and we may compare the architect to the beaver, the engineer to the bee and the ant, the weaver to the spider, the carpenter to the termite. The only characteristic of instinct wanting would be innateness. This hypothesis exhibits the metamorphosis of intellectual acts into instincts : we had only to restrict intelligence within narrow limits and to deprive it of consciousness ; we had to take away its suppleness and its manifold aptitudes, to impoverish, and, so to speak, to prune it.

But this is only an hypothesis which might properly enough be rejected. To look more closely at the question, we take a familiar fact, one known to all—somnambulism. The sleep-walker walks, runs, waits at table, like Gassendi's valet, writes verses, copies music, composes and revises sermons, solves problems, even writes pages of philosophy, like Condillac. All this is done as well as and even better than in the waking state, and with as remarkable steadiness as in the case of instinct. The somnambulist, moreover, during the crisis, performs only acts which are habitual with him : the poet does not compose music, the musician does not write verses, nor did Condillac ever awake and find himself embroidering. Finally, it also resembles instinct, in that all its acts are performed unconsciously. If somnambulism were permanent and innate, it would be impossible to distinguish it from instinct. The resemblance was pointed out by Cuvier. 'We can gain a clear notion of instinct,' he well observes, ' only by admitting that animals have in their sensorium images, or constant sensations, which determine their action, as ordinary and accidental sensations determine action in general. It is a sort of dream or vision, which haunts them constantly, and, so far as concerns their instinct, animals may be regarded as a kind of somnambulists.' ' The organization of animals,' says Müller, ' is singularly favourable to the realization of the images, ideas, and inclinations which appear in the sensorium. As the internal and the external depend upon one and the same final cause, the form of the animal perfectly corresponds with its propensities. Thus, the instinctive propensities of the spider represent to it, like a sort of dream, the theme of its actions—the construction of its web.'

Here, again, in the case of somnambulism, all that is needed in order to bring about the metamorphosis of intellectual into instinctive acts is, that intelligence should be reduced to a few special acts (making verses, composing music, or the like), and that it should become unconscious. The phenomena of habit, which have been so justly compared with those of instinct, exhibit equally the transformation of intelligence into instinct. So soon as any intellectual operation, by repetition (that is to say, by restricting its domain), has become automatic (that is to say, unconscious), then the act is habitual or instinctive.

Hence it is less difficult than is generally supposed to conceive how intelligence may become instinct : we might even say that, leaving out of consideration the character of innateness, to which we will return, we have seen the metamorphosis take place. There can, then, be no ground for making instinct a faculty apart *sui generis,* a phenomenon so mysterious, so strange, that usually no other explanation of it is offered but that of attributing it to the direct act of the Deity. This whole mistake is the result of a defective psychology, which makes no account of the unconscious activity of the souL

But we are so accustomed to contrast the characters of instinct with those of intelligence—to say that instinct is innate, invariable, automatic, while intelligence is something acquired, variable, spontaneous—that it looks, at first, paradoxical to assert that instinct and intelligence are identical.

It is said that instinct is innate. But if, on the one hand, we bear in mind that many instincts are acquired, and that, according to a theory to be afterwards explained, all instincts are only hereditary habits ; if, on the other hand, we observe that intelligence is in some sense held to be innate by all modern schools of philosophy—which agree to reject the hypothesis of the *tabula rasa,* and to accept either latent ideas or *à priori* forms of thought, or preordinations of the nervous system and of the organism—it will be seen that this character of innateness does not constitute an absolute distinction between instinct and intelligence.

It is true that intelligence is variable ; but so also is instinct, as we have seen. In winter, the Rhine beaver plasters his wall to windward : once he was a builder, now a burrower ; once he lived in society, now he is solitary.[1] Intelligence can scarcely be more variable. Of this we have elsewhere given other instances. Instinct may be modified, lost, and re-awakened.

Although intelligence is, as a rule, conscious, it may also become unconscious and automatic, without losing its identity. Neither is instinct always so blind, so mechanical, as is supposed, for at times it is at fault. The wasp that has faultily trimmed a leaf of its paper begins again. The bee only gives the hexagonal form to its cell after many attempts and alterations. It is difficult to believe that the loftier instincts of the higher animals are not accompanied by at least a confused consciousness. There is, therefore, no absolute distinction between instinct and intelligence ; there is not a single characteristic which, seriously

---

[1] *Bulletin de la Société d'Anthropologie,* 2° Série, tome I, p. 307.

considered, remains the exclusive property of either. The contrast established between instinctive acts and intellectual acts is, nevertheless, perfectly true, but only when we compare the extremes. As instinct rises, it approaches intelligence : as intelligence descends, it approaches instinct. This must not be forgotten ; and while differences are borne in mind, the resemblances also must be noted.

Intelligence is a mirror which reflects the universe. It is a wonderful instrument, and is in some sense infinite as the world itself, which it encompasses and measures. By the accumulated progress of generations it tends to correspond more perfectly with its object. In its development through time and space, and through the infinite variety of living creatures, it ever pursues its ideal, that is, to comprehend all things, from common phenomena up to the eternal and sovereign laws of the Cosmos. Instinct is much more humble : it reflects the world only at a small angle ; its relations are limited ; it is adapted to a restricted medium ; it is fitted only to a small number of circumstances. Instead of being an immense palace, whence a boundless horizon may be seen, it is a lowly cottage, with only one window. But if we look at both instinct and intelligence from without, their processes are the same.

Nor is it surprising that instinct should be always restricted to the same order of phenomena, since, being unconscious, it cannot compare, deliberate, select, or improve.

We have still to inquire whence comes the infinite variety of instincts; why each species views the world at one particular angle, and at no other. These differences are, no doubt, owing to the organization ; to enter on such inquiries here would carry us too far from our subject, to which we must return.

IV.

A far more difficult question than that of the nature of instincts is the question of their origin. Till now it has not been asked, and is only now logically proposed by the great scientific controversy on the origin and variations of species. It is clear that we cannot pretend to decide an open, perhaps unanswerable question, warmly disputed by great authorities. We only suggest an hypothesis; but as it is founded on heredity, and assigns to it a very prominent part, it is impossible not to state it.

The reader is aware that a theory sketched by De Maillet, Robinet, and especially Lamarck, accepted and modified by Darwin and Wallace in our own days, has gained the assent of many eminent men in England, Germany, and France. According to this theory, species are variable, and are formed by the accumulation of slight differences, which have been fixed by heredity. The genera and species now extant, however numerous they may be, are derived from three or four primitive types, perhaps from one only. It was only necessary that some variations should occur spontaneously. If these variations were adapted to new conditions of existence; if they gave to the individual one more weapon to fight the battle of life, and if they have been transmitted by heredity, then a new species has been formed, which, under the continued action of the same causes, has departed more and more from the primordial type. Spontaneous variations, the struggle for life, selection, time, and heredity—these are the factors by the aid of which can be explained the evolution of living creatures, the formation and disappearance of species.

This bold hypothesis has thrown an entirely new light on instinct. Since in all animals the physical and the mental constitution are, as we have seen, correlated, if there were originally none but rudimentary organisms, instincts must then have been very rude. And again, since instinct, like the organism, presents spontaneous variations, and like it is subject to the laws of the struggle for life and heredity, we must conclude that if these causes explain the formation of species, they will also explain the formation of instincts. If a physical modification, by adapting an animal to new conditions, produces a deviation that may become fixed, because it constitutes a progress from antecedent states, the same will be true of mental modifications. Every variation of instinct that puts the animal in a better position to defend itself against new enemies, or to capture some new prey, will make it likely to survive under more complicated conditions.

So long as species were regarded as fixed, the question of the origin of instincts could not be even raised. The matter appeared very simple : the species was sent into the world ready-made, with all its physical and moral characteristics. The Evolutionists, on the other hand, hold that instincts, as they now exist, are very complex, formed by the gradual accumulations of time and heredity. They must be subjected to a careful analytical process, each stratum must be taken apart; by comparison, induction, and analogy we must determine which are of more recent formation, and must descend from these, step by step, to the more ancient strata. Proceeding thus from the complex to the simple, we arrive at certain very lowly mental manifestations, which we may regard as the source from which the entire series is derived.

Thus we have, at the outset, a minimum of intelligence, a something which plays in mental life the part of the cell in physiological life; then come actions and reflex actions, which by constant repetition are changed into habits and fixed by heredity; next we have variations, also passing into habits, and similarly fixed by heredity—in short, we have a sum of hereditary habits. Such, according to the Evolutionist school, is the genesis of instincts.

Darwin has developed this theory with consummate science and ability. He has boldly addressed himself to the most complicated, the most wonderful, and the most inexplicable instincts; those, for instance, of the ant and the bee—has striven to show how these singular phenomena may have arisen, by selection and heredity, out of a few very simple instincts.

If we take the honey-bee as it now exists, without comparing it to any other animal; if we assume that from the first it constructed cells, as it does now, we are filled with astonishment, but cannot explain the fact. But if we recur to the principle of gradual transitions, and seek to establish a series of transitional steps, 'Nature will perhaps herself reveal to us her method of creation.' Let us, then, compare the bee with the melipona and the humble-bee.

The humble-bee exhibits only very rude instincts. It deposits its honey in old cocoons, with the occasional addition of short tubes of wax. Sometimes also it constructs isolated cells of an irregular globose shape.

Between the perfect cells of the honey-bee and the rude simplicity of those of the humble-bee stand the cells of the domesticated melipona of Mexico, as an intermediate degree. The melipona itself is, by its structure, intermediate between the honey and the humble-bee, though more closely allied to the latter. It constructs a comb of wax, almost regular, consisting of cylindrical cells, in which the larvæ are hatched, and a certain number of large cells to hold its store of honey. The latter cells are nearly spherical, and situated at a considerable distance from each other. Now, it has been calculated that if the melipona were to construct these cells at equal distances, and all of one size, if she were to arrange them symmetrically in two layers, the result would be a structure as perfect as the hive of the honey-bee. ' Hence we may safely conclude,' says Darwin, ' that if we could slightly modify the instincts already possessed by the melipona, and in themselves not very wonderful, this bee would make a structure as wonderfully perfect as that of the hive-bee.'

Since natural selection acts only by accumulating slight variations of organization or of instinct, which may be advantageous to the individual, the question arises, How comes it that the successive and gradual variations of the constructive instinct, rather than of any other instinct, should have by degrees formed the architectural talent of the honey-bee? Darwin's answer is—' The bee must consume a great amount of honey in order to secrete a small quantity of wax; and during the winter it lives on its honey. Whatever tends to make a saving of wax will also tend to save honey, and so will be of service to the future of the hive.' If, now, we suppose that the humble-bee hibernates, it will need a great quantity of honey; consequently every modification of instinct, which would lead them to construct cells so near each other as to have a parti-wall, would save some little wax, and so be of advantage to them. Hence it would continually be more and more advantageous to the humble-bees if they were to make their cells more and more regular, nearer together, and aggregated into a mass, like the cells of the melipona. ' So, too, it would be advantageous to the melipona if she were to make her cells closer together, thus approaching the perfect comb of the honey-bee. Thus the most wonderful of all known instincts, that of the hive-bee, can be explained by natural selection having taken advantage of numerous successive slight modifications of simpler instincts.'[1]

---

[1] *Origin of Species,* ch. vii.

Darwin has endeavoured to explain in the same manner the slave-making instincts of certain ants. From P. Huber's famous observations, we know that female ants carry off the larvæ of the black ants, which become their slaves. Incapable of any other work save that of warfare, they are fed, carried about, cared for, and even governed by the slave ants. In England, the *formica sanguinea,* too, has slaves ; these they employ in the labours of the ants' nest, but they also work themselves. This instinct may, according to Darwin, be explained as follows. First, these ants stole some eggs from a foreign nest for food ; some of the eggs were hatched, and the stranger ants did some service to the community as workers. Hence the instinct of going and capturing eggs with a view to having slaves. Then the masters, leaving a part of their toil to their slaves, like English ants, came finally to renounce labour altogether, like the Swiss ants.

The theory which refers instincts to hereditary habits has also been maintained in France, but only by naturalists who, like Darwin, have given special attention to physiological phenomena. The only author who, so far as we are aware, has put it forward under its psychological form is Mr. Herbert Spencer. He has endeavoured to show, not how such instincts—those of the cuckoo, the ant, and the beaver, for instance—have arisen, but to discover and describe, in a general way, the process of evolution which has deduced complex from simple instincts, by heredity and selection. Attacking the question of primal origin, which had been avoided by Darwin, Spencer has attempted to give the true and complete genesis of instincts. All we can do is to indicate the chief points of this difficult synthesis.

In the first place, from the author's special point of view—that of the unity of composition of psychological phenomena—instinct represents one of the first stages in the ascending evolution of mind. In the faculties of instinct, memory, reason, etc., as they are generally accepted, Mr. H. Spencer sees only a convenient way of grouping and naming phenomena, but no real difference. These phenomena form a series, in which there are only insensible transitions from class to class. In this ascending series, instinct occupies an intermediate place between reflex action and memory ; instinct may be regarded as a sort of organized memory, and memory as a sort of nascent instinct.

Instinct may be defined to be 'composite reflex action.' It springs from simple reflex action by successive complications. While in simple reflex action a single impression is followed by a single contraction; while in the most highly developed forms of reflex action a simple impression is followed by a combination of contractions, in those which we distinguish by the name of instinct a combination of impressions is followed by a combination of contractions. This is the case with the fly-catcher, which, immediately after it has left the egg, will seize an insect with its beak. The question of instinct is therefore reduced to this : How can reflex actions, which grow ever more and more complex, spring from simple reflex actions ?

In order to understand how this transition may be effected by means of an accumulation of experiences, let us, says Mr. Herbert Spencer, take some aquatic animal of a low order, provided with rudimentary eyes. This nascent vision being little more than anticipatory touch, the animal will be able to note the passage of opaque bodies through the water only when they are very near its eyes. Consequently, in most cases these bodies will come in contact with its organism, and will so produce a tactile sensation, which will be followed by contractions—the necessary effect of a mechanical derangement of the vital force. Hence in this kind of animals there constantly occurs this succession, viz., a visual impression, and a tactile impression, or contraction. 'But if psychical states which follow one another time after time in a certain order, become every time more closely connected in this order, so as eventually to become inseparable, then it must happen that if, in the experience of any species, a visual impression, a tactile impression, and a contraction are continually repeated in this succession, the several nervous states produced will become so consolidated that the first cannot be caused without the others following.'

If we now assume a more perfect vision in the animal, it will follow that the same bodies will be visible at a greater distance, and that smaller bodies will be visible at a less distance. In such a case, there will be no collision, or it will be slight, and only produced by the small and nearer object. Neither will there be any strong contraction, but a partial tension of the muscles, like that of an animal about to seize his prey. There will therefore be a visual impression, a tension of the muscles : the latter condition allows the animal either to seize a small object, if close to it, to retire into its shell, or to escape from an enemy by convulsive movements.

Let us go further, and suppose a further development of the animal's eyes, and a habit of moving about in the water. Of all the bodies in its vicinity those in front of it commonly make the strongest impression on it. These it first sees, and then often touches ; and this contact often brings near to its head and its tactile organs small bodies which may serve as food. The animal will experience the recurring succession of these psychical conditions : slight excitement of the retinal nerves ; excitement of the nerves of the prehensile organs ; excitement of a special set of muscles. These conditions must, by repetition in countless generations, become so closely combined that the first will of necessity call forth the others.

'Here, then, we see how one of the simpler instincts will, under the requisite conditions, be established by accumulated experiences. Let it be granted that the more frequently psychical states occur in a certain order, the stronger becomes their tendency to cohere in that order, until they at last become inseparable ; let it be granted that this tendency is, in however slight a degree, inherited, so that, if the experiences remain the same each successive generation bequeaths a somewhat increased tendency ; and it follows that, in cases like the one described, there must eventually result an automatic connection of nervous actions, corresponding to the external relations perpetually experienced. Similarly, if, from some change in the environment of any species, its members are frequently brought in contact with a relation having terms a little more involved ; if the organization of the species is so far developed as to be impressible by these terms in close succession ; then an inner relation corresponding to this new outer relation will gradually be formed, and will in the end become organic. And so on in subsequent stages of progress.' [1]

It is, moreover, clear, as the author remarks, that we are not to

---

[1] Herbert Spencer, *Principles of Psychology*, § 194—198, Second Edition.

see in what has just been said anything more than a probable outline of the development of instincts. It will always be impossible to explain instincts as they are, in their endless varieties and complications. The data are inaccessible, and even were they accessible, it would be impossible to grasp them in their entirety.

We need not here pass judgment on this theory of the origin of instinct : the matter is beside our purpose, as well as beyond our powers. Evidently, this question is connected with the origin of species ; and science has not yet solved it, if it ever will be solved. Should Darwin's doctrine be confirmed, it must then be admitted that all instincts have been acquired, and that what is now fixed was at first variable ; that all stability comes from heredity, which conserves and accumulates, and that in the formation of instincts heredity is supreme.

However alluring the hypothesis of evolution may appear by its simplicity and breadth, it is not without difficulties in the region of facts. It explains many of these, but there are others at which it stumbles. We need only consider the objection drawn from the existence of neuter insects, which, though possessed of a structure of their own, and of peculiar instincts, still, being sterile, cannot propagate their kind. The formation of the wonderful instinct of working ants cannot, on this hypothesis, be explained, for among neuters this instinct cannot have been developed by selection and heredity. Darwin strives to explain this very ingeniously, while he admits that at first the facts appeared to be full of so great difficulty as even to overturn his theory. In the present state of science, it is not possible to say whether an instinct is the result of hereditary habit, or a primitive, natural, and irreducible fact. There is no mark whereby we might make a distinction.

Restricting ourselves within the bounds of the question which immediately concerns us, we would remark that the conventional saying, that 'instinct is hereditary habit' is so vague and incomplete as to be inaccurate. Habit is a disposition acquired through the continuance of the same acts ; it therefore necessarily presupposes a primitive act or state, whereof it is a repetition. I possess the habit of painting, writing, calculating, only because at first I painted, wrote or calculated painfully and slowly, and by a special effort of my will. If instinct is a habit, it is a habit of something. It presupposes a primitive state anterior to the habitual state, and this evidently is one of the lowliest modes of mental activity ; it is that minimum of intelligence of which we have spoken already—including in intelligence sensibility and volition, which are confused together and involved in instinct. Thus, then, we are again brought back to our conclusion in regard to the nature of instincts. Here is need of caution ; if intelligence does not exist in germ, even in the lowliest psychological act, then all the transformations and evolutions in the world will never put it there ; or we shall be the dupes of continual illusion and endless trickery, which will make us suppose that we may produce from a thing what was never placed in it. If we admit at the outset ever so small an amount of intelligence, we may well understand how the amount may afterwards have become greater. The seed may easily enough become a tree, but without the seed there will be no tree. Hence it is strictly necessary to qualify the hereditary habit from which instincts spring by calling it a mental habit.

In a word, according to the hypothesis which regards instincts as either fixed, or as varying only within narrow limits, heredity is simply conservative.

In the hypothesis of evolution, heredity is really creative; for since, without it, it is impossible for any acquired modification to be transmitted, the formation of instincts, properly so called, however slightly complex, would be impossible.

Both hypotheses accord equally well with our solution of the nature of instinct. It matters not whether it be the minimum of intelligence developed by gradual evolution, or an inferior form of intelligence, invariable and for ever fixed and determined by the organs. And, from our point of view, it might be said that, since the heredity of instincts is established, the heredity of intelligence is established partially and in advance. But this we will consider more closely in another place.

CHAPTER II.

HEREDITY OF THE SENSORIAL QUALITIES.

PERCEPTION is a fact of mixed nature, at once physiological and mental ; it is begun in the organs, is perfected in the consciousness. The soundness of the common opinion which regards our sensations as simple, irreducible, ultimate phenomena, by means of which we know the material world as it is, is extremely doubtful. Setting aside the discussion of this broad question, it is only necessary to say that, taking for their basis physical and physiological discoveries, recent works on psychology—notably those of Bain and Herbert Spencer in England, of Helmholtz and Wundt in Germany, and of Taine in France — have shown that sensations supposed to be simple must be dealt with, as chemistry, at its rise, dealt with bodies, also supposed to be simple. These psychologists have shown that neither colours, nor sounds, nor heat, probably, indeed, none of the qualities of the external world, at all resemble the ideas vulgarly entertained with regard to them ; that perception is a state of consciousness that corresponds in us to realities external to ourselves, but which does not resemble them : so that this totality of attributes which we call the external world, and which, by a universal illusion, we think we see as it is in reality, is to a great extent the product of our own mind—a creation of which the external world furnishes only the raw material, which our senses then, after their own fashion, work up and complete.

Though we cannot have the slightest hesitation in choosing between these recent theories and the current opinion in regard to the perception of external objects, between that of the Scotch school and of the *sensus communis*—whose least defect is that it explains nothing ; yet, so far as the subject of heredity is concerned, the question has no interest. Whether the material world is perceived immediately as it is, or otherwise than as it is, by a synthesis of consciousness, matters not at all. The only problem we have to solve is whether the perceptive faculties, the modes of sensorial activity, are subject to heredity.

We will observe, in the first place, that, as regards specific qualities, the reply admits of no doubt. If we examine the animal scale, from the lowest organisms, possessed of no other sense than that of an obtuse, passive touch, up to those most highly sensitive, we see at once that each animal derives a certain number, and a certain kind of senses from its parents. Heredity governs both the quantity and quality of the perceptive faculties, so far as those general characters are concerned which we call specific.

Heredity also governs all that concerns race or variety. Thus, the dog inherits not only a very acute scent, but also the variety of scent which adapts him for hunting a definite kind of game. In the negro the acuteness of this same sense characterizes that variety of the human species.

Doubt, therefore, can arise only with regard to individual differences, and thus our original question is transformed into this: Is the transmission of secondary and individual characters governed by the same heredity which governs the transmission of the perceptive faculties, in their essential and fundamental features? The answer can only be given by facts; we shall see that heredity is usually the rule, even with what is individual, anomalous, and capricious.

We take, then, in order, the five senses as usually accepted. There is now a general agreement to recognize, under the name of vital sense, organic sense, or internal sense, a mode of sensation, without a special organ, diffused over the entire body, and which is, as it were, an internal Touch, whereby we are sensible of what takes place within us. But as this sense is entirely personal, making us acquainted with our own body, and not with the external world, and as it very nearly concerns our pleasures, our pains, our instincts, our passions, we will treat of it in another place, when discussing the modes by which our feelings act, and the heredity of these modes.

I.—OF TOUCH.

Touch is the universal, primary sense, possessed by every sentient animal. All the other senses are but a modification of touch, said one of the ancients. Mr. Herbert Spencer has shown how, by evolution and specialization, the other senses—sight, hearing, smell, taste—could have sprung from touch; and how touch is a universal language into which the other senses, which are special languages, would at first have to be translated in order to be understood. In this fundamental sense, which is at once the most essential and the most material, we distinguish tactile sensations, properly so-called (hardness, softness, elasticity, etc.), and sensations of temperature (heat and cold). Both are governed by heredity.

The extreme difference of tactile sensibility between northern and southern races has often been remarked. Among the latter it is exquisite and refined ; among the former, obtuse, or, at least, imperfect. The Lapp, who takes tobacco oil for colic, has a skin as little irritable as his stomach. In Lapland, as Montesquieu puts it, ' you must flay a man to make him feel.'

It has been observed, says P. Lucas, that parents transmit to their children the most singular perfections and imperfections of touch. There are, probably, in the skin no modes of hyper-æsthesia or of anæsthesia that could form an exception to this rule. A woman whose tactile sensibility was so exalted that for her the slightest hurt was an agony, married a man endowed in the highest degree with the opposite quality. He did not lack intelligence, but his heart and his skin were impassible. A daughter was born to them, and she is as insensible to external pain as her father himself. We have seen her endure without complaint, and even without appearing to notice it, pain which would have been very acute for ourselves.

A family from the South, says the same author, who was acquainted with the persons, came to Paris some time ago. Several of the children were born in Paris; but those born there, as well as those brought there from the South, were in childhood extremely sensitive to cold. One of the daughters married a man from the North, who is insensible to cold, provided it is not excessive. The child born of this union is more sensitive to cold than even its mother ; like her, he shivers at the slightest fall of temperature, and so soon as the air becomes cold, he is afraid of leaving the house.

One of the most familiar forms of hyper-æsthesia of the touch is the sensibility to tickling. There are whole families that are insensible to this, while others are so sensible to it that the slightest touch will produce syncope.

Some persons cannot bear the contact or even the near presence of certain objects, such as silk or cork. This morbid sensibility is often transmitted by one or other of the parents. 'We are acquainted with a family, several members of which, both boys and girls, experience instinctively, on touching cork, or the downy skin of a peach, such an internal sensation of shuddering repulsion that the very sight of the fruit is unendurable to them ; which, therefore, must be given them with the skin removed.'[1]

Here we may refer, in passing, to certain hereditary anomalies, such as polydactylism, and the warty membrane of Edward Lambert (of which we have already spoken), both of which cases belong rather to the physiological side of the question.

The hand, which is pre-eminently the organ of touch, is modified by heredity. 'That large hands are inherited by men and women whose ancestors led laborious lives ; and that men and women whose descent, for many generations, has been from those unused to manual labour commonly have small hands, are established opinions.'[2]

The same is true of left-handed persons. There are families in which the special use of the left hand is hereditary. Girou mentions a family in which the father, the children, and most of the grandchildren were left-handed. One of the latter betrayed its left-handedness from earliest infancy, nor could it be broken of the habit, though the left hand was bound and swathed.

II.—OF SIGHT.

Sight is the noblest, the most intellectual, of all the senses, and the most important for science and æsthetics. It is a known fact that accidental blindness may lead to insanity. Congenital blindness certainly influences the mind : the imagination of one born blind, which possesses only tactile sensations, cannot be anything like ours, in which visual sensations predominate. Hence, from a purely psychological point of view, the heredity of the sensorial modes of vision is worth studying.

The individual varieties of this sense may be classed under three heads, accordingly as they depend on mechanical causes, or

---

[1] Lucas, i. 481.   [2] Spencer, *Biology*, vol. i. § 82.

on anæsthesia or hyper-æsthesia of the nervous element. All anomalies are transmissible by heredity.

1. The peculiarities of vision which depend on mechanical causes are strabismus, myopia, and presbyopia. The transmission of these is very common. In general, it is to hereditary causes that we are indebted for the conformation of our visual apparatus, and, consequently, for our being far or near-sighted.

Portal, in his *Considérations sur les Maladies de Famille*, describes an imperfect form of strabismus, called the Montmorency sight, with which nearly all the members of that family were affected.

Darwin observed that the Fuegians, when on board his ship, could see distant objects far more distinctly than the English sailors, notwithstanding their long practice.[1] This is clearly an acquired faculty, accumulated and fixed by heredity.

One of the most striking cases of heredity of vision is the ever increasing number of the myopic among persons given to intellectual work. According to M. Giraud Teulon, continual application with the eyes near the object is the great cause of myopia.[2] Professor Donders, of Utrecht, while studying the statistical reports, was surprised to find that myopia is a disease of the wealthy classes, and that the inhabitants of cities are specially liable to it, while those of the country are almost exempt. In France the *Conseils de Révision* have noticed the same fact. In England, at the Chelsea Military School, among 1,300 boys only three were myopic. In the Universities of Oxford and Cambridge, however, the number of myopic subjects was considerable—at Oxford 32 in 127. In Germany the results are even more decisive. Dr. Colin, of Breslau, undertook the task of examining, in the schools of his own country, the eyes of 10,000 scholars or students. Among these he found 1,004 myopic—about ten per cent. In village schools they are not numerous—only a quarter per cent. In the town schools the number of the myopic increases with the grade—primary schools it is 6·7; middle schools, 10·3; normal schools, 19·7; gymnasia and universities, 26·2 per cent.

[1] *Variation, etc.,* ii. p. 223.
[2] *Revue des Cours Scientifiques.* 3 Sept. 1870.

3

This explains why, in Germany, myopia is not a reason for rejection by the examining boards. Since constant study creates myopia, and heredity most frequently perpetuates it, the number of short-sighted persons must necessarily increase in a nation devoted to intellectual pursuits.

2. Anæsthesia of the nerves of sight is transmissible in all its grades and in all its forms. It is a well-known fact that the sensibility of the eye to light is very different in different persons. It may vary as much as 200 per cent., and, of course, will pass through all the intermediate degrees. Heredity transmits these inequalities, from partial to total anæsthesia, or blindness, when the eye, incapable of noting form or colour, has only an indistinct perception of light.

Congenital blindness may run in families. Blind persons will sometimes beget blind children. A blind beggar was the father of four sons and a daughter, all blind.[1] Dufau, in his work on Blindness, cites the cases of 21 persons blind from birth, or soon after, whose ancestors—father, mother, grandparents, and uncles— had some serious affection of the eyes.

Amaurosis, nyctalopia, and cataract in the parents may become blindness in the children ; and such transformations of heredity are not rare in animals.

The incapacity to distinguish colours, known under the name of Daltonism, or colour-blindness, is notoriously hereditary. The distinguished English chemist Dalton was so affected, as were also two of his brothers. Sedgwick discovered that colour-blindness occurs oftener in men than in women. In eight families akin to each other, this affection lasted through five generations, and extended to 71 persons.[2]

It is readily understood that such an anomaly of vision is not without influence on the mind, at least from the æsthetic point of view. An old man, who had from childhood observed that he could not call the various colours by their names, was grieved because he saw nothing in paintings but what was gray and sombre—in a landscape only an obscure haze, in the sunrise and

[1] Lucas, i. 404.
[2] Darwin, *Variation*, etc., ii. p. 70.

sunset, in the brightest tints of the rainbow, and in the grandest scenes of nature, only a cold and dull sameness.

3. There are some persons who seem gifted with extraordinary —almost supernatural—powers of sight. Some cases of this kind are so well attested as scarcely to admit of doubt. Thus, sight at great distances and through opaque substances appears, in some cases, to be proved beyond the possibility of fraud. If there is any explanation of this and other like phenomena, it can only be on the supposition of hyper-æsthesia of the optic nerve.

P. Lucas gives a long account of Hirsch Daenemarck, a Polish Jew, who, about the year 1840, travelled over Europe, showing by decisive experiments that he could read in a closed book any page or line that might be desired.[1] This man's son perceived, at about the same age as his father (ten years), that he possessed this same faculty, and perhaps in a more remarkable degree.

It is hardly necessary to observe that heredity always governs vision in its specific form, and that the only room for doubt would be with regard to individual varieties. Thus, all species of animals, from the eagle to the owl—from the earth-worm with its eye-points, to the spider with its facet-eyes—possess a visual apparatus of a structure and optical power peculiar to them, which is preserved and transmitted by heredity like all other specific characters.

III.—OF HEARING

Though hearing does not possess the same scientific and æsthetic importance as sight, yet it is one of our principal senses. It is the basis of a science—acoustics—and of an art—music; and, what is still more important, on it depends the possibility of articulate language or speech, and, consequently, of deliberate thought. If there be no hearing, there is an end of speech; suppress speech, and thought also is suppressed, with all results.

Hearing, like sight, can have its hyper-æsthesia, its partial and total anæsthesia—deafness. As we have seen, there are eyes that cannot distinguish certain colours; in like manner there are ears that cannot hear certain sounds. Wollaston met with persons

---

[1] Lucas, i. pp. 413—419.

who were insensible to all sounds above and below the diatonic scale.

To be congenitally deaf and dumb exerts a well-known and unfortunate influence on the development of the intellect, for which the only remedy is found in the use of artificial signs. If this infirmity is transmissible, heredity may be said to penetrate into the very essence of intellect. But this form of heredity has been disputed.

Dr. Ménière, in a special work on this question, while admitting that in a certain number of instances the direct and immediate heredity of deaf-muteness has been established, says :—' Nevertheless, these facts must be held to constitute a rare exception ; habitually deaf-mutes married to deaf-mutes beget children who hear and speak. This is, of course, still more the case where the marriage is a mixed one, that is, where only one of the couple is deaf and dumb—though even in this case there are well-attested cases of heredity.'[1]   Darwin also says :—' When a male or a female deaf-mute marries a sound person, their children are most rarely affected ;   in Ireland, out of 203 children thus produced only one was mute.   Even when both parents have been deaf-mutes, as in the case of forty-one marriages in the United States, and of six in Ireland, only two deaf and dumb children were produced.'[2]

We would remark that the returns of the Deaf and Dumb Institution of London, from its foundation to the present time, are conclusive in favour of heredity. Among 148 pupils in that institution at one time, there was one in whose family were five deaf-mutes ; another in whose family were four. In the families of 11 of the pupils there were three each, and in the families of 19, two each.

It is quite possible that, in the case under consideration, the law of heredity is not so much at fault as is commonly supposed. The deaf-muteness of ascendants may, in their descendants, be transformed into an infirmity of some other description, such as hardness of hearing, obtuseness of the mental faculties, or

---

[1] *Recherches sur l'Origine de la Surdi-Mutité,* par le Docteur Ménière.
[2] *Variation, etc.,* ii. p. 22.

even idiocy. Of this the distinguished anatomist Menckel gives many instances. But we will consider hereafter this obscure point of the metamorphoses or transformations of heredity.

It has seemed to us more natural to discuss the heredity of the musical faculty under the head of imagination. As will be seen, there is perhaps no other artistic talent that presents more conclusive instances of hereditary transmission (the three Mozarts, the two Beethovens, the more than 120 members of the Bach family). Still, however important the part we assign to the influence of the imagination and of the intellectual faculties, it must be admitted that there can be no musical talent without a certain disposition of the organs of hearing. Here education does next to nothing, for it is nature that gives 'a good ear.' Hence the incontestable heredity of the aptness for music necessarily implies the heredity of certain qualities of hearing. This conclusion applies to performers as well as to composers.

IV.—OF SMELL AND TASTE.

It is hardly possible to separate here these two senses, which are so closely allied that smell may be called taste acting at a distance.

Man, no doubt, ranks below other animals as regards fineness of the sense of smell. Nowhere among the human family, even among the negroes, can be found a sense of smell as acute as that of dogs, of carnivorous animals in general, and of certain insects. Gratiolet, in his *Anatomie Comparée du Système Nerveux,* states that an old piece of wolf-skin, with the hair all worn away, when set before a little dog, threw the animal into convulsions of fear by the slight scent attaching to it. The dog had never seen a wolf; and we can only explain this alarm by the hereditary transmission of certain sentiments, coupled with a certain perception of the sense of smell.

It is notorious that, to a great extent, the value of the canine race depends on their native, and therefore hereditary, subtlety of scent.

If in animals so highly endowed in this respect we could note individual differences, we should probably see them trans-

mitted by heredity. But, unfortunately, we can study them only
under the specific form. There, however, there is no room for
doubt, for heredity transmits them all without exception.

In the human species, savage races have a characteristic
acuteness of smell which allies them to animals. In North
America the Indians can follow their enemies or their game by
the scent, and in the Antilles the maroon negroes distinguish
by the scent a white man's trail from a negro's.[1] The whole
negro race has this sense developed to an extraordinary degree.
Whether this results from a great development of the olfactive
membrane, or from the more frequent exercise of this sense, in any
case, this innate or acquired faculty is preserved by heredity.

The specific and individual varieties of taste are transmissible,
like those of smell. Hybridism gives curious examples of this
among animals. 'The swine,' says Burdach, 'has a very strong
liking for barley; the wild boar will not touch it, feeding on
herbage and leaves. From a cross between a domestic sow and a
wild boar come young some of which have an aversion for barley,
like the wild boar, while the others have a taste for it, like the
common hog.'

In man, anæsthesia of taste, and antipathy for certain flavours,
are hereditary. Schook, the author of a treatise entitled *De
Aversione Casei* belonged to a family to nearly all the members of
which the smell of cheese was unendurable, and some of whom
were thrown into convulsions by it.[2] Such antipathy is very often
hereditary. 'In a family of our acquaintance, the father and
mother like cheese; the grandmother had an extreme dislike for it.
Four of the children share in the same dislike.'[3]

An exclusive liking for vegetable food and repugnance to flesh
is of very rare occurrence, but it is transmissible. 'A soldier of
the Engineers, who derived from his father an invincible repugnance to all food composed of animal substances, was unable,
during the 18 months he spent with his regiment, to overcome
this aversion, and was obliged to quit the service.'[4]

Finally, P. Lucas, following Zimmermann and Gall, gives the

[1] *Dictionnaire des Sciences Médicales.* Art. 'Odorat.'   [2] *Ibid.*
[3] Lucas, i. 389.   [4] *Gazette des Tribunaux,* 21 Mai, 1844.

following surprising case. A Scotchman had an irresistible longing for human flesh, which led him to commit several murders. He had a daughter, who, though taken from her parents, who were burned at the stake, before she was a year old, and though she was brought up among respectable people, still succumbed, like her father, to the inconceivable desire for eating human flesh.[1]

There exists in some families a sort of natural hydrophobia. 'Three members of a family with which we are acquainted—the grandmother, the mother, and a daughter—eat their food without taking any liquid; they do not drink at all, we might say. Their repugnance to liquids is so great that they refuse to drink until they fall into a feverish state.'[2]

We have collected sufficient facts enough to show that there is such a thing as heredity of the perceptive faculties, even under the individual form. Thus, if we take an animal, as it is naturally constituted, with its sensorial organs, through which it comes in contact with the outer world, we may say that the quantity and quality of its perceptive faculties will be certainly transmitted in their specific form, and very probably too in their individual form; therefore, heredity is the rule.

Sensation, however, presents only the raw material of cognition, which the mind's own activity has to transform and elaborate. To the external element supplied by the material world must be added the internal element supplied by ourselves, in order to produce what is properly called cognition, and the development of the mind. Hence it might be said that the heredity of the perceptive faculties, as here considered, is in some manner external, and that our having established it is a physiological rather than a psychological result. In our opinion, however, this is not the case, nor would that objection be made if it were borne in mind that per-

---

[1] We state this case with great reserve, because its authenticity does not appear to be beyond question. It is not, however, more improbable than other cases of heredity. It is notorious that the inclination to cannibalism is extremely lasting. A New Zealander of great intelligence, half-civilized by a protracted sojourn in England, while admitting that it was wrong to eat a fellow-man, still longed for the time to come when he could have that pleasure. Lucas, i. p. 391.

[2] Lucas, ibid. 388.

ception is an act essentially active, into which the whole mind enters. But we need not dwell upon a point which would require a lengthy explanation, carrying us beyond the limits of our subject. We shall presently see whether the heredity of the intellectual faculties, in their highest forms, can be directly established.

CHAPTER III.

HEREDITY OF THE MEMORY.

I.

IF, in treating of Memory, we confine ourselves to a description of the phenomena, and the investigation of their organic conditions, our task is simple. Nothing is easier than to attribute recollection to a special faculty which knows the past as consciousness knows the present. Unfortunately, however, this supposed faculty adds nothing to our knowledge, and with it we are in possession of only what the phenomena gave us, with just a word over. On the other hand, when we go beyond mere description and verbal explanations, the problem of memory, simple as it appears, becomes very difficult. Yet since, in order to understand the relation between heredity and memory, it is necessary to have some precise notions about this subject, the problem must be attempted.

The phenomena of memory, considered in their *ultima ratio*, are explained by the law of the indestructibility of force, of the conservation of energy, which is one of the most important laws of the universe. Nothing is lost; nothing that exists can ever cease to be. In physics, this is admitted readily enough; the principle is well-established, and confirmed by so many facts, that doubt is impossible. In morals, the case is different : we are commonly so accustomed to regard all occurrences as the results of chance, and as subject to no laws, that many at least implicitly admit the annihilation of that which once was a state of consciousness to be possible. Yet annihilation is as inadmissible in the moral as it is in the physical world ; and but little reflection is needed to see that in all orders of phenomena it is alike impossible for something to become nothing, or for nothing to become something. Such a miracle is neither conceived by reason nor justified by experience. We may, indeed, state such a proposition verbally; but so soon as we pass from words to things, from vagueness to precision, from the imaginary to the real, we cannot form an idea of any such annihilation in external or internal experience.

Nor are the considerations in favour of the indestructibility of our perceptions and ideas merely of a theoretical nature; there are also facts which, however strange they may appear at first, are very simple, if we bear in mind that in the mental world, as elsewhere, nothing perishes. Works on medicine and psychology cite numerous instances where languages apparently altogether forgotten, or memories apparently effaced, are suddenly brought back to consciousness by a nervous disorder, by fever, opium, hasheesh, or simply by intoxication. Coleridge tells a story of a servant-maid, who, in a fever, spoke Greek, Hebrew, and Latin; Erasmus mentions an Italian who spoke German, though he had forgotten that language for twenty years; there is also a case recorded of a butcher's boy who, when insane, recited passages from the *Phèdre* which he had heard only once. All these facts are so well known that they need only here be cited; they, with many others, prove that in the depths of the soul there exists many a memory which seemed to have vanished for ever.

The physiological study of *perception* further shows that the production of the phenomena of consciousness is subject to the law of the transformation of force. Though this point is yet beset with difficulties, the works of Mateucci and of Dubois-Reymond show that electric currents are produced in the nerves, and are there in continual circulation. When sensation takes place, and in general whenever a nerve is active, there is produced a diminution of its special current, as is indicated by the needle of a galvanometer connected with the nerve. This diminution takes place because a molecular change is produced within the nerve, which, on reaching the muscles, produces a contraction, and on reaching the brain produces a sensation;—in other words, sensation is *work*, and to perform work a certain force has to be expended and transformed. The electrical forces which serve to produce the sensation could not, at the same time, either give motion to a magnetic needle or produce chemical decomposition, because, while per forming work within they cannot, at the same time, perform work without; and 'as the nerve cannot produce electricity without using up something, the ultimate source of the forces which the nerve transforms into electricity is the materials furnished by the blood. The nerve is nourished with these materials, as the pile is fed with zinc and acid.'[1] Thus perception—that is to say, the primary phenomena of consciousness—comes under the general law. It is impossible that it should come of nothing. We daily experience thousands of perceptions, but none of these, however vague and insignificant, can perish utterly. After thirty years some effort—some chance occurrence, some malady—may bring them back; it may even be without recognition. Every experience we have had lies dormant within us: the human soul is like a deep and sombre lake, of which light reveals only the surface; beneath, there lives a whole world of animals and plants, which a storm or an earthquake may suddenly bring to light before the astonished consciousness.

Both theory and fact, then, agree in showing that in the moral, no less than in the physical world, nothing is lost. An impression made on the nervous system occasions a permanent change in the cerebral structure, and produces a like effect in the mind—whatever may be understood by that term. A nervous impression is no momentary phenomenon that appears and disappears, but rather a fact which leaves behind it a lasting result—something added to previous experience and attaching to it ever afterwards. Not, however, that the perception exists continually in the consciousness; but it does continue to exist in the mind, in such a manner that it may be recalled to the consciousness.

It is not easy to say what it is that survives our perceptions and ideas. The least objectionable name for it is *residuum*, a term which does not imply any theory, because it only indicates an unquestionable fact of our mental life. It is not to be supposed that these *residua* are always present to the mind, so that the attention can at any moment be voluntarily directed to them. But it may be assumed that every mental act leaves in our physical and mental structure a tendency to reproduce itself, and that when-

---

[1] Wundt, *Menschen- und Thierseele*, 5th and 6th Lectures.

ever this reproduction occurs the tendency is thereby strengthened ; so that a tendency often reproduced becomes almost automatic. We might go somewhat further, and say that the relation subsisting between the actual perception and the residuum is the relation between the conscious and the unconscious. In the perception or the idea the consciousness perishes ; or, more accurately, there takes place a transformation, of which we can have no precise idea, but which must be very analogous to the transformations of the physical world (heat into motion, motion in light, etc.). Between these two worlds of consciousness and unconsciousness, there must exist such a correlation that to each mode of the one a mode of the other corresponds. Mental life is a constant transformation, the unconscious becoming conscious, and *vice versâ ;* but this transformation does not take place by chance : though the laws are unknown, it is not without laws. If we could say which form of the unconscious corresponds to each form of consciousness, we could say what relation subsists between a perception or an idea and its residuum.

This we cannot do. Herbart, and after him Müller, the physiologist, supposed they made some advance in the explanation of the phenomena by comparing ideas to forces which have their statics and dynamics. But, in the first place, it may be remarked that consciousness is *one*, and that therefore it can at each instant hold only one idea. Its form is that of a simple series ; and though certain states of consciousness seem to be simultaneous, they are, in fact, successive. It we try to think simultaneously cf a lion and a mountain, a cube and a sphere, it will be seen that one idea excludes the other, and that we can think of them only successively or alternately. From this it follows :—

That an idea which occupies the consciousness can be displaced only by a stronger idea. If the two mental forces which contend for the occupation of the consciousness are alike, and act in one direction, the result is a very intense state of consciousness. If the two forces are equal and contrary, they will be in equilibrium. If they are unequal and contrary, the one will over-master the other, but in doing so loses a part of its own force equivalent to that which it displaces. This is proved by the fact that an idea is perceived all the more vividly in proportion as the mind is less occupied at the same moment with anything else. When a person is deeply occupied, a new idea makes little impression on his mind, because before it can lay hold of the consciousness it has expended all its force. On the other hand, it is well known that persons who are altogether idle interest themselves much about trifling details, and that an empty mind breeds hypochondria.

An idea that has passed away from the consciousness is not destroyed, but only transformed. Instead of being a present idea, it becomes a residuum, representing a certain tendency of the mind exactly proportioned to the energy of the original idea. The existence of ideas in the unconscious state might, therefore, be regarded as a state of perfect equilibrium. 'Forgetfulness means that the idea of a thing is in equilibrium with other ideas, and recollection that this idea quits the state of equilibrium, and enters the state of motion. No idea is lost; and every operation of the mind in virtue of which a latent idea passes to the active state is a state of recollection.'[1]

Amid all these hypotheses, which the future, perhaps, will show to be truths, this remains certain and unquestionable,—that the phenomena of recollection are to be referred to the grand law of the conservation of force, of which it is only a particular case. If, now, we pass from this very general law to one that is less general—from a formula embracing all changes which occur in the universe to a formula restricted to the domain of life—we shall see memory under another aspect.

This biological law is habit. In the first place, habit, considered in its essence, is referable to the law of the conservation of force, for its cause is the primordial law or form of being—that is, the tendency of beings to persevere in the act which constitutes them. As has been already seen, every act leaves in our physical and mental constitution a tendency to reproduce itself, and whenever this reproduction occurs the tendency is strengthened; and thus a tendency, often repeated, becomes automatic. This automatism is the link between memory and habit, and gave rise

[1] Müller, *Psychologie*, ii. p. 517.

to the saying that *memory is only a form* of habit—a proposition which, with some restrictions, is true.

On the one hand, it is certain that the association of ideas (a current expression, but inexact, for association occurs also between perceptions, sentiments, motions, etc.) is the indispensable condition of memory. On the other hand, habit consists of automatic associations: an act does not become a habit until the various terms of the series which compose it are perfectly fused and integrated, so that one necessitates the others (as drilling, dancing, playing the piano). Not to inquire here whether association is to be referred to habit, or habit to association, it is clear that he who does not see the fundamental identity of these two modes of activity, and consequently of habit and memory, must be totally without the faculty of generalization.

But to confound them absolutely appears to us incorrect, for the following reasons. Habit is altogether unconscious and automatic; memory is so only in part. We do not attribute to memory those psychic states which are so well organized, and so incorporated in us, as to constitute a part of ourselves. We do not say we *remember* that an effect has a cause, that a body possesses extension, that a self-moving body is an animal. It would, therefore, be more exact to say that memory is an incipient habit. If we trace the evolution of mind—going from instinct, which is automatic, to reason, which is so no longer—we may say that memory is the transition from perfect to imperfect automatism. If we trace it in the reverse direction, then memory indicates the moment when what was free and conscious tends to become unconscious. 'Memory, then, appertains to that class of psychical states which are in process of being organized. It continues so long as the organizing of them continues, and disappears when the organization of them is complete. In the advance of the correspondence, each more complex cluster of attributes and relations which a creature acquires the power of recognizing is responded to, at first irregularly and uncertainly; and there is then a weak remembrance. By multiplication of experiences this remembrance is made stronger—the internal cohesions are better adjusted to the external persistences; and the response is rendered more appropriate. By further multiplication of experiences, the internal relations are at last structurally registered in harmony with the external ones; and so conscious memory passes into unconscious or organic memory.'[1]

II.

The foregoing remarks are all within our subject, though they may not seem so ; for, having now referred memory to habit, we will endeavour, in the conclusion of the work, to refer heredity also to habit, and to show that both are but one form of the universal mechanism—of that inflexible necessity which rules the world of life and even of thought, and of which memory itself is but one aspect. Without forestalling this conclusion, of which the value can only be appreciated when we have first studied the facts, the laws, and the causes, heredity may at least be compared with memory. Heredity, indeed, is a specific memory : it is to the species what memory is to the individual. Facts will hereafter show that this is no metaphor, but a positive truth. If these considerations seem too theoretical, it must be at least admitted that, memory being as closely and perhaps even more closely connected with the organism than any other faculty, the heredity of memory is implied in physiological heredity. Some recent authors, among them Dr. Maudsley, attribute a memory to every nerve-cell, to every organic element of the body. 'The permanent effects of a particular virus, such as that of variola or of syphilis, in the constitution, show that the organic element remembers, for the remainder of its life, certain modifications it has received. The manner in which a cicatrix in a child's finger grows with the growth of the body proves, as has been shown by Paget, that the organic element of the part does not forget the impression it has received. What has been said about the different nervous centres of the body demonstrates the existence of a memory in the nerve-cells diffused through the heart and the intestines ; in those of the spinal cord ; in the cells of the motor ganglia, and in the cells of the cortical substance of the cerebral hemispheres.'[2]

Still, when we search history or medical treatises for facts to

[1] Herbert Spencer, *Principles of Psychology*, 2nd Edition, § 202.
[2] Maudsley, *Physiology of Mind*, ch. ix.

establish the heredity of the memory in its individual form, we meet with little success. While such facts are numerous in reference to the imagination, the intellect, the passions, we find very few in favour of heredity of memory.

There is a mental disorder, however—idiocy—which presents some instances. This infirmity—an hereditary one, as we shall see, at least in the shape of atavism—presents, among other characteristics, an excessive weakness of memory. Idiots generally recollect only what concerns their tastes, their propensities, their passions. But, as this is doubtless the result of the feebleness of their sensorial impressions, this heredity is the effect of a more general hereditary transmission.

Aphasia, which is nearly always connected with paralysis of the right side, is produced by lesion of the anterior lobes of the brain (the third frontal convolution of the left side, according to Broca). Its psychological cause appears to be amnesia, or a loss of memory, an inability to find words in general, or some particular words. Although this disease has been studied with much care, no cases of heredity are cited.

History shows the same scarcity of instances. The almost fabulous powers of memory that are recorded (Mithradates, Hadrian, Clement VI., Pico de la Mirandola, Scaliger, Mezzofanti, etc.) seem isolated cases; at least, we cannot trace them up or down in the genealogical line. Yet some facts may be noted. The two Senecas were famed for their memory : the father, Marcus Annæus, could repeat 2000 words in the order in which he heard them ; the son, Lucius Annæus, was also, though less highly, gifted in this respect. According to Galton, in the family of Richard Porson, one of the Englishmen most distinguished as a Greek scholar, this faculty was so extraordinary as to become proverbial —the Porson memory. The case may also be noticed of Lady Hester Stanhope, the daughter of one of the most illustrious English families, who, under the name of 'the Sibyl of the Libanus,' led so strange and adventurous a life. Among many points of resemblance between herself and her grandfather she herself cites memory. 'I possess my grandfather's eyes, and his memory of places. If he saw a stone on the road he remembered it—it is the same with me ; his eye, which usually was dull and lustreless, lighted up, like mine, with a wild gleam under the influence of passion.'

It may be remarked that certain determinate forms of memory are hereditary in artist-families. It will be seen that the talents for painting and for music are very often transmitted. Now and then they persist through four or five consecutive generations ; and it is evident that no one can be a good painter without possessing a memory for forms and colours, or be a good musical composer without memory of sounds.

To sum up, it must be admitted that there are not many facts to show the heredity of memory ; but the conclusion is not thereby justified that this form of heredity is rarer than others. The opposite opinion is still tenable, and the lack of evidences can be explained.

Memory, with all its undoubted usefulness, plays in human life, and consequently in history, only a secondary and obscure part. It produces no works, like the intellect and the imagination ; nor does it perform any brilliant actions, like the will. It does not give material evidence of itself, like a defect of the senses. It does not come under the ken of the law, like the passions ; nor does it enter the domain of medicine, like mental disease. Since, then, it is so little tangible, the lack of evidences need not surprise us ; and there is still reason to hope that, in proportion as the subject of mental heredity, hitherto much overlooked, is better studied, attention will be directed to this matter, and will abundantly show that here, as elsewhere, heredity is the rule.

CHAPTER IV.

HEREDITY OF THE IMAGINATION.

I.

ALL psychologists distinguish two kinds of imagination : one reproductive, the other creative. Both of these are alike subject to the law of heredity ; perhaps, indeed, apart from instinct and perception, there is no faculty of which the transmission is so common. This is not surprising, if we remember the close relation between perception and imagination; that the latter, in its passive form, depends entirely on the nervous system and the organs, and in its active form is closely connected with them ; and that, consequently, psychological heredity implies mental heredity.

Passive imagination is the property by which our sensorial impressions tend to reproduce themselves, though in less vivid shape, in the absence of their object. In its highest degree it becomes hallucination, which makes our internal states objective, and presents them to us as external realities; and this gives ground for believing that passive imagination is, in its mechanism, a reversed perception—perception proceeding from without inwards, imagination from within outwards. The part played by imagination in insanity, sleep, drunkenness, hallucination, ecstasy, and various states called miraculous, has been profoundly studied in our time, in works on mental diseases. In these works are many important facts in the study of heredity. We propose to discuss these hereafter, and bring under one head all the phenomena of morbid heredity.

At present we deal only with active imagination—the imagination of the poet, the artist, and even of the man of science ; the imagination which creates and interprets an ideal conception by means of sensible forms. It is a complex faculty, presupposing, at least, taste and sentiment; yet, at bottom, it differs less than might be supposed from passive imagination ; nor is common parlance at fault when it confounds the two under one name. The essential characteristic of both is vivid representation, intense vision.[1] Hence it is that great artists have ever come so near to hallucination and madness, and hence many of them have overstepped the limits of sanity.

The history of art shows that creative imagination is transmissible by heredity. We often find families of poets, musicians, painters. Families of poets are, it would seem, more rare ; nor is the reason hard to find. No one can be a musician without an exquisite

---

[1] At the close of a conversation about family affairs, Balzac said to Jules Sandeau, 'Now let us come to reality'—meaning his novels. G. Flaubert, while describing the poisoning of one of his heroines, felt, as he himself says, all the symptoms of poisoning—the taste of arsenic, indigestion, and vomiting. —Taine, *L'Intelligence,* i. p. 94.

sensibility of ear, nor a painter without an innate gift for colour and form, which presupposes a certain conformation of the visual organ. These physiological conditions are not to the same degree necessary for the poetic faculty. Hence we may say that musical or plastic talent is more dependent than the poetic on the conformation of the organs. In the former case, psychological heredity is more closely connected with physiological heredity,, and this makes its transmission more certain; for, as will be shown, heredity is a form of necessity (in other words, of mechanism); and this is far more inflexible in the domain of life than in that of thought.

In the following list, and in all others of the same kind, it is, of course, not intended to give a complete enumeration of every case of heredity. We merely wish to place facts before the reader's eyes; we cite only well-known names, or thoroughly conclusive cases, judging that here, as in every experimental study, the important thing is not the quantity of experiences, but their quality. Although, too, much is to be allowed for education and tradition, in considering a talent hereditary in a family, we must not attempt to explain, by these external means, what we attribute to heredity. The creative imagination is probably, of all the faculties, the one that it is least possible to produce artificially. Perhaps the following summaries of historical facts will be found to embrace enough *experimenta lucifera* to justify the assertion that heredity is the rule, not the exception.

II.—POETS.

Poets are scarcely slandered, if it be said that as a rule they form a passionate, ardent, sensitive race; that is the very condition of the artistic temperament. Hence the disorders, extravagancies, and singularities of their lives. These conditions are not favourable to the foundation of a family. A great artist is only so by a mixture of qualities, which are, so to speak, extra-natural. This is a character which is produced only by a happy accident, and therefore its heredity must be very unstable.

And yet, in examining the families of the fifty-one poets named below, there will be found twenty-two who have had one or more distinguished relatives. Their names are given in CAPITALS.

LIST OF POETS.

Alfieri, Anacreon, ARIOSTO, ARISTOPHANES, BURNS, BYRON, Calderon, Camoens, CHAUCER, CHÉNIER, COLERIDGE, CORNEILLE, COWPER, Dante, Dryden, ÆSCHYLUS, EURIPIDES, GOETHE, Goldoni, Gray, HEINE, Horace, HUGO, Juvenal, La Fontaine, Lamartine, Lucan, Lucretius, Metastasio, MILTON, MUSSET, Molière, Moore, Ovid, Petrarch, Plautus, Pope, RACINE, Sappho, SCHILLER, Shakspere, Shelley, SOPHOCLES, Southey, Spencer, TASSO, Terence, TENNYSON, LOPE DE VEGA, Virgil, WORDSWORTH.

It will be observed that in this list, from which no poet of eminence is intentionally omitted, some might have been excepted whose genealogies are quite unknown—Sappho, Terence, and others, who left no family. In this way we reach the conclusion that upwards of twenty out of fifty poets (or forty per cent.) had illustrious relatives. We give some details on this point :—

ARIOSTO, while yet a child, wrote comedies. In his family we find—
His *brother* Gabriel, a poet of some distinction, who, after Lodovico's death, finished the comedy of *La Scholastica;*
His *nephew* Horace, Tasso's intimate friend, author of the *Argumenti*, and other works.

ARISTOPHANES. The talent of this famous comic poet is found in a minor degree in
His *son* Araros, author of five comedies, among which we may name the '*Kokalos*' and the '*Ailosikon;*'
Another *son*, Nicostratos, who wrote fifteen comedies ;
Perhaps also another *son*, Philippos.

BURNS appears to have inherited from his *mother* that excessive sensibility which made him one of the first poets of Britain.

BYRON. His genealogy is interesting.
His *mother* was an eccentric, haughty, passionate woman, and half insane. Hence a certain English author has said that 'if ever there was a case wherein hereditary influences could be pleaded as an excuse for eccentricity of character and conduct, that case was Byron's.' He was descended of a line of ancestors in whom, on both sides, was to be found everything that could destroy the harmony of character, as well as all peace and individual happiness.

His *daughter* Ada, Lady Lovelace, was distinguished for her mathematical abilities.

His *grandfather*, Admiral Byron, author of *Travels.*

His *father*, Captain Byron, a man of dissolute habits.

CHAUCER, the father of English poetry.

His *son*, Sir Thomas, speaker of the House of Commons, ambassador to the Court of France.

CHÉNIER, André, the most illustrious of his family ;

His brother, Marie-Joseph.

Both took after their *mother*, Santi Lomaka, a Greek by descent, and a woman of distinguished talent.

COLERIDGE—poet and metaphysician. The following abridged list of his descendants is taken from Galton :—

His *son* Hartley, poet, a precocious child, whose early life was characterized by visions. His imagination was singularly vivid, and of a morbid character.

His *son*, the Rev. Derwent, author, late Principal of the Chelsea Training College, the only survivor of the poet's children.

His *daughter* Sara possessed all her father's individual characteristics, and was also an author. Married her cousin, and of this union was born Herbert Coleridge, a philologist.

CORNEILLE, Pierre, with whom may be placed

His *brother* Thomas ;

His *nephew* Fontenelle, his sister's son. From this sister descended, in direct line, the celebrated Charlotte Corday.

ÆSCHYLUS numbered among his family

His *brother* Kynegiros, one of the heroes of Marathon ;

His *brother* Aminyas, who commenced the battle of Salamis.

His *son* Euphorion, and his *nephew* Philocles, seem to have possessed some talent as tragic poets. Philocles was victor in the contest at which Sophocles brought out his *Œdipus Tyrannus.*

GOETHE inherited his father's physical constitution, but his mother's character. As poet and physiological student, he thus notes these hereditary influences :—

> Vom Vater hab' ich die Statur,
> Des Lebens ernstes Führen ;
> Von Mütterchen die Frohnnatur,
> Und Lust zu fabu'iren.

> Urahnherr war der Schönsten hold,
> Das spukt so hin und wieder;
> Urahn frau liebte Smuck und Gold
> Das zuckt wohl durch die Glieder.

HEINE, Heinrich.

With him may be mentioned his *uncle,* Solomon Heine, the celebrated German philanthropist.

HUGO, Victor. Without noticing what he may have derived from his father or mother, may be named

His two *sons,* Charles-Victor and François-Victor;

His two *brothers,* both known as literary men, Eugène (died 1837), and Abel (died 1855).

LUCAN. His genealogy is given under the name of SENECA, his uncle.

MILTON.

His *father* was a man of great musical talent, whose songs are still known;

His *brother,* a judge, also took part in political life.

MUSSET, Alfred de. His talent is to some extent reproduced in

His *brother* Paul, novelist.

RACINE.

His *son* Louis, a 'good verse-maker.'

SCHILLER, like Burns, seems to have derived his extreme sensitiveness from his mother, who was a very extraordinary woman.

SOPHOCLES. Part of his tragic genius lived in

His *son* Iophon, of whom Aristophanes had a high opinion;

His *grandson,* Sophocles the younger, twelve times crowned.

TASSO, Torquato, who wrote his first poem, *Rinaldo,* at the age of seventeen, received his talent from

His *father,* Bernardo, a poet of merit, author of the *Amadis,* and from

His *mother,* Parzia di Rossi, a remarkable woman.

VEGA, Lope de, after a long life of adventure, died a priest. By Marcela he had

A natural *son,* who, at fourteen, had already gained some distinction as a poet. As fond of adventure as his father, he died young in battle.

WORDSWORTH, poet and metaphysician;

His *brother,* an ecclesiastical writer;

His three *nephews*, all distinguished scholars; one of them was senior classic at Cambridge in 1830.

III.—PAINTERS.

A glance at any history of painting, or a visit to a few museums, will show that families of painters are not rare. In England you have the Landseers; in France the Bonheurs. Every one has heard of the Bellinis, Caraccios, Téniers, Van Ostades, Miéris, Van der Veldes. In a list of forty-two painters—Italian, Spanish, and Flemish—held to be of the highest rank, Galton found twenty-one that had illustrious relatives.

LIST OF PAINTERS.

BASSANO, BELLINI, Buonarotti (Michael Angelo), CAGLIARI (Paul Veronese), CARACCI, Ludovico, and Annibale; Cimabue, CORREGGIO, Domenichino, Francia, GELÉE (Claude Lorrain), Giorgione, Giotto, Guido Reni, PARMEGIANO, Perugino, Sebastian del Piombo, Poussin, ROBUSTI (Tintoretto), Salvator Rosa, RAFAEL, Titian, Leonardo da Vinci.

MURILLO, Ribeira, Spagnoletto, Velasquez, Gerard Douw, A. Durer, the two VAN EYCKS, Holbein, MIERIS, VAN OSTADE, POTTER, Rembrandt, Rubens, RUYSDAEL, TENIERS, VAN DYCK, VAN DER VELDE.

BASSANO, Giacomo da Ponte (1510—1592), the greatest of his family;

> His *father*, Francisco, founder of the school which bore his name;
> His four *sons*, Francisco, Giovanni, Leandro, Girolamo, all distinguished painters. Francesco, who was of a melancholy temperament, committed suicide at the age of 49.

BELLINI, Giovanni, Venetian, was one of the first who painted in oils;

> His *father*, Jacopo, a celebrated portrait-painter.
> His *brother*, Gentile, one of the favourites of the Venetian senate.

CAGLIARI (Paul Veronese);

> His *father*, Gabriele, was a sculptor;
> His maternal *uncle*, Antonio, was one of the earliest among the Venetian painters who abandoned the Gothic style;

His *son*, Carletto, a painter of great promise, died at the age
of 26;

Another *son*, Gabriele, attempted painting, but without success.

CARACCI (Ludovico), founder of a school which bears his family
name;

His three *cousins-german*, Agostino, Annibale, and Francisco.
Agostino was remarkable as an artist, man of science and
poet;

His *nephew*, Antonio, was also a distinguished painter, but died
young;

Also his *father*, Pietro, a painter of no originality.

CLAUDE LORRAIN (Gelée) never married.

His *brother*, was an engraver on wood.

CORREGIO, Allegri, died young, leaving

An only *son*, Pomponeo, who painted fresco in his father's style.

EYCK, Jan van, and Hubert, two brothers whose names are
inseparable;

Their *father* was an obscure painter;

Their *sister*, Margaret, followed painting with zeal.

MIERIS, François, called the old;

His two *sons*, John and William, the latter scarcely inferior to
his father;

His *grandson*, François, called the younger, son of William.

MURILLO, Bartolome Esteban, was pupil of

His *uncle*, Juan of Castille, a painter of great merit. We may
also name his *uncle*, Augustino del Castillo, and his *cousin*,
Antonio del Castillo y Salvedra, both painters of merit.

OSTADE, Adrian van, whose name is almost inseparable from that
of his *brother*, Isaac, who died very young.

PARMEGIANO (Mazzuoli), a great colourist 'into whom' according
to Vasari ' Raffaelle's soul passed;'

His *father* Filippo, and his two *uncles*, Michael and Pietro,
painters of some note.

POTTER, Paul, the most celebrated animal-painter of the Dutch
School;

His *father*, Peter, a landscape-painter.

RAFAEL SANZIO.

His *father*, Giovanni Sanzio.

Robusti (Tintoretto), one of the most celebrated painters of the Venetian school;

His *daughter*, Marietta, famous as a portrait-painter;

His *son*, Domenico, a good portrait-painter.

Ruysdael, Jakob, and his *brother*, Salomon, both landscape-painters.

Teniers, David, called the younger, the most celebrated of his family;

His *father*, David the elder;

His *brother*, Abraham.

Titian (Vecellio). In his family were nine painters of merit, among them his *brother*, Francesco, and his sons, Pomponio and Horatio. The following is his genealogy from Galton.

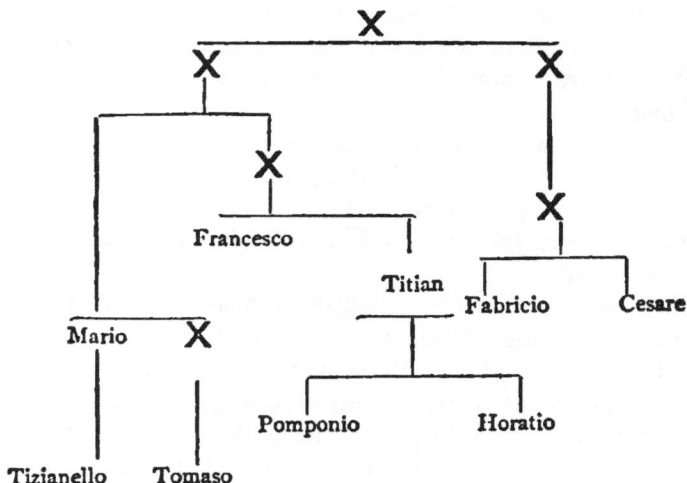

Van Dyck, Antony. His *father* was a painter, his mother worked landscapes on tapestry with wonderful skill.

Van der Velde, William (the younger), a master of marine landscape;

His *father*, Van der Velde the elder, and

His *son*, William, both marine painters;

Probably the two brothers, Isaiah and Jan van der Velde, born at Leyden, and Adrian, a native of Amsterdam, were of this family.

IV.—MUSICIANS.

The development of the art of music is far more recent than that of painting. It dates back no more than three centuries. Still we shall find that the heredity of this art is not rare : the family of the Bachs alone presents us with most singular evidence. Of great musicians who constitute exceptions to the law of heredity I find only Bellini, Donizetti, Rossini, and Halévy.

ALLEGRI, the famous composer of the Sistine Chapel *Miserere*, was of the same family as Correggio the painter.

AMATI, Andrea, the most illustrious member of a family of violinists at Cremona ;

His *brother*, Niccola, his two *sons*, Antonio and Girolamo, and his *grandson*.

BACH, Sebastian, the greatest of his family.

The Bach family is, perhaps, the most distinguished instance of mental heredity on record. It began in 1550, and continued through eight generations, the last known member being Regina Susanna, who was living in indigence in the year 1800. ' During a period of nearly 200 years this family produced a multitude of artists of the first rank. There is no other instance of such remarkable talents being combined in a single family. Its head was Weit Bach, a baker of Presburg, who used to seek relaxation from labour in music and song. He had two sons, who commenced that unbroken line of musicians of the same name that for nearly two centuries overran Thuringia, Saxony, and Franconia. They were all organists, church singers, or what is called in Germany Stadt-Musiker. When they had become too numerous to live near each other, and the members of the family were scattered abroad, they resolved to meet once a year, on a stated day, with a view to keep up a sort of patriarchal bond of union. This custom was kept up until nearly the middle of the 18th century, and often more than 100 persons bearing the name of Bach—men, women, and children—assembled.' In this family are reckoned twenty-nine *eminent* musicians. Fétis, in his *Dictionnaire Biographique*, mentions fifty-seven members of this family.

BEETHOVEN, Ludwig ;

4

His *father*, Johannes, was tenor in the choir of the Elector of Cologne;

His *grandfather*, Ludwig, was first singer, and then Kapell-meister in the same choir.

BELLINI, son and grandson of musicians of no great mark.

BENDA, Francisco (1709—1786), the principal member of a remarkable family of violinists;

His three *brothers*, Giovanni, Giuseppe, and Georgio;

His two *sons*, Federico and Carolo, and two *daughters;*

His two *nephews*, Ernest, son of Giuseppe, and Federico, son of Georgio.

BONONCINI. His *father*, Antonio, and his *son*, Giovanni; the latter was for some time in England, and the rival of Händel.

DONIZETTI, Gaetano;

His *brother*, Giuseppe, specially cultivated military music.

DUSSEK, Ladislas, a noted composer and performer;

His *brother*, Johannes, an organist of repute;

His *brother*, Franz, a good violinist;

His *daughter*, Olivia, inherited her father's talent.

EICHHORN and his two *sons*, who from their earliest years showed great talent as instrumentalists.

GABRIELLI, Andrea, and his *nephew* Giovanni.

HALÉVY. Of Jewish origin—a point worthy of note, to which reference will again be made;

His *brother*, Léon, literary man and poet.

HAYDN and his *brother*, who was a good organist and composer of church service.

HILLIER, Johann Adam—musical composition and works on music;

His *son*, Friedrich Adam (1768—1812);

His *grandson*, Ferdinand, 'now one of the best composers in Germany' in the opinion of Fétis.

KEISER, Reinhard, his *father* and his *daughter*.

MENDELSSOHN, of a Jewish family;

His *grandfather*, Moses, philosopher, wrote works on æsthetics;

His *uncle*, an author;

His *sister*, a distinguished woman, a clever pianist—she had a share in much of the work done by her brother.

MEYERBEER (Jakob Baer);

His two *brothers*, the one, Wilhelm, an astronomer, noted for his lunar chart, the other, Michael, a poet, who died young.

MOZART.

His *father*, Johann Georg, second Kapellmeister to the Prince-Bishop of Salzburg ;

His *sister*, whose success while yet a child seemed to give evidence of talent not realized in maturer years ;

His *son*, Carl, was an amateur musician ;

His *son*, Wolfgang, born four months after his father's death, gave evidence early in life of a happy turn for music.

PALESTRINA. His *sons*, Angelo, Rodolfo, and Sylla, who all died young, seemed to have inherited some of their father's talent, if we may judge by some of their compositions which have been preserved.

ROSSINI. His *father* and *mother* musicians at fairs.

CHAPTER V.

HEREDITY OF THE INTELLECT.

I.

THE faculty of knowing may be hypothetically divided into two parts : the one includes perception, memory, and imagination, of which we have now studied the heredity ; there will remain for the other a certain number of faculties which have for their object abstract and general conceptions, which we will here call intellect proper. We have now to consider if these last-named modes of knowing, which are the highest of all, are subject to the law of heredity.

First, it is evident that these manifestations of thought are indeed the higher forms of the human intellect—that is to say, of the highest intellect of which we are cognizant. Man can rise from the concrete and confused sensation to the simplicity of abstract notions ; he can reduce a countless mass of facts to one general idea, and denote it by an arbitrary sign ; he can, by ratiocination, arrive at the most remote, or the most complicated consequences, and divine the future from the past. It is because man can compare, judge, abstract, generalize, deduct, and form inductions, that sciences, religion, art, morals, social and political life, have sprung into being, and have continued their incessant evolution. So wonderful are these faculties, that, by their accumulated results, they have made of man, as it were, a being apart from all the rest of nature.

The inquiry, therefore, whether these faculties can be hereditary, is an inquiry whether psychological life, in its highest form, is subject to this law of biology. If we take a narrow and superficial point of view, it might appear as if, so far, we had at most proved the heredity of the lower forms of intelligence, and as if we had merely touched the outer margin of the subject; and it might be said that we have no right to argue from the less to the greater, from the lower to the higher. Now, however, we meet the difficulty face to face.

It cannot, however, be said that the controversy with regard to this point has been very keen. It could only have been maintained by metaphysicians who have for the most part shown the utmost indifference for this subject. The partisans of experience, physiologists and others, who have treated of heredity, have generally attributed to it the greatest degree of influence. Some, carried away by misdirected zeal, and more concerned about the hypothetical consequences of such a doctrine than about its intrinsic truth, have imagined a division of the intellectual faculties, and have withdrawn one portion of it from heredity. According to this theory, which claims the authority of Aristotle, we have two souls, the one sensitive or animal, transmissible like the body, and the other rational or human, 'not dependent on the act of generation,' and which would, therefore, lie wholly beyond the influence of heredity. This hypothesis, now wholly obsolete, needs no discussion. They who maintain it, and Lordat in particular, have shown so clearly that their preconceived opinion would not submit to facts, that criticism is quite superfluous.

The problem for us is this : Are the higher, like the lower, modes of intellect transmissible? Are our faculties of abstraction, judgment, ratiocination, invention, governed by heredity, as are our perceptive faculties? Or, in plainer terms, and in common parlance,—Are common sense, insanity, genius, talent, subtlety, aptitude for abstract studies, hereditary?

In order to reply, we will examine the question from the two-fold standpoint of theory and fact, of metaphysics and experience. Reason will show that the heredity of intellect is possible, experience that it is real.

If we admit the heredity of the lower modes of intellect—and facts are here decisive—logic alone ought to convince us that it extends to all intellect, for it is admitted by all schools of thought that this faculty is essentially one. Psychology has always distinguished different modes of the faculty of knowing, and, indeed, the analytical study of intellect is only possible on that condition. But these are but differences in the way of looking at them, not specific differences. In the same way, phrenologists have thought that they could assign to each faculty a special portion of the brain; but, even had their view been sustained, such localization would in no degree have invalidated the unity of the intellect itself. However far back the question may be carried, every inquiry into the ultimate nature of intellect must necessarily issue in one or other of these two conclusions: either it is an *effect*, of which the cause is the organism; or it is a *cause*, of which the effect is all that exists or can be known. The first hypothesis is called materialism, the second idealism. We shall see, taking our stand on reasoning only, that between these two hypotheses and the heredity of the higher modes of intellect there exists no contradiction, no logical incompatibility.

There is no difficulty in the materialistic hypothesis; for if it be admitted that thought is only a property of living matter, then, as heredity is one of the laws of life, it must therefore be also one of the laws of thought. Or, in more precise terms, intellect is a function whose organ is the brain; the brain is transmissible, as is every other organ, the stomach, the lungs, and the heart; the function is transmissible with the organ; therefore intellect is transmissible with the brain. Physiological heredity involves, as a necessary consequence, psychological heredity in all its forms.

On the other hand, the idealistic hypothesis seems to stand in utter opposition to heredity of intellect; but, as will be seen, this opposition is not so radical as would at first appear.

Idealism has recently found learned and able advocates; its details will hereafter be noticed. Enough here to explain, in a few words, that idealism is that metaphysical system which holds thought to be the only reality. Sometimes, regarding thought or intellect as a secondary and derivative mode of existence, it strives to ascend still higher, and to discover in will the first cause of all things, the supreme reality. Such is the position of Schopenhauer and his school, that is to say, the most philosophic form of contemporary idealism. Thus exalted, and under this exceedingly abstract form, idealism is as far removed as it well can be from experience, in the common acceptation of that term. To experience, however, it must come. This system, like all others, must account for the world of sense, for nature, and her phenomena and laws. There being no other absolute existence save thought, matter must be referred to thought. Matter, according to Schelling, can be nothing else but 'extinct or exteriorized mind.' Hegel defines it to be idea made objective to itself. It matters little what these theories are worth. Idealism has never explained the transition from the absolute to the relative, from mind to matter, except by metaphors,—a process, moreover, which it has in common with every other metaphysical system. It is enough that it admits the material world, with its laws, as a purely phenomenal existence. In this admission we find the basis for a reconciliation between idealism and heredity.

For if we hold, with Schopenhauer, that the will is the primitive element in everything and in every being, then intellect will be only a derived faculty, a first step toward materialization. Hence it will be subject to the mechanism of logic, emprisoned in the 'forms of thought,' in the categories discovered and analyzed by Kant, and, like all the rest of nature, it will have its laws. This admission is enough. Henceforth, between the idealists and ourselves there exists no real opposition. Their theory is that there are two distinct modes of existence : the noumenon in the will and the phenomenon in the intellect and in nature. To the mind, regarded as noumenon, none of our conceptions of laws, logical necessity, or categories are applicable; for all this only pertains to the mind considered as phenomenon. Consequently, since we restrict ourselves to the study of experience—that is to say, of facts and their laws—there can be no disagreement between us and the idealists. The difference between us springs, not from any diametrical opposition of doctrine, but from the fact that to the study of phenomena which both sides pursue, and to which we strictly confine ourselves, the idealist joins a metaphysical theory, which, in our eyes, has no scientific value, since it transcends science.

It is true that idealists hold that the laws of nature, and, generally, of internal or external experience, have only a relative phenomenal value; but we have never asserted that experience can give us the absolute. If the idealist admits, as he does, that in the order of physical, chemical, physiological, and psychological facts there are coexistences and sequences that can be reduced to fixed formulas, he has no fair grounds for refusing to concede to heredity a place among these empiric laws, though he may deny that it applies to the intellect considered as noumenon.

Thus the heredity of intellectual faculties can be reconciled with the most transcendental idealism. If, now, we examine the question in our own way, that is, without transcending experience, we say that intellect, in its inmost nature, appears to us as one of the manifestations of the unknowable. We may, indeed, as psychology and the sciences advance, determine its empiric laws and conditions more precisely; but we shall not arrive at its essential nature. It is indisputable that within the last thirty years English and German psychologists—and particularly Herbert Spencer, Bain, and Wundt—have, with a precision previously unknown, analyzed the modes of intellect and the conditions of its development. They have shown that all intellectual processes, ∨ from the highest and most complex down to the most elementary, consist in apprehending resemblances and differences. To assimilate and dissimilate, to integrate and disintegrate, to combine and differentiate—such is the fundamental process of the intellect, and it is found in all its operations, as well in the simplest as in the most complex. Yet this analysis, while it discloses to us in a striking way the 'unity of composition' of psychic processes, in reality only enables us to understand the mechanism of intellect and the laws of its empiric development. We may, indeed, reduce the infinite variety of the facts of thought to two simple facts, viz.

combination and differentiation; but it still remains true that these two facts themselves exist only *in* and *by* thought, and we do not know what thought is.   If we add that these phenomena are given us under the form of a sequence, or of simple series, and that succession is the essential condition of consciousness, we do but express the form of thought, not its nature, for things may be successive without being facts of consciousness.   Thought, therefore, is still impenetrable to us: it explains all things, but does not explain itself; it is one of those noumena wherewith we solve the enigma of the universe, but it is itself an enigma.

The unity of the intellect is an indisputable fact, established alike by consciousness, experience, and theory. Nothing, therefore, could be more chimerical that to suppose that given intellectual operations are, by their own nature, beyond the laws of heredity.   Logic rejects any such conclusion, and it is no less contradicted by facts.

It will, perhaps, excite surprise that, in the foregoing remarks, we have not named that highest mode of intellect which metaphysicians call reason.   This faculty—whose object, according to some, is the absolute, the infinite, the perfect, according to others, the necessary process of thought—is pre-eminently the metaphysical faculty.   It has its seat in that region of the impalpable and the invisible where we look for the ultimate reasons of things.   It lies so far above experience that, in a study on experimental psychology, we are almost obliged not to speak of it.   We need only declare our position with regard to every possible theory of reason.

Metaphysicians are by no means agreed as to the nature of this faculty.   In France, a theory, borrowed from Leibnitz, broadened and deepened by idealists in our own day, reduces reason to two constituent principles, viz. the principle of contradiction or of identity, and the principle of *raison suffisante*—both ultimately reducible to one.   The principle of identity, the last resort of logic and science, is subordinate to the principle of *raison suffisante*, which is the ultimate principle of all existences, because the latter accounts for all things, is not limited to the declaration that a thing is, but why it is, and what determined its existence; and this ultimate principle itself would not be explicable were it not that it implies the *summum intelligibile*, which is identical with the good.   All things, therefore, would be reduced to a moral principle. Logic, metaphysics, and morals are so thoroughly blended together, that the endless variety of human knowledge and of human actions would have but one origin, and, however unlike they may be to one another in their phenomenal multiplicity, they would be identical in their rational unity.

This coherent theory is, by its own nature, placed out of the reach of all experience and all verification. Attractive as it may be, it has the radical defect of all metaphysics, that we cannot say whether it has any objective, absolute value, or whether it is merely subjective. This, however, is clear, that between this theory and ours no opposition is possible, since each occupies a province of its own, and the world of pure reason begins only where the world of phenomena ends.

If from this strictly metaphysical theory of reason we descend to the usual doctrine, the joint product of the Scotch school and of French eclecticism, it will be found perfectly reconcilable with the heredity of intellect, even in its highest form. The one fixed and essential point in the vague, loose, and often contradictory system of Reid and Cousin is this, that reason is 'an impersonal, universal, and necessary' faculty. But it would hardly be possible to name any characters more in accordance with the law of heredity. Without stopping to inquire how the infallible transmission of these characters is explained—a question never so much as raised by the eclectic school—whether it is connected with some permanent state of the brain, or whether it results from some mysterious operation, it is enough that it is admitted that they are the same, everywhere, always, and in all men. Hence they are specific characteristics; that is to say, it is as much a contradiction in terms to think of a man without reason as of a vertebrate animal without a cerebro-spinal axis. But, as we shall see later, the special property of heredity is precisely this,—that it transmits, without exception, all specific characteristics. Thus, if we accept Cousin's theory, there is no faculty of man that is more certainly transmissible than the highest form of intellect—reason. For heredity, too, is impersonal, since it preserves the species; and universal, since it governs the whole domain of life; and it is one of the forms of inflexible necessity.

Thus, then, either we place intellect and reason, its highest form, beyond time and space, and then they have nothing in common with experience; or we consider them in their phenomenal manifestations, and then there is no logical ground for exempting them from the law of heredity.

II.

It must now be shown from facts that this transmission is not only possible, but actual. Here is a difficulty. Intellect—that is to say, the faculty of comparing, judging, reasoning—is found everywhere—in science, politics, art, industrial inventions, learning, history, etc. Is it, therefore, necessary to class under the head of intellect every case of heredity in politics, literature, and art? We must have recourse to an artificial process, and divide what in nature is united. Surrendering, therefore, to imagination all that concerns artists, and to active faculties all that has to do with politics, we here treat only of cases in which pure intellect—that is to say, reflection, taste, or criticism—predominates.

Still these cases are sufficiently numerous to make two categories. In the first we place men of science, philosophers, political economists, etc.; in the second, writers, properly so called, historians, critics, and novelists. This division is, of course, somewhat arbitrary, nor should any great stress be laid on it; but it will enable us to introduce more order into our arrangement.

MEN OF SCIENCE.

Families eminent in science are not rare. Many scientific men take after their fathers. The atmosphere of free inquiry in which they were brought up has not been without influence on their vocation. Still, education does not constitute genius; and in order to have a turn for scientific investigation, something more is required than the external transmission resulting from education. It has also been observed that the mothers or grandmothers of several men of science were remarkable women, as in the case of Buffon, Bacon, Condorcet, Cuvier, d'Alembert, Forbes, Watt, Jussieu, etc.[1] Heredity among philosophers is somewhat rare.

---

[1] Galton, who notes this fact, assigns for it a reason which to us seems very questionable. Women, says he, are blinder partisans and more servile followers of custom than men; and it is a great blessing for a child to have a mother

This will appear less surprising when we bear in mind that few philosophers have left any posterity. Thus, in modern times, Descartes, Leibnitz, Malebranche, Kant, Spinoza, Hume, A. Comte, Schopenhauer, etc., either never married or had no children.

The exceptions, real or apparent, to the laws of heredity are: Bacon (Roger), Berkeley, Berzelius, Blumenbach, Brewster, Comte, Copernicus, Descartes, Galen, Galvani, Hegel, Hume, Kant, Kepler, Locke, Malebranche, Priestley, Réaumur, Rumford, Spinoza, Young, etc.

AMPÈRE, André-Marie, mathematician, physicist, and philosopher ;
His *son*, Jean-Jacques, traveller, literary man, historian.

ARAGO, François ;
His three *brothers*, Jean, Jacques, and Etienne, authors and artists ;
His son, Emmanuel, lawyer, politician.

ARISTOTLE. Though ancient genealogies are difficult to make out, we may name
His *father*, Nicomachos, physician to Amyntas II., and author of medical works ;
His *son*, Nicomachos, held by some to be the author of the *Ethics* which bear his name ;
His *nephew*, Callisthenes, son of Hero, a cousin of Aristotle.

BACON, Francis ;
His *father*, Nicholas, Lord Keeper of the Great Seal ;
His *mother*, Ann Cooke, belonged to a highly-gifted family. She was a distinguished scholar, and was very well versed in Latin and Greek ;
His *brothers* were distinguished men ; among them, Nathaniel, a brother by another mother, who was a clever painter.

BENTHAM, Jeremy, logist and moralist ;
His *brother*, General Samuel Bentham, a distinguished officer ;
His *nephew*, George, an eminent botanist, president of the Linnæan Society.

BERNOUILLI, Jacques, of Swiss origin, was the first to establish the reputation of this family, which is famous for the number of

that approves its free inquiry into truth. We will come back to this point when treating of the *Laws* of Heredity.

mathematicians, physicists, and naturalists it has produced. The following is a list of this family. Each of the members mentioned was distinguished in some branch of science.

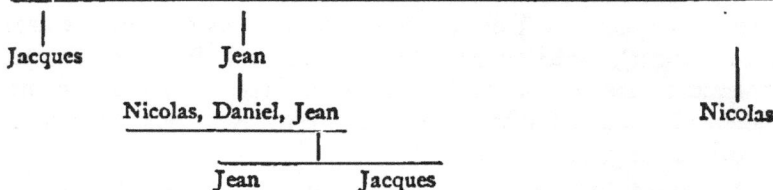

```
     |                    |
  Jacques              Jean                              |
                         |                               |
              Nicolas, Daniel, Jean                   Nicolas
                         |
              ┌──────────┴──────────┐
             Jean              Jacques
```

In our own century there yet remained in Switzerland descendants of this family : Christophe Bernoulli (1782—1863), Professor of Natural Science in the University of Bâle ; Jerôme Bernouilli (1745—1829), chemist and mineralogist.

BOYLE, Robert. In his family we count no less than seventeen notable members, most of whom gained distinction in political life.

BRODIE, Benjamin, one of the most celebrated surgeons in England. His family reckons six distinguished members.

BUCKLAND, William, geologist ;
His *son*, Frank, naturalist, well-known for his popular writings.

BUFFON. His views on heredity will be hereafter stated. He used to say that he derived all his mental qualities from his *mother;*
His *son*, a man of good endowments, guillotined as an 'aristocrat.'

CASSINI, Jean-Dominique, a celebrated astronomer, the first remarkable member of a family which might be compared with that of the Bernouillis ;
His *son*, Jacques Cassini, astronomer ;
His *grandson*, Césare-François Cassini de Thury, became a member of the Académie des Sciences at the age of twenty-two ;
His *great-grandson*, Jacques-Dominique, Director of the Observatory at Paris, completed the topographical chart of France ;
His *great-great-grandson*, Henri-Gabriel (1781-1832), naturalist and philologist, died of cholera.

CONDORCET, mathematician and philosopher, seems to have derived much of his mental qualities from his *mother;*
His *uncle*, a bishop, was a relative of the Cardinal de Bernis.

CUVIER, Georges, naturalist;
His *mother*, an accomplished woman, took great pains with his
   education;
His *brother*, Frédéric, naturalist. *Researches on Instinct.*
D'ALEMBERT, was a natural son of Destouches, inspector of
   artillery, and of Mdlle. de Tencin;
His *mother* was noted for her wit, and belonged to a family
   that counted among its members the Cardinal de Tencin,
   Pont de Veyle, a dramatic author, and d'Argental, the corres-
   pondent of Voltaire.
DARWIN, Erasmus, author of *Zoonomia ;*
His two *sons*, Charles and Robert, physicians of note, of whom
   Charles died very young;
His *grandson*, Charles, the celebrated author of the *Origin of
   Species ;*
In this family we mention only those most worthy of note.
DAVY, Humphrey, chemist, and his brother John, physiologist.
DE CANDOLLE, Augustin-Pyrame, and his *son*, Alphonse, both
   celebrated botanists.
EULER, Leonhard. His *father* was a mathematician;
His three *sons*, Johann, Carl, and Christoph, astronomers,
   physicists, and mathematicians.
FRANKLIN, Benjamin.
Two *great-grandsons*, authors of works on the natural sciences,
   on chemistry and on medicine.
GALILEO-GALILEI ;
His *father*, Vicenzo, wrote a theory of music;
His *son*, Vicenzo, was the first to apply to timepieces his father's
   discoveries as to the pendulum.
GEOFFROY SAINT-HILAIRE, Étienne ;
His *brother*, an officer highly esteemed by Napoleon, died of
   fatigue after the battle of Austerlitz;
His *son*, Isidore, a naturalist.
GMELIN, Johan Friedrich. The *father*, two *uncles*, a *cousin*, and a
   son of this famous German chemist, were known by their works
   on botany, medicine, and chemistry.
GREGORY, James. The most distinguished of a family of mathematicians and physicists, which reckons no less than fifteen

remarkable members, among them his *son* and his two *grand-sons.* Thomas Reid was the son of one of his nieces.

HALLER, Albrecht, regarded as the founder of modern physiology;
His *father*, learned in the law;
His *son*, a literary man and historian.

HARTLEY, David, philosopher and physician;
His *son*, a member of Parliament, a correspondent of Franklin, and one of the plenipotentiaries at the Peace of Paris.

HERSCHEL, Sir William;
His *father* and *brother* are specially noted as musicians—musical talent was hereditary in the family;
His *sister*, Caroline, aided him in his astronomical labours, and received a gold medal from the Royal Society;
His son JOHN, one of the greatest astronomers of this century;
Two *grandsons*, also astronomers.

HOOKER, William, and his *son*, Joseph D., botanists.

HUMBOLDT, Alexander, and his *brother* William.

HUNTER, John, the famous English anatomist;
His *brother* William, and his *nephew* Matthew, were also distinguished anatomists.

HUYGHENS, a Dutch astronomer;
His *father*, a mathematician and statesman;
His *brother* was engaged in public life, and followed William III. to England.

JUSSIEU, Bernard de, may be regarded as the most eminent of a family of botanists, whose genealogy is as follows:—

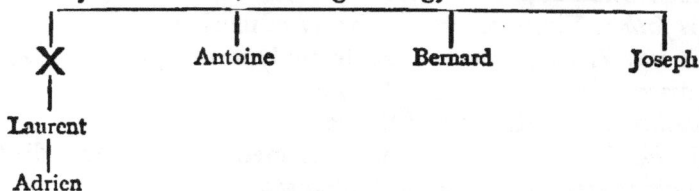

```
  |        |         |          |
  X      Antoine   Bernard    Joseph
  |
Laurent
  |
Adrien
```

LEIBNITZ. His *grandfather* and his *father* professors of jurisprudence at Leipzig.

LINNÆUS. The talent of this great botanist is found, though in a lower degree, in his *son* Charles.

MILL, John Stuart.
His *father*, James, was well-known for his works on psychology and political economy.

NEWTON, like many men of genius, stands alone. Galton, however, thinks Charles Hutton, the mathematician, and James Hutton, the geologist, were his remote descendants.

ŒRSTED, Danish physicist;
His *brother* and his *nephew* were statesmen;
His *son*, a naturalist and traveller

PLATO left no children;
His *nephew*, Speusippos, was head of the Platonic school after the master's death.

PLINY (the Elder), naturalist;
His *nephew*, Pliny the Younger.

SAUSSURE, Swiss geologist and physicist;
His *father*, author of works on agriculture and statistics;
His *son*, a naturalist.

SAY, Jean-Baptiste, his *son*, Horace, and his *grandson*, Léon, a family of political economists.

STEPHENSON, George, and his *son* Robert, both celebrated engineers.

WATT, James. His *mother*, Agnes Muirhead, was a superior woman;
His *grandfather* was a humble professor of mathematics;
His *father* was baillie of Glasgow for twenty years;
One of his *sons*, who died at the age of twenty-seven, gave great promise as a geologist, and was the friend of Sir Humphrey Davy.

AUTHORS AND MEN OF LETTERS.

ADDISON, one of the best prose writers of England, minister in the reign of George I.;
His *father*, a very learned divine and author.

ARNOLD, Thomas, Head-Master of Rugby School, one of the reformers of public instruction in England;
His *son*, Matthew, poet and critic.

BOILEAU, Nicolas, falls rather under this category than under that of imagination;
His two *brothers*, Jacques, Doctor of the Sorbonne, and Gilles, both authors.

BOSSUET. We may, perhaps, class with him
His *nephew*, Bishop of Troyes, who edited his uncle's works.

BRONTĒ, Charlotte, published, under the name 'Currer Bell,' *Jane Eyre* at the age of twenty-two. Her *sisters*, under the names Ellis and Acton Bell, published remarkable novels.

CASAUBON, Isaac, and his *son* Méric, scholars and philologists.

CHAMPOLLION, J.-François, the earliest interpreter of hieroglyphics;
His *son*, Jean-Jacques, historian and archæologist.

ÉTIENNE, a family of literary men and scholars, whose principal members were—Robert, who printed the Bible ;
His *brother* Charles, scholar and man of science ;
His *son* Henri, author of the *Greek Lexicon;*
Another *son*, Robert.

FÉNELON, Archbishop of Cambrai.
His *nephew*, ambassador in Holland, author of diplomatic memoirs. Also two *great-nephews* were remarkable men.

GRAMMONT, DE, author of the famous *Mémoires ;*
His *father*, Philibert, a courtier of much wit, and an author;
His *grand-uncle*, Richelieu (*vide* Richelieu).

GROTIUS, founder of international law ;
His *grandfather*, a scholar;
His *father*, curator of the University of Leyden;
His *uncle*, Cornelius, professor of philosophy and jurisprudence ;
His *son*, Petrus, diplomatist and scholar.

HALLAM.
His *father*, Dean of Bristol, and his *mother* are both spoken of by the biographers as remarkable persons ;
His *son* Arthur, who died at twenty-three ; the subject of Tennyson's *In Memoriam ;*
His other *son*, Henry, died at twenty-six ; was a young man of great promise.

HELVETIUS, author and philosopher ;
His *father* and *grandfather* were distinguished physicians, and inspectors general of the hospitals of Paris.

LAMB, Charles, whose name is always inseparable from that of his *sister* Mary.

LESSING, Gottlieb Ephraim, had two *brothers*, Karl and Johann, both distinguished as men of letters.

MACAULAY, Thomas Babington.
His *grandfather*, minister of Inverary, was an eloquent preacher;
His *father*, a brilliant writer and zealous abolitionist ;

Two *uncles*, one of them a general, long governed a portion of the Madras Presidency; the other was tutor to the Princess Caroline of Brunswick.

NIEBUHR, the Roman historian;
His *father*, traveller and author.

PALGRAVE, Sir Francis, author of erudite works on Anglo-Saxon history. Two *sons*, one a scholar, the other a traveller and orientalist.

PORSON. A family of classical scholars. We have already mentioned the 'Porson memory.'

ROSCOE, well-known by his historical studies on the period of the Renaissance, had
Three *sons*, political writers and poets.

LE SAGE, novelist. With him may be named
Two *sons*, dramatists and actors.

SCALIGER, Julius Cæsar, first made his mark as a scholar at the age of forty-seven;
His *son* Joseph, a scholar, like his father.

SCHLEGEL, Wilhelm, and his *brother*, Friedrich;
Their *father* was a well-known preacher, who also wrote some poems;
Two *uncles*, one dramatic poet and critic, the other historian to the King of Denmark.

SENECA, Lucius Annæus.
His *father*, Marcus, a rhetorician, had a prodigious memory;
His *brother*, Gallio, Proconsul of Achaia, considered as one of the most accomplished Romans of his day;
His *nephew*, Marcus Annæus Lucan, the poet.

SÉVIGNÉ, the Marquise de;
Her *son* was, as her letters show, a man, though dissipated, of considerable wit;
Her *cousin*, Bussy-Rubutin, was of similar character.

STAËL, Madame de.
Her *grandfather*, Charles Frédéric Necker, was professor of law at Geneva, and wrote on that subject;
Her *father*, minister of Louis XVI., and an author;
Her *uncle*, Louis Necker, professor of mathematics at Geneva;
The *son* and *grandson* of the latter, Jacques and Louis Necker, professors of natural science at Geneva.

SWIFT. The poet Dryden was his *grand-uncle.*
TROLLOPE, Mrs., the novelist;
Two *sons*, Anthony and Thomas, novelists.

The list might easily have been extended, but the names here given are probably sufficient for our purpose.

CHAPTER VI.

HEREDITY OF THE SENTIMENTS AND THE PASSIONS.

I.

MAN is situated in the midst of the universe, which acts upon him only by its properties. Colours, odours, savours, forms, resistances, movements, become modes of our organism, producing therein a shock to the nerves. Then all these peripheric impressions pass to the brain, probably into the optic thalami; and, being thence transmitted to the cortical substance of the brain, they are transformed, we know not how, into facts of consciousness: the physiological phenomenon becomes psychological, constituting that state of the mind which we denominate cognition. But this is not all. The nerve-vibrations produced by material objects not only make us acquainted with something outside of us, but they also produce within us a certain agreeable or disagreeable state, which we call feeling. If there were no such reverberation of pleasure or pain within us, then our experiences of the external world would be, as Bichat says, ' only a frigid series of intellectual phenomena.'

Those phenomena of sensation of which the subjective character is opposed to the objective character of the phenomena of cognition may have an ideal as well as a real cause. Experience shows that pure concepts—simple ideas—may not only be acts of consciousness, but may also produce in us agreeable or painful conditions. Thus, whoever conceives the ideal of a future state of society, with a larger measure of justice, morality, science, and happiness, simultaneously with his perception of this fair vision is pleasurably affected by the sight of what might be, painfully by the sight of what is.

If we add that pleasure and pain may be excited in us either by some state of our organs dependent on the vital processes, or by recollections suggested by memory, we have enumerated every mode of cognition which can produce phenomena of sensation. Causes—real and ideal—present and past—all these elements are added to each other, placed in juxtaposition and fusion, and neutralize each other, so as to produce these complex sensations, which make their appearance very slowly, both in the individual and in the species. Thus, the sentiment of nature in a poet of the nineteenth century, a Byron or a Goethe, is the result of so great a number of actual perceptions, recollections, and ideas blended together, that it defies the analysis of the most accomplished psychologist. The psychology of the sentiments, moreover, is far from being as advanced as that of the intellect.

In studying the sentiments, we may do so either as naturalists or as metaphysicians. In the former case, we describe and classify the various phenomena of sensibility; this is the work of the psychologist. In the other case, we strive to reduce all these phenomena to their law, their ultimate cause ; and this is the work of the philosopher.

The descriptive method is much indebted to contemporary physiologists and psychologists, and particularly to Mr. Bain in his great work, *The Emotions and the Will.* Still, there is no definite classification of phenomena of the affections, for this can only be founded on an embryology of the sentiments, which has, as yet, no existence. Every naturalist knows that a natural classification is based on anatomy, physiology, and embryology. So, too, in psychology, until we have investigated and described the manifestations of sentiment in the animal kingdom, and in the lower races, with a view to a comparative psychology ; until we have traced the evolution of the sentiments, in the individual and in the species, in order to ascertain its genesis, it will be impossible to arrive at a natural, objective, stable classification.

Since Spinoza, no essential contribution has been made to a philosophical study of the ultimate reason of sensible phenomena. Physiologists—those, at least, who are acquainted with philosophy— appear to have the same opinion ; for Müller copies the third book of Spinoza's *Ethics,* and Dr. Maudsley, in his recent work,

The Physiology and Pathology of Mind, says 'the admirable explanation of the passions given by Spinoza has never been surpassed, and certainly it will not be easy to surpass it.'

As the author of the *Ethics* profoundly observes, the ultimate explanation of all sensible phenomena is found in the fact of desire, 'desire meaning appetite with self-consciousness,' and appetite being 'the very essence of man, in so far as it is directed to acts which tend towards his conservation.' Desire is the physical and moral constitution of man, inasmuch as it strives towards being and well-being, towards existence and development. It has its ultimate root in the region of the unconscious; nor do we know how it becomes conscious, under that form of tendency which characterizes it. Desire is, like thought, one of the forms of the unknowable : it is the unknown quantity, the x which serves to explain for us all phenomena of the affections. We may, indeed, reduce the endless variety of passions, emotions, and sentiments to two very broad states, viz. pleasure and pain—that is to say, an augmentation or diminution of being—but the cause of the two states is desire. It is just because there are in us tendencies that may be satisfied or opposed, that we feel pleasure or pain. In fact, when we experience pleasure or pain, we wish to preserve the one and to destroy the other; but this conscious desire, sometimes regarded as the effect of the primitive unconscious desire, is, in reality, only a continuation of it. That state of tension which we call *desire*, and which lasts as long as we live, is modified each instant—and hence our joys and our sorrows; these are but moments of a continuous process, and desire is, as it were, the woof on which the chances of life embroider all our emotions.

In sensibility everything tends first of all and directly towards ourselves; later and indirectly towards others. 'The love of self is the root of all the passions; it is the supreme law of sensibility, the nature of which is to look only to its own good.' We love only ourselves; or, in others, that which is like ourselves. Our sympathetic tendencies, manifold and strong though they be, are derived from, and may be ultimately reduced to, love of self without egotism. Sympathy being, in its genuine sense, 'the tendency of one individual to fall in with the emotional or active states of others,'[1] to have a community of sentiments with a man or an animal is to resemble him in one respect; it means being at once ourselves and another. Our selfish and our sympathetic tendencies are, therefore, both equally natural, but the former are based upon our own nature, the latter on an analogy with it. The admirable researches of physiologists on the sympathetic contagion of nervous diseases, may some day serve as the basis for new studies on the emotions. This is not the place to enter on them; we would merely show that phenomena of the affections pertain to our inmost being. By this fact of cognition the outer world is let in upon us, and is reproduced in miniature, for thought is nothing but existence arriving at self-consciousness; but our feeble personality is associated with this impersonal state by the pleasures and pains it produces in us; for sensation and volition make us what we are. The modes of sensibility are so intimately connected with the organs, and with the whole constitution, that, *a priori*, we might conclude that they are transmitted by heredity. Experience will be found to verify this hypothesis.

II.

We can cite only striking facts—that is to say, passions so violent or so extravagant as to attract the attention of the physician or the historian; yet any one, by questioning his own memory, may easily see that certain modes of sensation, and, consequently, of action, may be preserved hereditarily in families too obscure for notice.

First, then, in animals the transmission of individual character is a fact so common as scarcely to need illustration. 'A horse that is naturally vicious, sulky, and restive,' says Buffon, 'will beget foals with the same character.' Every horse-breeder has verified this fact in regard to his stud.

'Heredity,' says Girou de Buzareingues, 'may, even in animals, extend to their most whimsical peculiarities. A hound taken from the teat, and bred far away from either parent, was incorrigibly obstinate and gun shy in circumstances where other dogs were

---

[1] Bain, *The Emotions*, ch. xii., 'On Sympathy.' The entire chapter should be studied.

eagerly excited. When a bystander expressed his surprise, he was told that there was nothing remarkable, "his father was the same."'

Nor is the transmission of characters less striking when races and species are crossed. As we have seen, when the domestic pig and the wild boar, or the wolf and the dog are crossed, some of the progeny inherit the savage, and others the domestic instincts. Similar facts have been observed by Girou in the crossing of different races of dogs and cats. 'Lord Orford, as is well known,' says Darwin, 'crossed his famous greyhounds, which failed in courage, with a bull-dog—this breed being chosen from being deficient in the power of scent. At the sixth or seventh generation there was not a vestige left of the form of the bull dog, but his courage and indomitable perseverance remained.'[1]

The heredity of propensities, instincts, and passions in animals is very good evidence for this form of heredity in man, inasmuch as it does away with all superficial explanations drawn from education, example, habit, and all those external causes which are supposed to stand in lieu of heredity. And we may remark that this circumstance shows the value of a comparative psychology.

If, now, we consider man, the first phenomena of the affections with which we meet are those of organic sensibility, or cœnæsthesis, a kind of inner sense of touch whereby we are cognizant of the state of our organs, of the tension of our muscles, and of all muscular exertion in general, of the state of weariness, of pleasure, etc. This universal consciousness of existence, this *Gemeingefühl*, is the result of an infinite number of internal sensations proceeding from the nerves, the muscles, the circulation, the nutrition—in a word, from all those functions the sum of which constitutes what we call our manner of being.

It cannot be doubted that heredity transmits these sensations; and it is probably in them that we must look for the true source of all resemblances of character. But these internal states are of so indeterminate a nature that it is almost impossible to prove their transmission. Nevertheless, we believe that the heredity of certain strange propensities, instincts, and dislikes, may

---

[1] *Variation, etc.*, i. 57.

be referred to these unconscious modes, which underlie all consciousness and all thought.

Thus, families have been known in the members of which the smallest doses of opium produce a convulsive state. Zimmermann speaks of a family on whom coffee had a soporific effect, acting like opium, while opium itself produced no effect. Some families can hardly endure emetics, others purgative medicines, others blood-letting.

Montaigne, who took an interest in the question of heredity, because he derived from his family a tendency to stone, inherited also an invincible repugnance for medicine. 'The antipathy,' he says, 'is hereditary. My father lived seventy-four years, my grandfather sixty-nine, and my great-grandfather almost eighty, and never tasted nor took any kind of physic, and for them anything not in common use was a drug. My ancestors, by some secret instinct and natural inclination, have ever loathed all manner of physic—the very sight of drugs was an abomination to my father. The Seigneur de Gerviac, my paternal uncle, who was an ecclesiastic, and sickly from birth, and who, notwithstanding, made his weak life to hold out to the age of sixty-seven, falling once into a high protracted fever, the physicians had word sent to him that he must surely die if he would not take some remedy. The good soul, affrighted as he was at this horrible sentence, said, ''Then it is all over with me.' But God soon after made their prognostications to prove vain. Possibly I have received from them my natural antipathy to physic.' [1]

When, from the organic sensations diffused over the whole body, we pass to the wants and inclinations which have their seat in a special organ, it is easy to give indisputable instances of passions hereditarily transmitted. This we propose to show with regard to the three chief physical wants, viz. thirst, hunger, and the sexual appetite.

The passion known as dipsomania, or alcoholism, is so frequently transmitted that all are agreed in considering its heredity as the rule. Not, however, that the passion for drink is always transmitted in that identical form, for it often degenerates into mania,

---

[1] Montaigne, *Essays,* ii. 37.

idiocy, and hallucination. Conversely, insanity in the parents may become alcoholism in the descendants. This continual metamorphosis plainly shows how near passion comes to insanity, how closely the successive generations are connected, and, consequently, what a weight of responsibility rests on each individual. 'A frequent effect of alcoholism,' says Dr. Magnus Huss, 'is partial or total atrophy of the brain : the organ is reduced in volume, so that it no longer fills the bony case. The consequence is a mental degeneration, which in the progeny results in lunatics and idiots.'

Gall speaks of a Russian family in which the father and grand-father had died prematurely, the victims of this taste for strong drink. The grandson, at the age of five, manifested the same liking in the highest degree.

Girou de Buzareingues knew several families in which the taste for drink was transmitted by the mother.

In our own times, Magnus Huss and Dr. Morel have collected so many facts bearing on the heredity of alcoholism, we need only select a few instances :—

A man belonging to the educated class, and charged with important functions, succeeded for a long time in concealing his alcoholic habits from the eyes of the public ; his family were the only sufferers by it. He had five children, only one of whom lived to maturity. Instincts of cruelty were manifested in this child, and from an early age its sole delight was to torture animals in every conceivable way. He was sent to school, but could not learn. In the proportions of the head he presented the characters of microcephalism, and in the field of intellectual acquisition he could only reach a certain low stage, beyond which further progress was impossible. At the age of nineteen he had to be sent to an asylum for the insane.

Charles X——, son of an eccentric and intemperate father, manifested instincts of great cruelty from infancy. He was sent at an early age to various schools, but was expelled from them all. Being forced to enlist in the army, he sold his uniform for drink, and only escaped a sentence of death on the testimony of physicians, who declared that he was the victim of an irresistible appetite. He was placed under restraint, and died of general paralysis.

A man of an excellent family of labouring people was early

addicted to drink, and died of chronic alcoholism, leaving seven children. The first two of these died at an early age, of convulsions. The third became insane at twenty-two, and died an idiot. The fourth, after various attempts at suicide, fell into the lowest grade of idiocy. The fifth, of passionate and misanthropic temper, broke off all relations with his family. His sister suffers from nervous disorder, which chiefly takes the form of hysteria, with intermittent attacks of insanity. The seventh, a very intelligent workman, but of nervous temperament, freely gives expression to the gloomiest forebodings as to his intellectual future.

Dr. Morel gives the history of a family living in the Vosges, in which the great-grandfather was a drunkard, and died from the effects of intoxication ; and the grandfather, subject to the same passion, died a maniac. He had a son far more sober than himself, but subject to hypochondria, and of homicidal tendencies ; the son of this latter was stupid, idiotic. Here we see in the first generation, alcoholic excess ; in the second, hereditary dipsomania; in the third, hypochondria ; and in the fourth, idiocy, and probable extinction of the race.

Trélat, in his work, *Folie Lucide,* states that a lady of regular life and economical habits was subject to fits of uncontrollable dipsomania. Loathing her state, she called herself a miserable drunkard; and mixed the most disgusting substances with her wine—but all in vain, the passion was stronger than her will. The mother and the uncle of this lady had also been subject to dipsomania.

Quite recently, Dr. Morel had again an opportunity of proving the hereditary effects of alcoholism, in the 'children of the Commune.' He inquired into the mental state of 150 children, ranging from ten to seventeen years of age, most of whom had been taken with arms in their hands behind the barricades. ' This examination,' he says, ' has confirmed me in my previous convictions as to the baneful effects produced by alcohol, not only in the individuals who use this detestable drink to excess, but also in their descendants. On their depraved physiognomy is impressed the threefold stamp of physical, intellectual, and moral degeneracy.' [1]

---

[1] For all the facts here cited, see Morel, *Traité des Dégénérescences,* p. 103 ; Dr. Despine, *Psychologie Naturelle,* tome ii. 525—528 ; tome iii. 142 ; see also Lucas, i. 476, *seq.*, and ii. 776.

As regards those passions which have their origin in the desire of eating, it is impossible to cite facts to prove their heredity so remarkably. Gluttony and voracity seldom lead to such deplorable results as alcoholism. It is not, however, difficult to find families in which voracity is inherited. This has been observed in the Bourbons. Saint-Simon informs us that Louis XIV. was a man of extraordinary greediness, and the same was the case with his brother. Nearly all this king's sons were gourmands and great eaters, and this passion has been transmitted to their descendants.

A more curious case, and one comparable to alcoholism, owing to its morbid character, is the fact of cannibalism which we have elsewhere cited, on the authority of Gall, Lordat, and Prosper Lucas. These authors tell of a Scotch family possessed of an instinctive propensity to cannibalism, which persisted through several generations : sundry members of this family paid the penalty of this with their lives, and others had to be placed under surveillance.[1]

It is probable that the children of cannibals, brought up in Europe, would exhibit the like tendencies in the midst of our civilization. Although no facts of this kind are recorded, it must be admitted that the incurable love of a wandering life manifested by these civilized savages, and their inability to adapt themselves to our usages—instances of which will elsewhere be given[2]—somewhat justify these presumptions.

Earth-eating, which A. von Humboldt met with in all tropical countries, presents a curious instance of morbid heredity. 'The people,' says this naturalist, 'have an odd and almost irresistible liking for a kind of greasy potter's clay with a strong, unpleasant smell. The children have often to be locked up to prevent them from running out after recent rain and eating clay.' He states that the women who are engaged in the potteries on the Rio Magdalena swallow great lumps of clay. At the mission of San Barjo, he saw an Indian child who, according to the statement of its mother, would hardly eat anything but earth ; the child, in consequence, looked like a skeleton. The negroes of Guinea have the same propensity ; they swallow a yellowish kind of earth which

---

[1] Lucas, i. 391, 497.   [2] See Part Fourth, ch. ii.

they call caouac, and when transported as slaves to America they try to procure a similar clay.

There is scarce need to insist on the heredity of all that is connected with the sexual appetite. This passion is associated with an organ which depends on the law of heredity. A multitude of names famous in history offer themselves in support of our position. Augustus and the two Julias; Agrippina and Nero; Marozia and Benedict IX. ; Alexander VI. and his children; Louise de Savoie and Francis I., etc. In all classes of society analogous facts may be found, and any one may know families in which this unfortunate disposition is hereditary.

' I knew,' says Prosper Lucas, ' a very handsome man, of an excellent constitution, but possessed of an unbridled passion for wine and women. He had a son, who, while yet but a lad, carried both these vices to excess. He carried off a mistress from his father, who never forgave the offence to the day of his death. This was the outset of his career ; he was afterwards ruined, and reduced to the utmost penury by harlots. *His* son died young, but incorrigible; and from the same vices as his father and grandfather.'

' But here,' says the same author, ' is a fact perhaps still more instructive. A man-cook, of great talent in his calling, has had all his life, and has still, at the age of sixty years, a passion for women. To this passion he adds unnatural crime. One of his natural sons, living apart from him, does not know even his father, and, though not yet quite nineteen, has from childhood given all the signs of extreme lust, and, strange to say, he, like his father, is equally addicted to either sex.' [1]

There are also well-authenticated instances of a heredity of a propensity for rape. The *Droit* (newspaper) states that in 1846, at Pontoise, a father, named Alexandre de M——, was so unfortunate as to have his eldest son, barely sixteen years of age, violate and murder his cousin ; and recently his second son attempted to violate a little girl. The punishment of these youths was mitigated, because it was proved at the trial .that they were under the influence of hereditary insanity.[2]

---

[1] P. Lucas, i. 479.   [2] Ibid. i. 504.

III.

If from propensities which, in their origin at least, are purely physical, we pass to the consideration of more complex passions, independent, or rather seemingly so, of the organism—for example, gambling, avarice, theft, and murder—we shall find these also subject to the law of heredity.

The passion for play often attains such a pitch of madness as to be a form of insanity, and, like it, transmissible. 'A lady of my acquaintance,' says Da Gama Machado, 'and who possessed a large fortune, had a passion for gambling, and passed whole nights at play. She died young, of pulmonary disease. Her eldest son, who was very like his mother, had the same passion for play. He, too, like his mother, died of consumption, and at about the same age. His daughter, who resembled him, inherited the same taste, and died young.'[1]

Avarice produces the same consequences. 'In several instances,' says Maudsley,[2] in his *Physiology and Pathology of the Mind,* 'in which the father has toiled upwards from poverty to vast wealth, with the aim and hope of founding a family, I have witnessed the results in a mental and physical and mental degeneracy, which has sometimes gone as far as the extinction of the family in the third or fourth generation. When the evil is not so extreme as madness or ruinous vice, the savour of a mother's influence having been present, it may still be manifest in an instinctive cunning and duplicity, and an extreme selfishness of nature—a nature not having the capacity of a true moral conception or altruistic feeling. Whatever opinion other experimental observers may hold, I cannot but think that the extreme passion for getting rich, absorbing the whole energies of a life, does predispose to mental degeneration in the offspring,—either to moral defect, or to intellectual and moral deficiency, or to outbreaks of positive insanity under the conditions of life.'

The heredity of the tendency to *thieving* is so generally admitted that it would be superfluous to bring together here facts which abound in every record of judicial proceedings. One, but that decisive, may be cited from Dr. Despine's *Psychologie Naturelle,* the genealogy of the Chrétien family.

[1] Da Gama Machado, p. 142.   [2] Maudsley, p. 234.

Jean Chrétien, the common ancestor, had three sons—Pierre, Thomas, and Jean-Baptiste. 1. Pierre had a son, Jean-François, who was condemned for life to hard labour for robbery and murder. 2. Thomas had two sons: (1) François, condemned to hard labour (*travaux forcés*) for murder, and (2) Martin, condemned to death for murder. Martin's son died in Cayenne, whither he had been transported for robbery. 3. Jean-Baptiste had a son, Jean-François, whose wife was Marie Tauré (belonging to a family of incendiaries). This Jean-François had seven children: (1) Jean-François, found guilty of several robberies, died in prison; (2) Benoist, fell off a roof which he had scaled, and was killed; (3) X——, nicknamed Clain, found guilty of several robberies, died at the age of twenty-five; (4) Marie Reine, died in prison, whither she had been sent for theft; (5) Marie-Rose, same fate, same deeds; (6) Victor, now in jail for theft; (7) Victorine, married one Lemaire: their son was condemned to death for murder and robbery.[1]

We have given this instance because it cuts short all explanations drawn from the influence of education and example. Doubtless it is difficult in many cases to determine what is due to education, and what to nature; and the children of thieves are not very likely to be trained to honesty by their parents; but still nature is always the stronger agency. Sundry authors, and among them Gall, have given instances of a disposition to thieving, where any parental influence was impossible. He gives one instance still more curious—that of two conflicting heredities: one good, from the mother, and one bad, from the father.

In 1845, the *Cour d'Assises* of La Seine condemned to severe and degrading penalties three out of the five members of a family of thieves. The father of this family had not found in his children the dispositions he desired. He had been compelled to use compulsion with *his wife and his two eldest children*, but they, to the last, refused to obey him. His eldest daughter, on the other hand, trod instinctively in her father's steps, and was passionate and

---

[1] Despine, tome ii. p. 410. Several facts of a like kind may be found in this work. Observe the tendency of such families to unite, thus conferring the hereditary transmission. See also Lucas, i. p. 480, *seq.*

violent like him. She took after her father, the rest of the children after their mother.

We may apply to the instinct for murder what we have just said of thieving. Instances of hereditary transmission are equally conclusive and equally numerous. We have already seen the heredity of homicide added, in a portion of a family, to the heredity of theft; and it is needless to cite cases that may be found in abundance on all sides.[1] Here, however, are two instances, in which the circumstances of the crime remove all doubt as to its hereditary transmission.

In the *Annales Médico-Psychologiques* for 1853 we read that two girls, Adèle and Lucie H——, aged thirteen and seventeen, were bound apprentices at Paris. Adèle was of remarkably gentle manners, and industrious; but Lucie was of an unsociable disposition, and disagreeable to her mistress and her companions. Enraged at her state of isolation, she endeavoured by threats and caresses to persuade her sister to murder their mistress. As Adèle refused, Lucie passed a stay-lace round her neck, intending to strangle her. Adèle cried out, and the mistress came to the spot. Lucie, disappointed in her hope of an accomplice, resolved to take her vengeance herself. She collected bits of glass and ground them to a powder; this she mixed with her mistress's dinner. The latter for several days suffered internal pain, the cause of which was unknown, until she discovered the pounded glass in Lucie's hands. The girl was arrested, but on her trial it was proved that her grandfather had, during his life, made many attempts at murder, and at last strangled his wife. His children never showed the least symptoms of homicidal mania; it reappeared, as we have seen, in the second generation.

In all cases where hereditary transmission takes the form of atavism, it is clear that the influence of education has no weight. The same may be said of all precocious homicidal acts, and of those committed out of frivolous motives, like the following :—

A boy of fourteen, one of a family in bad repute, went, armed with his bow, to a neighbouring village feast. He met on the way a little girl of six, who had in her hand thirty sous to buy bread,

---

[1] See Lucas, i. 504, 520; Despine, ii. 281, 283; Mireau, *Psychologie Morbide,* 319, 321.

knocked her down, strangled her, threw her body into a field at a distance from the road, took the thirty sous, and went on to the village feast to spend the money and enjoy himself.

The innate, incurable taste for a vagabond life shown so strikingly in inferior races, and in the gypsies, is also unquestionably a consequence of heredity. These facts will be considered from the social standpoint in the fourth part of this work.

The conclusion, perhaps unexpected, to which we are led by all the foregoing arguments, is this—that insanity very much resembles passion; and this statement is to be taken in the strict sense of the words. The common opinion readily enough admits that both obscure the intellect and paralyze the will, but is loth to admit that a violent passion is, in its generating causes, identical with insanity. When, however, we read judicial records, and especially medical annals, in search of facts to show the heredity of homicide, theft, or alcoholism, then, side by side, with the somewhat homogeneous facts wherein we see the passions of ancestors transmitted in identical form to descendants, we find other heterogeneous facts, in which what is passion in the former becomes insanity in the latter, and *vice versâ*. Such facts are very numerous. We have not cited any of these, though they are excellent instances of heredity. As we restrict ourselves to facts that are absolutely incontestable, we have put aside from consideration the whole question of heredity by metamorphosis.

We do not maintain that every violent passion or every crime is only a variety of insanity, but only that in many cases the conditions which produce both are identical. ‘Nothing in Nature is limited and isolated : all things are connected together by intermediate links, which attentive observation sooner or later discovers, where, at first glance, they were not even suspected. It were to be wished, in the interest of science, that inquiries should be made as to the progenitors of criminals for at least two or three generations. This would be an excellent means of demonstrating the kinship which exists between those cerebral infirmities which produce the psychic anomalies leading to crime, and the pathological affections of the nerve centres, particularly the brain. The fact, demonstrated by Drs. Ferrus and Lélut, that insanity is much more frequent among criminals than other persons, goes far to prove that crime and insanity are closely connected.'[1] The number of criminals whose ancestors have given signs of insanity is very great. Verger, the assassin of the Archbishop of Paris, was of this number. His mother and one of his brothers perished, prior to his crime, the victims of suicidal mania.

Dr. Bruce Thompson, in his recent work on *The Hereditary Nature of Crime*, adopts this conclusion, and supports it by figures. Of 5,432 prisoners, he found 673 whose mental state appeared to him to be unsound, though, according to the general opinion, they were not subjects for a lunatic asylum. Out of 904 convicts in prison at Perth, 440 were recommitted, thus showing the fatal power of the passions. In a house of detention there were 109 prisoners belonging to only 50 families ; among them were eight members of one family, and several families were represented by two or three members.

It is beyond our purpose to inquire to what extent passion shares in the fatal character of insanity, or to ascertain the practical consequences of this. The argument simply shows that (1) passions which are inexplicable, so long as they are studied in the isolated individual, find their explanation so soon as we have studied them in their metamorphoses through generations, and brought them under the great law of heredity ; (2) that passion is so near insanity that the two forms of heredity are really one : so that the preceding section is, as it were, a chapter, detached and in advance, on morbid heredity.

CHAPTER VII.

HEREDITY OF THE WILL.

I.

THE title given to this chapter is hardly exact, and is only selected for want of a better. Yet it seems to us that in the statesmen and great soldiers of whom we are about to speak, the will must be regarded as the dominant faculty. They must, no

---

[1] Despine, *Psychologie Naturelle*, ii. 983.

doubt, furthermore, possess a broad and penetrating intellect, passion to rouse men and enforce obedience; but their distinguishing characteristic is action, and that strong, bold nature which commands. It is only through the will one man gains an irresistible influence over others. A lofty intellect excites admiration, but it is only a strong will that demands obedience.

The word 'will' is here used, of course, in its ordinary sense, and as commonly employed. We lay aside for the moment all those philosophical discussions about free-will and its relations to heredity,[1] and here consider the will only as the active faculty, without inquiring whether the tendency to action be the result of individual inclination, of a fixed idea, or of an invincible passion.

The ancient moralists distinguished three kinds of life, according as pleasure, action, or contemplation was looked on as the end of man; they thought that a choice must be made between the three. They all, or nearly all, agreed in placing the life of pleasure in the lowest rank; but they long discussed the question whether the active life or the contemplative were preferable. This discussion is infinite, for every man decides according to his tastes, his temperament, and his habits. Men of action and men of thought contribute, each in his own way, to the common weal—the former sway the present, the latter prepare the future. The distinction, however, which lies at the base of this discussion is founded on a true observation of human nature. Except the mere sensualist, every man, from the highest to the lowest, is either active or contemplative: every one is a Cæsar or a Plato, as far as his intellect will allow. He who in some obscure village, in some remote land, takes trouble to conduct some small business, is akin to those who govern great states, or who win great battles. He who prefers leisure, who loves to dream and meditate, who aspires to some rude education as his ideal, is akin to great thinkers and great poets. The more closely we study men, the better we see that they may be brought under these two categories. Even where the contrast is not striking, it still exists, and we detect it when we observe more deeply. 'The keener the mind, the more men of originality will it discover.'

---

[1] See Part Second, ch. iii.

We have already seen that the contemplative faculties—imagination and simple intellect—are transmissible by heredity. History must answer whether it is the same with the active faculties. However, we must first consider what is meant by active faculties.

So far, we have employed a method of analysis, which, though really artificial, was necessary and sufficiently exact. We have been enabled to examine instinct, perception, imagination, memory, intellect, sentiments, and have inquired whether each of these modes of mental life, taken separately, is hereditary. In the present instance, the analytical method is impossible. With the statesman, the soldier, and, generally, with those who are called men of action, the play of the various faculties must be simultaneous. Their processes are essentially synthetic. In them, the work of each faculty counts only in so far as it concurs in the general result; the aim to which all means are subordinate. In the statesman, moreover, the mental activity must be exerted in every direction. M. Guizot somewhere observes that public life is ' the highest occupation of man's faculties.' If we reflect on the conditions it demands, and the faculties it requires, we may, perhaps, agree with him. The great advantage of public life is that it develops simultaneously our various faculties, and that it is, as has been said, of a synthetic nature. A thinker, a man of science, may isolate himself in the highest regions of intellect, but may be without sentiment, and unsuited for action. An artist may, by his imagination, be enchanted with the most delightful dreams, and yet know nothing of the real world. For politics, on the other hand, is required an intellect capable of grasping at once the universal and the particular, the abstract and the concrete. Is a statesman incapable of generalization?—he can have no broad views, and is the slave of routine. He cannot, moreover, like the man of science, content himself with general results: he must decide particular and definite cases; hence he must be able to grasp at once the whole, and its details. Furthermore, his reflections must of necessity result in acts. He is no speculative theorizer: for him theory is but a means, action alone is his end. Hence he is characterized by a strong power of will, always exercised, as also by the qualities which this implies; viz. boldness, courage, self-confidence, and mastery over the timid and irresolute

Thus, a talent for observation at once minute, broad, and rapid; a ready and faithful memory, recalling with exactitude and without hesitation the results of theory; a great presence of mind, not to be disconcerted by unforeseen circumstances; an energetic will; and, as a basis, physical strength, and certain bodily qualities —such are the faculties which must be combined, and act simultaneously, with the rapidity and certainty of instinct.

History shows that this sum of qualities is transmissible, as a whole or in part—for it sometimes happens that the original combination is broken up in passing to the descendants, who can collect but fragments (as Pitt and his grand-daughter). Like every other faculty, strength of will may be hereditary. This was observed by Voltaire with regard to the Guises. ' The physical, which is " father of the moral," transmits the same character from father to son for ages. The Appii were ever proud and inflexible; the Catos always austere. The whole line of the Guises was bold, rash, factious, full of the most insolent pride, and of the most winning politeness. From François de Guise down to that one who, all alone, and unexpectedly, put himself at the head of the people of Naples, they were all—in look, courage, and character— above ordinary men. I have seen full-length portraits of François de Guise, of Balafré and his son : they were all six feet high, and they all possess the same features—there is the same courage, the same audacity on the brow, in the eyes, and in the attitude.'[1] We know not how the will is thus transmitted; but when we see that its energy and its weakness are connected with certain states of the organism, and that physical strength commonly renders men bold and courageous, while physical weakness makes them timid, we can scarcely doubt that this transmission takes place by means of the organs, and that it is, in fact, physiological.[2]

Not to dwell on this point, we now proceed to note the most important cases of the heredity of the active faculties, quoting historical facts. These fall naturally under the two categories of statesmen and soldiers, though many men have been both. Here

---

[1] Voltaire, *Dictionnaire Philosophique*, Art. ' Caton.'
[2] Concerning the will as groundwork of the personality and character, see Part Fourth, ch. iii.

we must guard against the error of taking high official position as a proof of personal merit. In letters, science, or art, where every one is judged directly by his works, this illusion is impossible. In political life, the fame of ancestors, alliances, and power previously acquired, count for much, and sometimes supply the lack of all else. To avoid the danger of confounding an external and conventional heredity with that which is internal and natural, we cite none but the most indisputable cases.

II.—STATESMEN.

ADAMS, John (1785, 1826), second President of the United States;
His *son*, John Quincey, sixth President of the United States ;
His *grandson*, Charles Francis, American Minister to England, author of a *Life of John Adams.*

ANTONIA (the Gens Antonia) reckoned among its most distinguished members Marcus Antonius, the orator, Marcus Antonius, the critic, and Mark Antony, the rival of Cæsar.

ARTEVELD, Jacques, the famous brewer of Flanders ;
His *son*, Philippe, who continued his father's political work.

BENTINCK, William, Duke of Portland, Prime Minister of England, 1783, 1784, and 1807—1810 ;
His *son*, Henry, Governor-General of India ; he introduced there the freedom of the press and abolished Suttee ;
His *grandson*, member of Parliament, eminent financier, and a leading statesman.

CÆSAR. He might equally have been ranked among the soldiers, but is placed here on account of his family ;
His *mother*, Aurelia, seems to have been no ordinary woman. His *daughter*, Julia, who married Pompey and died prematurely, was remarkable for her wit and beauty. Historians have observed the transmission of certain hereditary characters in the family of the Cæsars. ' There existed in all the Cæsars,' says J.-J. Ampère, 'a morbid principle. The first was epileptic; his nephew (the Emperor Augustus) was a life-long valetudinarian ; an acrid humour disfigured the countenance of Tiberius ; Caligula was extraordinarily pale, slept little, and was constantly delirious; Claudius was physically inclined to imbecility ; Nero gave unequivocal indications of insanity ; Tiberius, adopted stepson of Augustus, ' had fine and noble

features, and was remarkably like his mother, Livia. His thin, dry lips show his crafty and ruthless soul.' The mother of Mark Antony belonged to the Julian family.

CHARLES THE FIFTH. There is a curious similarity between this sovereign and Don Carlos. On comparing Don Carlos with his celebrated grandfather, we discover such striking features of resemblance between them, that we cannot but see here an instance of reversional heredity, or atavism.

Don Carlos was the son of Philip II. and Dona Maria of Portugal. His mother, who died four days after giving him birth, appears in history only as an insignificant personage. As for the father, he was in nearly every respect the antithesis of his sons.[1] The character of Don Carlos, his temperament and his physical habit, are inexplicable unless we go back to Charles V.

Charles V. was slow in his development, and grew old early. He was nearly twenty-one before he could grow a beard. He was rather below the medium stature, his health was feeble, and his face long and sad in expression ; he spoke slowly, and stammered. The development of his intellect was as slow as that of his body. He remained for a long time absolutely dependent on Chièvres, his tutor. His phlegmatic temperament saved him from excesses, although his gluttony is well known. ' Before getting up, a capon was usually served to him, dressed with sugar, milk, and spice. He dined at noon, off a large number of dishes. Soon after vespers he took another meal, and for supper, later in the evening, he would take anchovies, or other strong, gross food. Even at the monastery of San Yuste he ate with avidity, before the eyes of his physician, frogs' legs and eel pies.'[2]

Don Carlos, according to the account of the Venetian envoys, and of the imperial ambassador at Madrid,[3] was a prince of very inferior stature—his features ugly and disagreeable. His temperament was melancholy, nor had he any taste either for study or for manly exercises. He spoke with difficulty

---

[1] See the contrast in Gachard, *Don Carlos and Philippe II.*, p. 237, *seq.*
[2] Prescott, *Reign of Philip II.*, vol. i. ch. 9.
[3] Gachard and Prescott, vol. iv.

and slowly, and his words were disconnected. 'His voice is thin and shrill; he is embarrassed when he begins to speak, and the words come with difficulty. He pronounces his *r*'s and his *l*'s badly.' At the age of twenty-one he had his tongue-string cut. He had little desire for women, but was a glutton, like his grandfather. In his prison, he brought on his own death by his excess in eating. He took to a diet consisting of partridge pie, pie-crust, spiced meats, and iced drinks. And he began these excesses very early in the day. ' He eats so much, and with such ravenousness,' writes the imperial ambassador, 'as to surpass belief; scarcely has he finished one meal when he is ready for another.'

The reader will observe that in the foregoing comparison we have not mentioned Don Carlos's violence of temper, which, also, we incline to think hereditary. As an infant, he would bite the breast of his nurse; there were three of them bitten so severely by him as to have their lives endangered. His short life is full of cruel acts. He used to beat his servants; he made an unskilful shoemaker eat a pair of boots; he wanted to burn down a house because a drop of water fell from it on his head. Later, while in prison, he would have the floor of his chamber flooded with water, and then would walk about barefooted and almost naked on the icy boards. Several times during the night he would have a pan full of ice and snow brought to his bed, keeping it there for hours. (Prescott, vii. 12.)

These, and sundry other acts, show mental derangement. If now, the reader will bear in mind that Charles V.'s mother was Juana the Mad,[1] Queen of Castille, he will see in Don

---

[1] According to recent investigations, the restraint of Juana was in a great measure due to political reasons ; but even if her insanity has been exaggerated, it must be admitted that she had a strange disposition, and a morbid sensibility. She was subject to 'frightful hallucinations.' (See Hildebrand, *Revue des Deux Mondes*, 1866, June 1.) Diseased, trembling with fever, and crippled by gout, he (Charles V.) nevertheless dragged his bones from place to place, disquieting the whole world by his own unrest, till an evil trick of fortune drove so wise a man into the convent of San Yuste, and afflicted him with the madness of Jane the Mad and Charles the Bold. Michelet, *Histoire de France*, vol. vii.

Carlos's insane acts fresh proof of reversional heredity. This same observation was made at the time by the Venetian ambassadors. ' He has been suffering almost uninterruptedly during the past three years from quartan fever, attended at times by mental alienation—a thing the more worthy of note, inasmuch as he seems to have inherited this disorder from his grandfather and great grandmother.'

CONDÉ. Of the family of Condé we will speak hereafter.

COLBERT, Jean-Baptiste. The family of this celebrated minister reckoned several distinguished members ;

His *brother*, Charles, statesman and diplomatist ;

His *son*, Jean-Baptiste, commanded the expedition against Genoa, in 1684 ;

Another *son*, Jacques, archbishop, member of the French Academy ;

A *nephew*, Charles's son, diplomatist.

CORNELIA (the Gens Cornelia). This family, which we shall meet again under the head of the Scipios, reckoned from P. Cornelius Scipio, Magister Equitum in 396, to Scipio Nasica, who died in 56, without issue, nineteen consuls, one dictator, two tribunes (the Gracchi), two quæstors, one ædile, one censor, two magistri equitum. To this family belongs the famous Sylla.

CROMWELL. His direct descendants are mediocre ; but we may mention with him two collaterals—the patriot Hampden, uncle's son to Oliver ; and Edmond Waller, the poet, Hampden's nephew.

DISRAELI, Benjamin, novelist, Prime Minister of England in 1868 ;

His *father*, Isaac, author of *Curiosities of Literature*, etc.

FLAVIA (the Gens Flavia) had for its principal representatives Vespasian, Titus, Domitian. Vespasian's avarice was hereditary. ' The founder of this family was a Cisalpine, Petro by name, a centurion under Pompey, who afterwards called himself Titus Flavius Petronius, and became a banker's clerk. His son, Flavius Sabinus, a tax collector in Asia, afterwards followed the trade of a usurer in Helvetia. One of *his* sons was Vespasianus, Proconsul of Africa. He bought, and sold and sold again horses and mules, and hence his nickname, "the Jockey."'

Fox, Charles James, Pitt's rival;

His *grandfather*, a statesman;

His *father*, Lord Holland, Secretary at War;

His *brother*, Stephen, statesman, and leader of the House of Commons;

Several *nephews*, statesmen, authors, and generals.

Grenville, George, Premier in 1763. Galton reckons twelve notable members in this family.

Guise, François, Duc de;

His *brother*, Charles, Cardinal de Lorraine;

His *son*, Henri, assassinated at the assembly of the States at Blois;

His *son*, the Cardinal, killed at the same time;

His *grandson*, Charles, who, with his *uncle*, the Duc de Mayenne, fought against Henri IV.;

His *great-grandson* conspired against Cardinal Richelieu.

Lamoignon, a celebrated family of magistrates, 'one of those families whose members seem born only to practise justice and charity, wherein virtue is transmitted with the blood, is upheld by good counsels, and is exalted by great examples.' (Fléchier.) Charles de Lamoignon, born 1514, was about to succeed to the chancellorship when he died, in 1572. He had twenty children, among whom were Pierre, a wonderful child, who died prematurely, and Chrétien, who was *Président à mortier*. Chrétien had a son, Guillaume de Lamoignon, First President of the Parliament, and the most celebrated of his family; Fléchier preached his funeral sermon. His son, Chrétien-François, *Président à mortier*, was an associate of Boileau, Racine, etc. His brother, Nicolas, was Intendant at Montauban, Pau, Poitiers, and Montpellier; he was implicated in the Dragonnades, but displayed great ability. Guillaume, son of Chrétien-François, First President, exiled by Maupéou. Chrétien-François II., great grandson of Boileau's friend, Chancellor in 1787. Malesherbes was of this family.

Medici. The following is their genealogy, abridged. The family was of middle-class origin ; in the fourteenth century, Silvestro was Gonfaloniere, or head of the Florentine Republic.

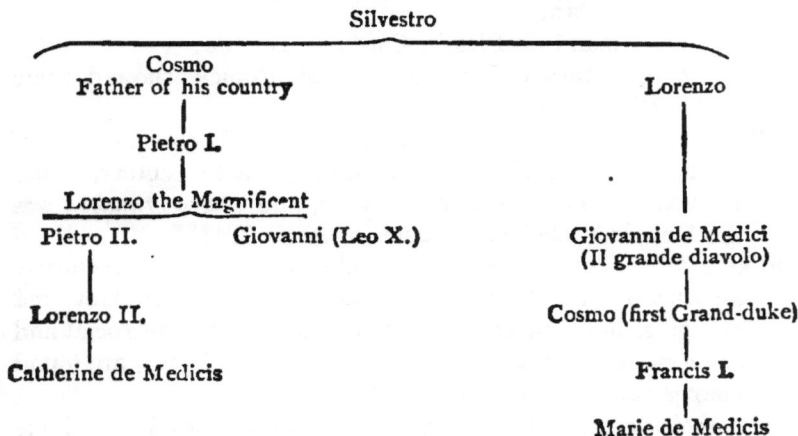

Silvestro

Cosmo Father of his country		Lorenzo

Cosmo, Father of his country
   Pietro I.
   Lorenzo the Magnificent

Pietro II.	Giovanni (Leo X.)

Pietro II.
   Lorenzo II.
   Catherine de Medicis

Lorenzo
   Giovanni de Medici (Il grande diavolo)
   Cosmo (first Grand-duke)
   Francis I.
   Marie de Medicis

As regards the relations of the Medicis to the three kings of France, Francis II., Charles IX., and Henry III., see Michelet, *Histoire de France,* vol. ix. He gives some very ill-digested physiological details.

MIRABEAU. In the opinion of his father, the ' Friend of Man ' (*ami des hommes*), possessed ' all the vile qualities of his maternal stock.'

' The correspondence of the great tribune's father and uncle, and the notice on the life of his grandfather, give evidence of a peculiar race, and exhibit the characters of a grand and lofty originality. Our Mirabeau needed but to descend from such stock, in order to spread himself abroad, to shower down as he has done, and to give of himself to all, so that we might name him the *enfant perdu,* the *enfant prodigue et sublime* of his race.' (Ste.-Beuve.)

PEEL, Sir Robert, thrice Premier ;
His *father*, a great manufacturer, founded the family ;
Two *brothers* and three *sons* of Peel's have held high judicial or administrative positions.

PITT, William, Lord Chatham, Premier in 1766, married a Grenville. (See Grenville.)
His *son*, William, Premier at twenty-five, the famous rival of Fox;

His *grand-daughter*, Lady Hester Stanhope, the 'Sibyll of the Libanus.' We shall meet with this family again, when we speak of the law.

RICHELIEU, Armand du Plessis, Cardinal, Duc de;

His *father*, François, Grand-Prévôt of France, showed some diplomatic ability;

The grandson of his *brother* Henri, Duc de Richelieu, one of the most curious characters of the eighteenth century, whose *son* was the famous Duc de Frousac, and whose *grandson* was the Duc de Richelieu, Minister of Louis XVIII.

SHERIDAN. 'The name of Sheridan,' says Galton, 'is peculiarly associated with a clearly marked order of brilliant and engaging, but "ne'er-do-weel," qualities. Brilliant social and conversational qualities, with a dash of profligacy, are found among numerous members of this family;

His *father* wrote a dictionary, and was manager of Drury Lane Theatre;

His *grandfather*, friend and correspondent of Swift;

His *son*, 'a Sheridan all over;'

His *grand-daughter*, Caroline, Mrs. Norton, poetess and novelist.

TEMPLE, Henry, Lord Palmerston. This family has had many remarkable members, among whom we may name Palmerston's great grand-uncle, Sir William Temple, author and statesman.

THEODOSIUS, Roman Emperor. In this family talent and vigour seem to have descended particularly to the female members.

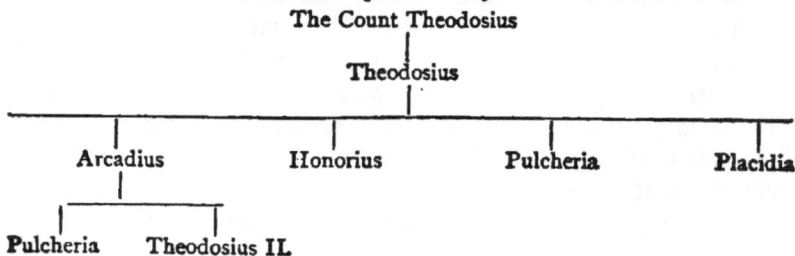

The Count Theodosius
|
Theodosius
|

| Arcadius | Honorius | Pulcheria | Placidia |

Arcadius
|

Pulcheria   Theodosius II.

WALPOLE, Sir Robert, Premier, 1721-42;

His *father*, Sir Edward, a distinguished member of Parliament in the reign of Charles II.;

His *brother*, Horace, a diplomatist of great ability;

Two *sons*, Edward, in government employ, and Horace, a man of letters. Byron calls him ' the incomparable.'

WITT. John de Witt and his brother Cornelius.

III.—SOLDIERS.

ALEXANDER THE GREAT, died at the age of thirty-two, had but one posthumous son, who was assassinated at the age of twelve ;
His *mother*, Olympias, an ambitious, intriguing woman ;
His *father*, Philip, King of Macedon ;
His *brother* (half-brother) Ptolemy, Philip's son by Arsinoe, though this filiation is very questionable. The family of the Ptolemies will hereafter be mentioned.
His *grand-nephew* (or great-grand-nephew ?) Pyrrhus, King of Epirus, whose resemblance to Alexander was long since noticed.

BERWICK, Duke of, natural son of James II. and Arabella Churchill ;
His *maternal uncle*, John Churchill, Duke of Marlborough.

BONAPARTE, Napoleon. The genealogy of this family is so well known, that the mere mention is enough.

CHARLEMAGNE. The direct succession is noteworthy ;
His *great-grandfather*, Pepin d'Heristal ;
His *grandfather*, Charles Martel ;
His *father*, Pepin the Short.

COLIGNY, Admiral Gaspard de, murdered in the massacre of Saint Bartholomew ;
His *father*, Gaspard, Marshal of France, gained distinction during the wars in Italy ;
His *uncle*, Duc de Montmorency, Constable of France.

DORIA, Andrea, Genoese admiral and statesman;
His *nephew*, Filippino, succeeded him as admiral and defeated the French.

EUGÈNE, Prince, ranked by Napoleon with Turenne and Frederick the Great;
His *grand-uncle*, Cardinal de Mazarin.

GUSTAVUS ADOLPHUS. Equally remarkable as statesman and general; spoke French, Italian, Latin, and German ; restored the University of Upsala ;

His *daughter*, Christina, who induced Grotius, Descartes, and Vossius to reside at Stockholm;

His *great-grandfather*, Gustavus Vasa. The latter had a daughter Cecilia, who was in many respects very like Christina;

His *grand-nephew*, the romantic Charles XII.

HANNIBAL, the greatest of a distinguished family of soldiers;

His *father*, Hamilcar Barca;

His *brothers*, Hasdrubal and Mago.

MAURICE OF NASSAU, one of the greatest captains of his time, was Governor of the Low Countries;

His *father*, William of Orange, 'the Silent;'

His *grandfather*, Maurice, Elector of Saxony;

His *brother*, Frederick William, Statholder;

His *great-nephew*, William III., Statholder, and King of England;

His *nephew*, Turenne.

NAPIER, Sir Charles, conqueror of Scinde;

His *great-grandfather* invented logarithms, and the family reckons eight members distinguished as generals or statesmen.

PTOLEMIES, the family of the Lagidæ;

The founder of this dynasty was Ptolemy Soter, son of Lagos, or, according to some, of Philip and Arsinoe. There were in this family three distinguished men: Ptolemy Soter; his *son*, Ptolemy Philadelphus, and his *grandson*, Ptolemy Euergetes.

The rapid decline of the Lagidæ seems to be the result of heredity, produced by intermarriage. Ptolemy II. married first his niece and then his sister; Ptolemy IV., his sister; Ptolemy VI. and Ptolemy VII. brothers, both married, consecutively, the same sister; Ptolemy VIII. married two of his sisters; Ptolemy XII. and Ptolemy XIII. married their sister, the famous Cleopatra.

SAXE, Marshal, natural son of Augustus II., King of Poland; he was great-grandfather of Georges Sand.

SCIPIO, P. Cornelius (Africanus Major) the greatest soldier of the Gens Cornelia, of which we have already spoken;

His *father*, who was conquered by Hannibal;

His *grandfather*, drove the Carthaginians out of Corsica and Sardinia;

His *daughter*, Cornelia, mother of the Gracchi;

His two *grandsons*, Tiberius and Caius Gracchus.

TROMP, Marten, and his *son*, Cornelius van Tromp, famous Dutch admirals.

TURENNE, probably the greatest general produced by France, prior to Napoleon ;

His *father*, Henri, Duc de Bouillon, pupil of the École de Henri IV., was leader of the Huguenots ;

Turenne's relationship to the house of Orange has been already mentioned.

It would be easy, by searching history, to collect a far larger number of cases of heredity. Those here given are sufficient to disprove all idea of accidental coincidence. It is not surprising that cases of heredity seem to be rarer among great soldiers than elsewhere. Many soldiers gifted with great natural abilities must have died before they could attain to fame or found a family.

CHAPTER VIII.

HEREDITY AND NATIONAL CHARACTER.

I.

WE have thus hastily traversed the field of history, noting a few important cases of mental heredity in families of artists, men of science, literary men, soldiers, and statesmen. Considerations of this nature are so foreign to most historians that their works afford but little aid in our present study. They care little for details, which are 'beneath the dignity of history,' and disregard those little, precise, and trivial facts which teach us more about a character than ten pages of vague phrases. From biographies and memoirs we may learn more, though in them little attention is bestowed on physiological data. The day will, perhaps, yet come when such history will not be so disregarded and so rare, and when it will be seen that the infinitesimally small plays, in the evolution of humanity, the same latent and incessant part as in the evolution of nature. Then history, without neglecting the study of great facts and their connection—which is its chief purpose—will furnish the psychologist with materials both numerous and precise. Since, in the absence of such works, our researches would necessarily be long, tedious, and often without result, all that we have been able to do here is to indicate roughly the part of heredity in history, as a physiological and psychological law. We have had to content ourselves with showing its existence, for we have no means of telling, save in a vague way, in what measure a given quality has descended from one generation to another, whether it has varied, or why it has varied.

We have now to treat of the influence of heredity, not on individuals, but on masses. We shall see how it transmits and fixes certain psychological characters in a people as in a family.

The habit of our times is to regard the State as an organism. Herbert Spencer has even shown that this simile holds good at every point ; that there is in nature a hierarchical series of organisms parallel to the hierarchical series of states, the one from the protozoon to man, the other from the savage tribes of Australia to the most highly civilized nations of Europe ; and that in the organism, as in the State, progress consists in division of labour, and in the increasing complexity of functions. The organism subsists only by a continual assimilation and disassimilation of molecules : the State by continual gain and loss of individuals. But amid this incessant whirl, which constitutes their life, there is ever something fixed, which is the basis of their unity and their identity. In a people, that sum of psychical characteristics which is found throughout its whole history, in all its institutions, and at every period, is called the national character.

The national character is the ultimate explanation, and the only true one, of the virtues and vices of a people, of its good or bad fortune. This truth, simple though it is, is hardly yet recognized. The successes and reverses of a people do not depend on their form of government, but are the effect of their institutions. Their institutions are the effect of their manners and their creeds; their manners and creeds are the effect of their character. If one people is industrious, another indolent ; if the one has an internal, moral religion, and the other an external, sensuous religion, the cause is to be looked for in their habitual mode of thinking and feeling—that is to say, in their character. Nor can it be seriously doubted that character itself is also an effect. It is extremely probable that every character, individual or national, is the very complex result of physiological and psychological laws. But sociology is a science so little advanced that we dare not risk a judgment on the causes of the formation of national characters, and hence we must provisionally regard character as an ultimate cause. On this basis, let us see what part is played by heredity in the formation of national character.

It is usual to explain the history of a people by their institutions, which, in one sense, is true, though institutions themselves are but an effect. In the social and political order, effects and causes are not presented under the form of a simple series, as in the physical order; we rather find a reciprocity of action between them. The character produces the institutions, and they in turn form the character; thus, after several generations, the two are but one, the institutions are but the character rendered visible and permanent. Still, we must not forget that the institutions are only an external cause, which is sustained by an internal cause—character—and this is transmitted hereditarily. Take a people in its earliest period—the Romans under the kings, or the Gauls before Cæsar's time—the grand outlines of its character are already traced. They are probably the result of its physical constitution, and of the climate. And as a people is perpetuated by generation; as it is a law of nature that like shall produce like; as the exceptions to this law tend to disappear when large masses instead of particular cases are examined, obvious facts point out how national character is preserved by heredity.

This is, after all, only to assert that physical transmission is as much the law for obscure individuals as for famous men. In the preceding chapters we have taken our examples from history, because such examples are known to all. But every one is aware that the various modes of imagination, intelligence, and sensibility may be preserved by heredity in ordinary, obscure families. Every one might readily find in his own experience instances to confirm this. The permanence of national character is at once the result and the experimental proof of psychological heredity in the masses.

If we had any true science of ethnographical psychology, we should more clearly perceive the part played by heredity in the formation of the character of a people. Such a science may one day exist; at present we have but fragments. In France, M. Taine has based on the law of heredity his studies on the literature, the constitution, and the manners of England, considered as an expression of national character—he has shown how firmly the old Germanic and Scandinavian groundwork was established, and sees in Lord Byron a true descendant of the Berserkers.

In Germany, Lazarus and Steinthal have laid the foundation for a psychology of nations, 'of which the object is to determine the nature of the mind of a people, and to discover the laws which govern its internal, intellectual, or ideal activity in life, in art, and in science.'[1] Even in the absence of such scientific researches, based on exact criticism, historians have long been accustomed to express decided judgments upon national character, and the impossibility of altering it. Thus, the French of the 19th century are, in fact, the Gauls described by Cæsar. In the *Commentaries*, in Strabo, and in Diodorus Siculus we find all the essential traits of our national character : love of arms, taste for everything that glitters, extreme levity of mind, incurable vanity, address, great readiness of speech, and disposition to be carried away by phrases. There are in Cæsar some observations which might have been written yesterday. 'The Gauls,' says he, 'have a love of revolution ; they allow themselves to be led by false reports into acts they afterwards regret, and into decisions on the most important events; they are depressed by reverses; they are as ready to go to war without cause as they are weak and powerless in the hour of defeat.'[2]

But it is, perhaps, among that people which has borne successively the names of Ancient Greeks, Byzantines, and Modern Greeks that we must look for the most striking instance of the tenacity of character. 'Amid all these vicissitudes,' says Ampère, 'the fundamental character of the Greek has not changed ; he has now the same qualities, the same defects, as of old.' Pougueville found in the Morea Apelles's and Phidias's models; and, what is

---

[1] *Zeitschrift für Völkerpsychologie und Sprachwissenschaft,* band i.

[2] Cæsar, *De Bello Gallico,* iv. 5. See also Strabo, iv. 4. Diodorus Siculus, v. ; Michelet and H. Martin, tome i. ; and Carlyle, *French Revolution,* vol ii. book iii. ch. 2.

of more interest to us, he shows that the chief traits of the national character and habits have been transmitted; thus, the Arcadians still lead a pastoral life, and the inhabitants of Sparta, their neighbours, have a love for fighting, and an excitable, quarrelsome temper. In the middle ages the Byzantine possessed all the essential characteristics of his ancestors.

If the reader will examine with us the ponderous, but scarce known, volumes of the histories of the Lower Empire, he will find that this people which called itself Roman[1] remained thoroughly Greek, notwithstanding their Latin traditions, their imperial routine, their manners imported from the East—such as eunuchs, the dress and worship of the emperor, etc.—and their narrow Christianity. There is here a curious study in historical psychology which we would one day willingly attempt. From the Greek the Byzantine derived, besides language and literary traditions, a subtlety which, for want of mental force to strengthen it, degenerated into low cunning. The love of the Greek for rhetoric and brilliant conversation became the braggart self-assertion of the Byzantine; the subtle sophistry of the philosophers degenerated into the empty scholasticism of the theologians; and the versatility of the *Græculus* into the perfidious diplomacy of the Emperors. The Byzantine is the Greek of Pericles' time, but in a dry and withered old age.

Similar observations might be made on any nation whatsoever, but it is enough to direct the reader's attention to this subject. To sum up, every people has its own physiognomy, and this results (1) from certain primary characteristics, considered here as final causes; (2) from external conditions, or the influences of circumstances; (3) from heredity, which maintains the primitive characteristics. To this last factor, so often overlooked, we will now attend.

II.

It may be further observed that crossings and alliances take place between different nations—to their advantage, say some, to their great disadvantage, say others. This, at least, is certain, that such intermingling of blood must, to some extent, modify

[1] 'Οι Ρωμαῖοι : so the Byzantines always designated themselves.

the national character, which remains intact where there is no such intermixture. But there are very few nations indeed that have been able to survive and gain civilization without fusion with others. Though it has been held that the superior races are those which have ever been exclusive—a proposition which we will hereafter examine in detail—still it is difficult to see how, under such conditions, a people could acquire that variety and that complexity of elements without which civilization is impossible. A great, simple civilization is a contradiction in terms, so that we have but little chance of reaching a conclusion. One of two things must always take place : either a people remains intact, and then its development is inconsiderable ; or it develops only by intermingling with other races.

Yet, after having spoken of nations among whom the primitive national character, in its struggle with foreign elements, must have been in some degree modified, we turn to some which have been at least relatively exclusive. Were China better known, that country would probably offer a curious subject of study. We take for examples the Jews, the Gypsies, and the Cagots.

THE JEWS.

The Jewish people is, perhaps, the only one that has played a part in history, while jealously guarding its purity of race. It is not, however, quite unmixed. From the psychological point of view, it is not easy to decide how far its character has been modified by Persian doctrines after the Babylonian captivity, by Greek and Egyptian manners from Alexander to Philo, and, in the middle ages, by the hard condition of its very existence. According to Munck, 'the commercial spirit of the modern Jew is not a heritage from his ancestors, but the result of the oppressions to which they were subjected, and of their exclusion from every other trade.' It will, however, be generally admitted that, notwithstanding a few physical and moral variations from which no living thing is free, the Jewish nation has preserved better than any other its distinctive character : in other words, that in them heredity is better seen than elsewhere.

But when we attempt to determine the physical and moral characteristics of this race, not in vague and general phrases, but in definite points, there is considerable difficulty.   Here, however, are a few.

The Jews are usually to be distinguished by their black hair and beards, their long eyelashes, thick, prominent, arched eyebrows, their large, dark, bright eyes, their dark complexion, their strongly aquiline noses.   In the east there are fair or red Jews : or, as they are called, German Jews.   They seem to result from a crossing of German or Sclavonic races with the original Jews.[1]   There are, also, black Jews settled in India from time immemorial, who possess very many of the physical characters of the Hindus, owing to the influence of the climate, of circumstances, and perhaps of cross-breeding.   Still, they have a remote resemblance to the Jews of Europe.   Nott and Gliddon, after having studied the question profoundly, conclude that 'all Jews possess some identical features.'

According to the statistical tables of France, Algeria, and Prussia, it would appear that this race is remarkably long-lived.[2] In the various countries of Europe they increase more rapidly than the Christian populations.   Thus, in Germany, twenty-five per cent. of Christians die before they are six months old ; twenty-five per cent. of Jews before they are twenty-eight years and three months ; fifty per cent. of the Christian population die before they are twenty-eight, while fifty per cent. of the Jews exceed fifty-three years.

As regards moral qualities, the Jewish race is presented in history as possessed of very definite characters, viz.—a pre-dominance of sentiment and imagination ; and this it is that has given that nature its aptitude for the creation of religion, poetry, and music.   We need not dwell upon the religious importance of a nation from which have sprung Judaism and Christianity, and which alone among the nations of antiquity rose to Monotheism. Nor can their poetic eminence be called in question, though this race has a poetry of its own—passionate, convulsive, abrupt, and full of imagery.   Though among the Jews we find very few painters and sculptors, their aptitude for music is remarkable : no other

---

[1] *Bulletins de la Société d'Anthropologie*, tome ii. p. 389.
[2] *Ibid.* vol. i. p. 180.

race has given to the world so high a proportion of musicians. We need only mention the names of Mendelssohn, Halévy, and Meyerbeer.

On the other hand, they are but ill-endowed with all that relates to scientific culture. 'A race incomplete by reason of its very simplicity, it has neither plastic art nor rational science, nor philosophy, nor political life, nor military organization. The Semitic race has never understood civilization in the sense which we attach to the word; no great organized empires, no public spirit are found in its womb. The questions of aristocracy, democracy, and feudalism, which constitute the whole secret of Indo-European history, have no meaning for the Semitic race. Their military inferiority is the result of their utter incapacity for discipline and organization.' (Renan.)

To these general considerations may be appended a few more precise facts. Heredity seems to have exerted on the Jewish race a baleful influence, by sowing the seed of sundry mental disorders, the result of intermarriage. The number of Jewish deaf-mutes is enormous. Idiocy and mental alienation are also very frequent. According to the German statistics, there is one *idiot*

In Silesia	to	580	Catholics, to	408	Protestants, to	514 Jews.
In Wurtemburg	to 4,113	,,	to 3,207	,,	to 3,003	,,

And one *lunatic*

In Bavaria	to	908	,,	to	967	,,	to	514	,,
In Hanover	to	528	,,	to	641	,,	to	337	,,
In Silesia	to 1,355	,,	to 1,264	,,	to 624	,,
In Wurtemburg	to 2,006	,,	to 2,028	,,	to 1,544	,,

(*Bulletins de la Société d'Anthropologie,* tome iv.)

THE GYPSIES.

The Gypsies, called in different countries by the names of Bohemians, Zingari, Zigeuner, and Gitanos (*Egyptians*), afford a striking example of the hereditary conservation of certain psychological characteristics.

According to Pasquier, they first appeared at Paris in 1427. Accused of palmistry and sorcery, they were excommunicated, expelled the country, threatened with death and the galleys. At present Gypsies are to be found in most European countries. In Turkey and in Hungary they are smiths, tinkers, musicians

In England they are tinkers and horse-dealers. In Transylvania, Moldavia, and Wallachia, they have their own chiefs, and enjoy a fair share of the comforts of life. In Russia there are some Gypsies that are rich and respected. But the classic land of the Gypsies is Spain. Seville, Cordova, the caves of Monte Sagro, near Grenada, and the forests of Andalusia, the cellars and attics of Madrid, swarm with them. They live in squalid huts, surrounded by all the paraphernalia of sorcery, and their only business is thieving, dancing, and fortune-telling. An English missionary, Mr. Borrow, who succeeded in overcoming their abhorrence of all Christians, who lived with them and spoke their language, has given us valuable particulars as to their habits and usages.[1]

It is generally believed that the Gypsies are of Hindu origin ; that they may have passed through Egypt, but do not spring from it ; that they were a despised caste, probably expelled from India, unless, indeed, they left it after the conquest of Tamerlane. Their true and sacred name is *Romi.* ' All the world over,' says Borrow, ' their usages are the same, and they employ the same words.' When we compare sundry terms of their idiom with the corresponding Sanscrit words (especially those denoting number), the analogy is striking.

Undoubtedly the physical and mental constitution of Gypsies is the same in all countries. It is, no doubt, somewhat difficult to decide how much is due to education, that is to say, to tradition ; and how much to heredity. To the latter, however, these facts seem due.

As regards physical constitution, Borrow finds in all Gypsies hard, sharp features, jet black hair, fine, white teeth, bright eyes, and the ' fascinating ' glance.

As regards their intellect, they appear to be as thoughtless and frivolous as children. ' Nothing makes a lasting impression on the Gypsy's mind ; it is as restless as running water, and reflects all images alike. The Gypsy believes everything and nothing, or, rather, believes only in the sensation of the moment ; a sensation that is past is for him only a fable. Hence he is sceptical, not only as regards moral and social ideas, but even with

---

[1] *An Account of the Gypsies of Spain.* By G. Borrow.

regard to his own impressions. He abandons himself to a
blind trust in fleeting emotions, just as, in the ordinary course of
life, he gives himself up to all the chances of vagabondage. One
impression is driven out by another. In him simple animalism is
supreme. Emotions—of whatever kind, gross or poetical, grovel-
ling or exalted—are the rule, and, as it were, the motive power of
his mind.' Their poetry, specimens of which Borrow gives, is
prosaic, rude, vulgar, and childish rather than artless.

As their mind, so their manners : with childish ideas they have
a childish morality. If children had a morality of their own, it
would be a very bad morality. Hobbes was right when he said :
Homo malus, puer robustus. What specially characterizes the
Gypsy is his love, his inborn need, of vagabondage, and an
adventurous life. He abhors civilization as slavery, and despises
all sedentary and regular occupation. Marriage is but a temporary
union, concluded in presence of a few members of the tribe.
Gypsies usually live organized into corporations or tribes, under
the authority of an elective chief—a very primitive form of polity.
Hating, as they do, all civilized peoples, they have certain vices to
which they cling as to an hereditary creed, and these they love and
uphold as a religion. Thus, their highest ambition is to steal from
the Christians ; and mothers teach their children thieving as the
noblest of virtues. They are, moreover, like children, less violent
than tricky, incapable of lofty thoughts, and unaffected in their
superstitions. Borrow having translated into Romany the
Gospel according to St. Luke, the Gypsies accepted the book,
and, regarding it as a talisman, carried it about their persons when
they went to thieve.

This race offers a curious instance of a native incapacity, preserved and transmitted by heredity, for adaptation to civilized life.
The Gypsies are in our moral and social world what the dodo and
the ornithorhynchus are in our physical world, the survivors of a
past age. Civilization is a very complex condition, a moral atmosphere to which man has to become acclimatized. There must be
a correspondence between the moral man and his moral conditions, as between the physical man and his physical conditions.
Whoever cannot adapt himself to new conditions of social life
must die out—gradually, perhaps, yet surely. If he disappears

but slowly, he remains only as a curious and useless thing, picturesque to an artistic eye ; but he is ill adapted to his circumstances, and certain sooner or later to vanish.

THE CAGOTS.

The various names of Cagots, Agots, Capots, Gahets, and Caqueux, are given to races which subsisted down to the present century in Guyenne, Gascony, and Béarn, on the northern side of the Pyrenees, in Navarre and Guipuzcoa, and even in Maine and Brittany.[1] They formed a population apart, separated from the other inhabitants by the aversion with which it was regarded. Popular tradition confounded these people with lepers. It was said that they might be distinguished by their dull-gray eyes, and by the shortness of the lobe of the ear. 'They are,' says an author of the 16th century, 'comely men, industrious, skilful mechanics ; but in their countenances and in their acts you always detect something that makes them worthy of all the abhorrence wherewith they are universally regarded. Furthermore, be they as comely as they may, they have all, men and women alike, a stinking breath, and when you come near one of them you experience a certain unpleasant odour emanating from their flesh, as though some curse descending from father to son had fallen upon this miserable race of men.'

Though, like the population amid which they lived, they were Catholics, still they were not allowed to mix with 'their co-religionists. Their hovels stood at some little distance outside the villages ; they could enter the parish church only through a narrow doorway exclusively reserved for them ; they took the holy water from a special stoup, or received it from the point of a stick; and in the church they had a corner where they were obliged to

---

[1] During the Reign of Terror there were yet to be found many of the Caqueux in Finistère. M. Francisque Michel states that in a commune of the canton of Accous, arrondissement of Oléron, a Cagot was, about the year 1817, nominated for maire of the commune, to the great scandal of the people of the place. Protests were sent in from all sides to the préfet, but he did not heed them. Still the complaints did not cease, they continued to be made till 1830, when the electors forced the maire to retire into his former privacy. —*Histoire des Races Maudites,* i. 127.

keep apart from the rest of the faithful. Down to the end of the
17th century they were required by the legislation then in force
to wear a distinctive mark, called 'the goose's foot,' or 'the
duck's foot' (*pied d'oie, pied de canard*) in the decrees of the par-
liaments of Navarre and of Bordeaux.

Of course these outcasts intermarried, as a general rule, and
marriages between Cagot families held to be 'pure' were very
rare. Hence this race remained under much the same conditions
as the Jews—in a state highly favourable to hereditary transmission. It is to be observed that many of those who have spoken of
these Cagots from personal observation, and particularly the
physicians of the 16th and 17th century, whose remarks are given
in M. Michel's work, noticed the fact of heredity. On the other
hand, the same author tells us that a modern writer says, 'I distrust external signs as means of distinguishing Cagots from people
of other races.' Perhaps these opinions might be reconciled, if
we observe that the Cagots do not appear to have been a race
strictly distinct, like the Jews and the Gypsies. While the origin
of the last-named races is known, that of the Cagots is extremely obscure. All sorts of conjectures have been made,
ranging from the one which would have them to be the descendants of a servant of the prophet Elijah, down to that which sees
in them a remnant of the Goths.[1] If, then, between the Cagots
and the surrounding population there were no diversity of race, all
external differences would gradually disappear under the influence
of identical conditions.

Still, during their pariah period the Cagots would have been a
curious object of study from the standpoint of psychological and
moral heredity. But unfortunately the data are totally wanting.
We only know that in Guyenne and in Gascony they were all
coopers or carpenters; and that in Brittany they were all rope-
makers; and were considered very expert in their trade. But this
fact seems to us to be far less the result of heredity than of the
caste-rule to which they were subjected. They were accused of
being presumptuous, arrogant, braggart—defects which may be
explained as well by the attitude of permanent hostility in which

---

[1] *Races Maudites,* i. 266.

they stood with regard to all other men, as by the organic transmission of quality. There is one simple fact, insignificant enough
in itself, respecting an hereditary taste and talent for music: 'Navar-
reins has seen the Campagnets hand down through three or four
generations a highly prized violin. No holiday was happily spent
where the violin or the flute of the Campagnets did not contribute
to the mirth.' [1]

CHAPTER IX.

MORBID PSYCHOLOGICAL HEREDITY.

I.

AT the commencement of this work, in the introduction
devoted to physiological heredity, we showed briefly that diseases
are transmissible, like all the characteristics of the external or
internal structure, and all the various modes of the organization in
a normal state. The same question now arises in the psychological order. Are the modes of mental life transmissible under their
morbid, as they are under their normal form? Does the study of
mental diseases contribute its quota of facts in favour of heredity?
The answer must be in the affirmative. The transmission of all
kinds of psychological anomalies—whether of passions and crimes,
of which we have already spoken, or of hallucinations and insanity,
of which we are next to speak—is so frequent, and evidenced by
such striking facts, that the most inattentive observers have been
struck by it, and that morbid psychological heredity is admitted
even by those who have no suspicion that this is only one aspect
of a law which is far more general.

In considering hereafter the direct causes of mental heredity,
we shall endeavour to establish this important proposition : that
in man, to every psychological state whatsoever, corresponds
a determinate physiological state, and *vice versâ*. Here this
question is presented incidentally, for it has been much debated
whether mental diseases have or have not an organic cause.

---

[1] *Ibid.* i. **41.**

If we restrict ourselves to palpable, visible, demonstrated, and accepted facts, we meet with two sorts of cases : those in which disorders of the intellect have corresponding to them evident changes of the tissue of the nerve-centres, and those in which the brain presents no appreciable degeneration.

Taking their stand on facts of the second of these categories, some writers on insanity, of whom the most celebrated is Leuret, have held that insanity may proceed from purely psychological causes. ‘ Physiology,’ says he, ‘ pathology, acquaintance with the facts and the laws of thought and of passion, clinical and microscopic observations, therapeutical experiments—all concur to negative the absolute proposition that insanity always and necessarily has its rise in an affection of the organs. While everything contributes to bestow the character of evidence upon the following definition of insanity : ‘ Insanity consists in the aberration of the understanding . . . and the causes that produce it mostly belong to an order of phenomena that have nothing to do with the laws of matter.’ Notwithstanding these categorical affirmations, Leuret’s view finds daily fewer adherents. The reason of this is, that it really rests only on our ignorance and impotence. It simply affirms that in many cases there exists no physical cause, since we discern none. But beyond the limits that cannot be passed by the microscope, there exist phenomena which, though inappreciable to our senses, are nevertheless material. Electricity, magnetism, and all the various physical and chemical agencies, produce in our inmost organs molecular changes which elude our methods of investigation, but of which the consequences may be fatal. Moreover, the idea of a mental disease independent of all organic cause is a theory so unintelligible that the Spiritualists themselves have rejected it, and it is now generally admitted that the cause of madness is always to be found in a diseased state of the organs : insanity, like other maladies, is a disease physical in its cause, though mental as regards most of its symptoms.[1]

---

[1] See Lemoine, *L'Aliéné*, p. 105—137. The hypothesis of purely psychological causes of insanity led Heinroth to pen the following absurdities which are worth quoting :—

‘ Insanity is the loss of moral freedom ; it never depends on a physical cause ;

Since the direct cause of insanity is some morbid affection of the nervous system, and as every part of the organism is transmissible, clearly the heredity of mental affections is the rule. It makes little difference whether we regard thought as simply a function of the nervous system, or the nervous system as a simple condition of thought. Our experimental psychology, which deals only with facts, remands to metaphysics all researches into first causes. The metamorphoses of heredity are still more perplexing. Nervous disorders are often transformed in their transmission. Convulsions in the progenitors may change to hysteria or to epilepsy in the descendants. A case is cited where hyperæsthesia in the father branched out in the grandchildren into the various forms of monomania, mania, hypochondria, hysteria, epilepsy, convulsions, spasms. Facts of this kind are very numerous. To confine ourselves to psychological metamorphoses, nothing is more frequent than to see simple insanity become suicidal mania, or suicidal mania become simple insanity, alcoholism, or hypochondria. ' A goldsmith, who had been cured of a first attack of insanity, caused by the revolution of 1789, took poison ; later, his eldest daughter was seized with an attack of mania, passing into dementia. One of her brothers stabbed himself in the stomach with a knife. A second brother gave himself up to drunkenness, and ended his career by dying in the streets. A third, owing to domestic annoyances, refused all food, and died of anæmia. Another daughter, a woman of most capricious temper, married, and had a son and daughter: the former died insane and epileptic; the latter lost her mind during her lying in, became hypochondriac, and wished to starve herself to death. Two children of this same woman died of brain fever, and a third would never take the breast.' [1] This is one of the most instructive cases we have.

---

it is not a disease of the body, but a disease of the mind, a sin. It neither is, nor can be hereditary, because the thinking *ego*, the soul, is not hereditary. What is transmissible by way of generation is temperament and constitution, and against these he must react whose parents were insane, if he would not himself become lunatic. The man who, during his whole life, has before his eyes and in his heart the image of God, need never fear that he will lose his wits,' etc.

[1] Piorry, *De l'Hérédité dans les Maladies*, p. 169. See also Maudsley, *Pathology of Mind*, 244—256.

There are others of a more obscure nature, which give us a glimpse of the curious relations between talent and insanity. Long before Moreau of Tours' celebrated thesis in regard to genius, Gintrac had noticed the following fact : a father touched with insanity had able sons, who filled public situations with distinction. Their children appeared at first sensible, but at the age of twenty became insane. In twenty-two cases of hereditary insanity, Aubanel and Thoré have noticed two facts of this kind.

Deferring, for a while, the difficult question of the metamorphoses of heredity, we here give only similar, and, consequently, the most indisputable, cases, and they also are the most frequent. There are families the members of which, with few exceptions, are all subject to the same kind of insanity. Three relations were placed at the same time in a lunatic asylum at Philadelphia. In a Connecticut asylum there was once a lunatic the eleventh in his family. Lucas mentions a lady who was the eighth. More curious still, this infirmity often appears at the same period of life in successive generations. All the scions of a noble family at Hamburg, distinguished through four generations for great military talents, went mad at the age of forty : there remained but one member, a soldier like his father, and he was, by decree of the senate, forbidden to marry ; the critical period came, and he also went mad. (Lucas.) A Swiss merchant saw two of his children die insane both at the age of nineteen. A lady went mad at the age of twenty-five after childbirth ; her daughter became insane at the same age, also after childbirth. In one family the father, son, and grandson committed suicide at about the age of fifty. (Esquirol.)

II.

We now proceed to show from examples that the chief varieties of mental malady are transmissible. In the absence of any universally accepted classification, we group our facts under the following heads : Hallucination, Monomania, Suicide, Mania, Dementia, Idiocy.

Hallucination assumes two principal forms. Sometimes it results from the automatic action of the nerve-centres, and is compatible with perfect reason ; hallucination in this case does not imply error of judgment: it is recognized as an illusion, nor is the subject of the hallucination at all deceived. In the other case, the hallucination is complete, and then the patient believes in the objective reality of his imaginary perceptions, and acts accordingly. Under this form, hallucination is one of the first symptoms of insanity. It is hereditary in both shapes.

'We cannot establish by statistics,' says the author of one of the best treatises on this subject, 'the power of heredity on hallucinations, because they almost always exist with insanity. In order to thoroughly appreciate this influence, it should be studied in individuals who have only simple hallucinations, and in those monomaniacs, subject to hallucination, who have a very decided form of insanity. It is undeniable that they often occur in the sons of those who have presented this double condition.

' The father of Jerome Cardan used to see apparitions ; so also did his son. Catherine de Medicis had an hallucination, as Pierre de l'Estoile relates ; and her son, Charles IX., had one the very night of the massacre of Saint Bartholomew.' [1]

Abercrombie cites a case of hereditary hallucination where the reason remained intact. ' I know a man,' says he, 'who all his life has been subject to hallucination. This disposition is of such a nature that if he meets a friend in the street, he cannot tell at once whether it is an actual person or a phantasm. By dint of attention he can make out a difference between the two. Usually he connects the visual impressions by touch, or by listening for the footfalls. This man is in the flower of his age, of sound mind, in good health, and engaged in business. Another member of his family has had the same affection, though in a less degree.'

Here is a case no less curious. A young man of eighteen, neither enthusiastic, nor superstitious, nor fanciful, lived at Ramsgate. Happening one evening to enter a village church, he was terror-stricken at seeing the ghost of his mother, who had died some months before. Having witnessed this same apparition many times, he fell sick, and returned to Paris, where his father lived. He did not venture to speak to him of this apparition.

Being obliged to sleep in the same room as his father, he was surprised on seeing that, contrary to his former habit, the latter

---

[1] Brierre de Boismont, *Des Hallucinations*, p. 431.

always kept a light burning through the night. As this trouble-some light prevented the son from sleeping, he put it out one night, but his father, much agitated, bade him light it again.

At length the young man went to visit a younger brother, who was at school in a small town some fifty miles from Paris. The schoolmaster's son said to him, almost at once : ' Has your brother ever given any signs of insanity ? Last night he came downstairs in his shirt, quite beside himself, declaring that he had seen his mother's ghost.' [1]

This fact can only be explained by supposing that the sons derived from their father a tendency to hallucination under the influence of their deep regret for their loss.

A man in the Lyons hospital was subject simultaneously to hallucinations of taste and smell; tormented by disgusting odours and tastes, he spent whole hours in blowing his nose and spitting. His father had died in the same hospital from the effects of mania with hallucination.

We might also cite the famous Seeress of Prevorst, Frederika Hauffe, whose life, together with a collection of her visions, was edited by Kerner. This faculty of ' talking with the spirits ' was shared by most of the members of the Hauffe family. Her brother, in particular, possessed this gift, but in a lower degree, and without the complication of the phenomena of ecstasy and cata-lepsy which characterized the seeress.[2]

III.

Among the morbid psychological affections to which Esquirol gave the name of monomania, there is none the heredity of which is better proved than that of suicide. Voltaire was among the first to call the attention of physicians to this subject.

' I have with my own eyes,' he writes, ' seen a suicide that is worthy of the attention of physicians. A thoughtful professional man, of mature age, of regular habits, having no strong passions, and beyond the reach of want, committed suicide on the 17th ot October, 1769, leaving behind him, addressed to the council of his

---

[1] Brierre de Boismont, *Des Hallucinations*, p. 57.

[2] Lucas, ii. 769.

native city, an apology for his voluntary death, which it was not thought advisable to publish, lest men should be encouraged to quit a life whereof so much evil is spoken. So far there is nothing extraordinary, since instances of this kind are everywhere to be found ; but here is the astonishing feature of the case :—

' His father and his brother had committed suicide at the same age as himself. What hidden disposition of mind, what sympathy, what concurrence of physical laws, caused this father and his two sons to perish by their own hand and by the same form of death, just when they have attained the same year of their age ?' [1]

Since Voltaire's day, the history of mental disease has registered a great number of similar facts. They abound in Gall, Esquirol, Moreau of Tours, and in all the writers on insanity. Esquirol knew a family in which the grandmother, mother, daughter, and grandson committed suicide. 'A father of taciturn disposition,' says Falret, 'had five sons. The eldest, at the age of forty, threw himself out of a third story window; the second strangled himself at the age of thirty-five ; the third threw himself out of a window ; the fourth shot himself; a cousin of theirs drowned himself for a trifling cause. In the Oroten family, the oldest in Teneriffe, two sisters were affected with suicidal mania, and their brother, grand-father, and two uncles put an end to their own lives.[2] One of the most singular combinations of related suicides on record is this . ' D——, son and nephew of suicides, married a woman who was daughter and niece to suicides. He hanged himself, and his wife married a second husband who was son, nephew, and first-cousin of suicides.'

The point which excited Voltaire's surprise, viz. the heredity of suicide at a definite age, has been often noticed. 'M. L——, a monomaniac,' says Moreau of Tours, 'put an end to his life at the age of thirty. His son had hardly attained the same age when he was attacked with the same monomania, and made two attempts at suicide. Another man, in the prime of life, fell into a melancholy state and drowned himself; his son, of good constitution,

---

[1] Voltaire, *Dictionnaire Philosophique*, Art. 'Caton.'

[2] *Annales Medico-Psychologiques*, 1844. Several other facts will be found in Lucas, ii. 780, and in Moreau, *Psychologie Morbide*, 171—174.

wealthy, and father of two gifted children, drowned himself at the same age. A wine-taster who had made a mistake as to the quality of a wine, threw himself into the water in a fit of desperation. He was rescued, but afterwards accomplished his purpose. The physician who had attended him ascertained that this man's father and one of his brothers had committed suicide at the same age and in the same way.'

This identity of the manner of suicide is another point worthy of notice, as tending to show the automatic character of the heredity. We have given several cases in point, and the data with regard to this matter show that the same manner of death is often traditional in a family : some drown, others hang, or strangle themselves, others throw themselves out of window.

With suicidal may be ranked *homicidal monomania,* of which we have already spoken under the head of passions, and which is also hereditary. We need here give only one instance of this form of morbid heredity, but it is one that by itself is more convincing than a host of others. We take it from the *Annales de Henςke,* 1821.

A woman named Olhaven fell ill of a serious disorder, which obliged her to wean her daughter, six weeks old. This complaint of the mother began by an irresistible desire to kill her child. This purpose was discovered in season to prevent it. She was next seized with a violent fever, which utterly blotted the fact from her memory, and she afterwards proved a most devoted mother to her daughter.

This daughter, become a mother in her turn, took two children to nurse. For some days she had suffered from fatigue and from 'movements in the stomach,' when one evening as she was in her room with the infants, one of them on her lap, she was suddenly seized by a strong desire to cut its throat. Alarmed by this horrible temptation, she ran from the spot with the knife in her hand, and sought in singing, dancing, and sleep, a refuge from the thoughts that haunted her. Hardly had she fallen asleep, when she started up, her mind filled with the same idea, which now was irresistible. She was, however, controlled, and in a measure calmed. The homicidal delirium recurred, and finally gave way, only after many remedies had been employed.

A form of monomania which has now disappeared, but which was in a highly flourishing state three hundred years ago, is the monomania of possession, or dæmonomania. In our day, the narratives of demoniacal possession read like dreams; but in the times when they had a place outside of the world of fiction, when they were a cruel and absurd reality, and when possession was a crime having its tribunals, its code of procedure, and its punishments, this mental affection, then qualified as supernatural, was transmitted by heredity.

Writers on possession are unanimously of opinion that from generation to generation the members of a family were bound to the devil, or were sorcerers. Two high authorities on the question—Bodin, in his *Démonologie,* and Sprenger, in his *Malleus Maleficorum*—lay down this principle as a rule that has no exception. Bodin says: 'When the father or mother is a sorcerer, the sons and daughters are sorcerers.' Sprenger says that the accused must always be carefully questioned, ' *si ex consanguinitate sua aliqui, propter maleficia, fuissent dudum incinerati, vel suspecti habiti,*' for witchcraft commonly infects the whole race. The accused were themselves the first to admit this.

In our times, persons who think themselves possessed are merely sent to a lunatic asylum, and sometimes several members of one family will be found there affected with this form of monomania. A mother and her daughter believed themselves to be under the special protection of spirits, which they called Airs. A lady of B—— believed herself to be a fantastic being whom she called Solomon, and who was, for her, the Genius of Evil, and the author of all her torments. Her father attributed to a sylph named Stratagème everything that happened to him.[1]

With dæmonomania may be classed the epidemic choreæ of the middle ages, which, according to mediæval authors, were hereditary in some families. So, too, with the convulsionaries of the seventeenth century: during the epidemic of ecstasy mingled with convulsions, which broke out among the Protestants of the Cévennes, children of four or five years, and even of eighteen months, were affected with the prevailing disorder. Sympathy

---

[1] Moreau, *Psychologie Morbide,* 171.

and nervous contagion certainly contributed to produce this phenomenon, but there is no doubt that it is to be in a great measure referred to heredity.

Another mental affection, known as melancholia and lypemania, by some authors identified with hypochondria, but by others held to be a distinct complaint, though it much resembles it in its psychological effects, while differing in its organic causes, is also hereditary. 'Lypemania,' says Esquirol, 'is most commonly hereditary; lypemaniacs are born with a particular temperament, the melancholic, and this predisposes them to lypemania.'

Cases are on record of families, all of whose members are tormented with the fixed idea that people want to murder them or poison them. A woman affected with lypemania was sent, at the age of forty-two, to an asylum, and there died. It was discovered that her grandfather and her mother had been insane; and her son, barely fifteen years of age, already gave signs of lypemania.[1] In 482 cases of this disorder, Esquirol found 110 to be hereditary.

With this form of morbid heredity we may couple the heredity of presentiments. The following curious case is taken from Brierre de Boismont. If we accept the anecdote as true, we must, says Dr. Delasiauve, recognize the principal cause of the phenomena in the heredity of a nervous affection.

'Marshal de Soubise related, in presence of Louis XIV., that as he was one day conversing in his cabinet with an English lady, he all at once heard the lady utter a shriek, and saw her rise to go away and fall unconscious at his feet; this without any external cause. Filled with surprise and concern, the Duke de Soubise rang the bell. The servants ran in and attended on the fainting lady, who soon came to herself. " Do not detain me," she said to the Marshal, excitedly; " I shall scarcely have time to put my affairs in order before I die."

'She then told M. de Soubise that both sides of her family had the gift of divination: every member of it had been able to name the very hour of their deaths a month beforehand. She added

---

[1] *Gazette des Hôpitaux,* 19 October, 1844. See also Moreau, 192; Maudsley, 376.

that, in the midst of the conversation she had held with M. de Soubise, her own double had appeared to her in the mirror before her. She saw herself wrapped in a shroud, over which was a black cloth sprinkled with white tears : at her feet was an open coffin.

'A month after this occurrence, M. de Soubise received a letter informing him that this mysterious premonition had been proved true by the event.'[1]

It is natural to suppose that these sudden visions are due to a certain mental constitution hereditarily transmitted : imagination does the rest, and on the appointed day brings about the catastrophe, which is thus an effect, not a cause.

IV.

Mania consists in a total derangement of the intellectual and affective faculties. 'The maniac,' says Esquirol, 'only lives in a chaos. His wild and menacing purposes show the disordered state of his mind; his actions are mischievous; he would injure or destroy everything; he is at war with every one. To this pitiable state, if the patient does not recover, succeeds a calm that is a thousand times more painful to behold : the maniac becomes demented; he drags out stupidly the remnant of material life, without thought, without desires, without regrets, sinking gradually into death.' 'Chronic mania,' adds the same author, 'is a chronic affection of the brain, ordinarily unattended by fever, and characterized by perturbation and exaltation of sensibility, intellect, and will. Maniacs are noted for their illusions and hallucinations, and for their faulty associations of ideas, which spring up with extreme vivacity, and without any coherence.'

The heredity of this mental affection is very frequent: according to figures collated by Esquirol, about fifty per cent. of the cases are hereditary. At the Salpêtrière, in 220 cases he found 88 hereditary; and in his own establishment 75 out of 152 cases were hereditary.

The mental diseases that remain to be considered represent the extreme forms of intellectual decay, viz. dementia, general paralysis, and idiocy.

---

[1] Brierre de Boismont, *Des Hallucinations*, p. 536.

Dementia and *general paralysis* are the usual, or, at least, the
possible termination of all kinds of insanity. Hence their
hereditary transmission does not properly constitute a particular
case to be considered separately. Sometimes the dementia of
progenitors is reproduced in the same form and at about the same
age in the descendants. Esquirol saw it appear at the age of
twenty-five in a young sculptor, whose family was subject to this
disease. At other times the simple insanity of parents is meta-
morphosed, and becomes dementia or general paralysis in the
children. Thus individuals have been seen, born of parents affected
with mental diseases, to reach the age of forty or fifty without
appreciable signs of mental disease, and then fall into dementia
without any apparent cause, and even contrary to all expectations.

In *idiots* and *imbeciles* the mental activity has suffered such an
arrest of development that some of them adopt the habits of the
mere animal. This disease is incurable, since to cure it we should
have to create a new brain. As Esquirol ingeniously remarks, the
demented subject is a rich man that has become poor; the idiot,
a pauper who can never attain to wealth.

As the sexual appetite is mostly very keen in idiots, the consequence being an unhappy fertility, it is easy to show the heredity
of idiocy. Cases of the *direct* heredity are numerous. Thus,
Esquirol saw at the Salpêtrière an idiot woman, the mother of two
daughters and a son, all of them idiots.[1] But idiocy appears to
be transmitted rather in the collateral form; or if in the direct
line, then it disappears for a generation or two. Haller was the
first to note this in the case of two noble families in which idiocy
had appeared one hundred years before, and it was found to
reappear in the fourth or fifth generation. In our own time,
Dr. Séguin, who is a good authority on the question, remarks :
' I have not, to my knowledge, ever had to attend an idiotic son
of an idiot, or even the son of a man of weak intellect; but I have
often found in the family of one of my pupils an aunt, an uncle,
or oftener a grandfather afflicted with idiocy, alienation, or, at
least, imbecility.'

In conclusion, we could wish that we could answer here two

---

[1] Further facts in Lucas, ii. 787.

questions that are unfortunately very obscure. The first is this : What rank must we assign to heredity among the causes of insanity? Good statistical documents alone can afford the answer ; but the various tables agree but little with one another. Cases of hereditary insanity are, according to Moreau of Tours, nine-tenths of the whole number ; according to other writers they are only one-tenth. According to Maudsley they are more than one-fourth, but less than half : in 50 cases of insanity carefully examined by him, 16 were hereditary, or one-third. In 73 cases given by Trélat in his *Folie Lucide,* 43 are represented as due to heredity. From a report made to the French Government in 1861, it appears that in 1000 cases of persons of each sex admitted to asylums, 264 males and 266 females had inherited the disorder. Of the 264 males, 128 inherited from the father, 110 from the mother, and 26 from both. Of the 266 females, 100 inherited from the father, 130 from the mother, and 36 from both. Hence we should hardly be in error were we to say that the cases of hereditary insanity represent from one-half to one-third of the total number.

The second question is this : To what form of mental heredity must hereditary insanity be referred? In the first place, as regards mere, simple hallucination, it is plain that it is only a form of heredity of the sensorial faculties. As for insanity, properly so called, since it assumes every possible shape ; since it presents, now separately, now collectively, perversion of the sentiments and instincts, loss of intellect, and weakness of will ; and since it has never been found possible so far to trace back all the psychological phenomena of insanity to one cause, we may affirm that the foregoing facts are a fresh demonstration, in extenso, of psychological heredity under all its forms.

PART SECOND.

THE LAWS.

Quel monstre est-ce, que cette goutte de semence, de quoy nous sommes produicts, porte en soy les impressions, non de la forme corporelle seulement, mais des pensements et inclinations de nos pères ?—Montaigne.

CHAPTER I.

I.

SCIENCE begins only with the investigation of laws. All that precedes has one only object, to prepare the way for this investigation. Unless we hoped that out of the mass of facts drawn from animal and human psychology, from pathology and history, some fixed and certain rule would arise, our store of materials were valueless, a mere collection of curious anecdotes, which would afford the mind nothing like true science. We believe that the facts we have cited are not to be thus lightly esteemed. It is the privilege of the experimental method—which is so often charged with creeping on the ground, with being tied down to facts, and restricted within narrow boundaries without a horizon—to reveal to us what is universal, to exhibit to us laws in facts, and to demonstrate for us the seeming paradox, that in the world for the scientific mind there are no facts, but only laws.

If we take any simple fact of the inorganic world—a stone, a liquescent gas, a falling drop of water—and consider these phenomena, as do people in general, with the eyes and not with the mind, they will be a complete reality, and whatever is not visible and tangible will be but a vain abstraction. But science analyzes these facts into laws of gravity, heat, molecular attraction, affinity, etc., secondary laws which may themselves be referred to more general laws—and, perceiving that these laws are found everywhere in the organic world, science concludes that they it is that are real. Group these laws, and we have facts ; group different kinds of laws, and we have different kinds of facts. It follows that to know a fact thoroughly is to know the quality and the quantity of the laws which compose it, to know that a given fact is resolvable into given laws of heat, gravity, etc., and into a given amount of heat,

7

gravitation, etc. But in this analysis the fact has crumbled away, vanished, ceased to be, and has left in its stead nothing but a group of laws.

If we take a biological fact, a flowering plant, a respiratory animal, there again we find only a sum of laws. First, there are the laws of inorganic matte1 ; and, indeed, if we reduce life to pure mechanism, there are no others. But if, on the contrary, we hold that physics and chemistry fail to explain life in its entirety, we bring in other laws, those governing assimilation, disintegration, generation, and all the vital processes ; and although we have as yet no precise knowledge of these laws, we do not doubt that they exist.

So, too, with the moral world. A passion, a poem, a historical event, a revolution, result from the grouping of an almost infinite number of laws. For, beyond the physical and biologic laws which they presuppose, they imply also psychological, economical, and social laws. The simplest moral fact presents such a complication, such a tangle of laws, themselves but ill-understood, that many men, unable to recognize them, have chosen rather to deny them. But each new advance of science discredits this solution ; and, although it is possible that beyond this general reference to law there may exist something which is not subject to it, still we may affirm that every fact, considered as such, is a grouping of laws.

Let us suppose all the facts of the physical and moral universe reduced to a thousand secondary laws, and these to a dozen primitive laws, which are the final and irreducible elements of the world ; let us represent each by a thread of peculiar colour, itself formed of a collection of finer threads ; a superior force—God, Nature, Chance, it matters not what—is ever weaving, knotting and unknotting these, and transforming them into various patterns. To the ordinary mind there is nothing besides these knots and these patterns ; for it these are the only reality—beyond them it knows nothing, suspects nothing. But the man of science sets to work: he unties the knots, unravels the patterns, and shows that all the reality is in the threads. Then the antagonism between fact and law disappears ; facts are but a synthesis of laws, laws an analysis of facts.

Thus a scientific idea of the world is formed. The experimental method appeared to be imprisoned in the raw material of the fact, when all at once its range of vision is enlarged, its horizon recedes almost immeasurably, to that mysterious limit where the world of laws comes to an end; observation attains to the universal, and experience gains the almost idealistic conclusion that facts are but appearances, laws the reality.

II.

We must now inquire whether, among the many threads the inter-weaving of which constitutes the facts we have cited, any one is common to this entire group. To speak more clearly, the question is whether heredity is a law of the moral world, or whether the many instances already quoted are only isolated cases resulting from the fortuitous concurrence of other laws.

It may be surprising why, after what has been already said, the question is now raised. But the perfect indifference of most psychologists with regard to heredity would seem to show that they do not recognize in it a psychical law. The doctrines of those physiologists who have bestowed more attention on the subject are by no means harmonious on this point, and many of them have roundly denied moral heredity. It is, therefore, important that the question should be studied. To speak frankly, the objections brought against psychological heredity do not appear to be very formidable; they would, indeed, be often inexplicable, did we not know the motive which has inspired them. This is the fear, whether with or without reason, of the consequences which may result from it; but such a prejudice is neither scientific, since it proceeds arbitrarily, nor moral, because it does not prefer truth to all else.

Thus it is not possible to accept the doctrine of which Lordat is the most illustrious exponent, and which, while unreservedly subjecting to the laws of heredity the 'dynamism' (or the various modes of psychic activity) of the animal, exempts from them the 'dynamism' of man. The author's intention is too plain.[1] He

---

[1] 'If the laws,' says he, 'are identical in the two orders (animal and human), analogy would lead us to suppose that the dynamism of brutes is like our own, and that man is only a nobler and better-developed animal, as Gall and his

would place between man and animals a chasm which has no existence. From either the physical or the mental point of view it is impossible to make man a being apart, to set up a 'human kingdom.' It is, no doubt, too daring to say, as some have done in our own time,[1] that there is nothing in man which is not found also in the animal, whether it be language, or the faculty of counting (the magpie counts up to seven), or moral ideas, or the sentiment of veneration and awe, which is the basis of the religious sentiment. But setting aside these hypothetical assertions, and these exaggerations in the opposite sense, which always characterize a reaction, it is certain that, in the transition from the animal to the human, the axiom of Linnæus remains true, *Natura non facit saltus.* Heredity is a biological law, which itself results from another law—that of the transfer, by generation, of the attributes of physical and mental life : and the laws of generation govern everything that lives—the plant as well as the animal, or as well as man. As we shall see hereafter, there is not one part of the domain of life subject to the laws of heredity and another part exempt from them.

So chimerical is Lordat's hypothesis that, even in a psychological study of heredity, we must not think of separating the animal from the man. We must take one after another all the modes of mental life, and see how they are influenced by heredity, as well under the lower, or animal form, as under the higher, or human form. This we have tried to do here, but very roughly, since this work is but an essay ; yet, in the absence of a comparative psychology which might serve as a basis and plan for our exposition, we are compelled to grope our way.

Another doctrine, maintained by Virey, holds that we must distinguish 'between the moral qualities which appertain to the body, and the moral qualities which belong to the soul :' the former are transmissible by heredity, the latter are not. And Lordat defends a similar thesis. 'In man,' he says, 'heredity

followers have so persistently taught. But if these two heredities present different laws, we are justified in questioning the identity of the two dynamisms.'

[1] See the *Bulletins de la Société d'Anthropologie,* 1ʳᵉ série, vol. vi., et 2ᵉ série, vol. i.

controls everything relating to vital force, but does not control the indigenous or exotic qualities of the inner sense : or, in plainer language, unconscious modes of vital activity are hereditary; not so the conscious modes.'

The objection so formulated is vague, and has but little force if closely pressed; it rests on the idea of an absolute distinction between body and mind—an idea which, if it were admissible in Descartes' day, is so no longer.   But if we look less at the letter than at the spirit of the objection—less at what it says than at what it means to say—we must acknowledge that it raises a nice question, on which now we do but touch, but which will hereafter be discussed.

Among the 'moral qualities' appertaining to the body are reckoned in the first rank sensations and perceptions.

The organism is inherited, and with it the organs of sense and their functions.   But the imagination depends in great measure on our faculty of sense, and sensations with sensorial images are the raw material of cognition.   It is no longer maintained that they are sufficient to constitute it.   We know that the mind adds somewhat, and that the phenomena are moulded by causality, time, and space.   These conditions of all thought—the subjective forms of the mind, according to Kant ; the preformations of the organism, according to the physiologists—are universal, common to all men, and consequently, without exception, hereditary.

If we set aside for the moment the question of intellectual activity, and consider only the sentiments, emotions, and passions ; we may yet be justified in placing these among those 'moral qualities which appertain to the body.'   It will be readily admitted that the emotions differ accordingly as the person who experiences them is of lymphatic or nervous, of bilious or sanguine temperament : and these original dispositions are the source whence afterwards spring our most complex sentiments.

Hence, when closely examined, this assumed difference between the 'moral qualities which appertain to the mind,' and those which 'appertain to the body,' entirely disappears.   We seek it, and find it not—for it is not.   Heredity has been willingly admitted in regard to certain inferior psychical conditions, and it was supposed that thus full justice was rendered to this principle ; but, logically and necessarily, it has invaded the entire field of psychology. This was but the natural consequence of a vague, loose, inconsistent hypothesis, totally at variance with facts. Yet, as we have said, there is perhaps some ground for this distinction. This, then, is the important point, which the objection has not sufficiently declared or explained.

Suppose that it has been distinctly proved that all modes of psychical activity—the senses, memory, imagination, reasoning, sentiments, instincts, passions, normal or morbid dispositions—are transmissible: is the aggregate of these modes the whole sentient and conscious being; or is there, besides these, a *nescio quid* called the *I*, the person, the genius, the character, that inner power which in its own way elaborates all these materials of sentiment and cognition, and impresses on them its own peculiar stamp? Must it be considered that the various modes of psychical activity, by varied inter-relations, constitute *in themselves* the personality; or is there something else? Is the I a result or a cause? If we consider that like impressions are felt and transformed in widely different ways by different individuals, and that between genius and idiocy are found all possible shades of mental activity, one may be inclined to regard as reasonable the hypothesis of a principle of individuation, which explains these differences. And then would arise the question: Is the I, the personality, the constituent element of the individual, transmissible by heredity, as are the various modes of mental activity?

Such is, it would seem, the only true way in which to put this objection: and under this form it cannot be denied that it raises a grave difficulty. We do not, however, now discuss it: a better occasion for so doing will hereafter present itself.

The part played by psychological heredity has been doubted not only by physiologists, but also by so great a philosophic historian as Buckle. It is surprising that so clear a mind, which brought to the investigation of historic phenomena a rare penetration, originality of method and scientific exactitude, should have misconceived a fact of such significance.

We often hear of hereditary talents, hereditary vices, and hereditary virtues; but whoever will critically examine the evidence will find that we have no proof of their existence. The way in which they are commonly proved is in the highest degree illogical; the usual course being for writers to collect instances of some mental peculiarity found in a parent and in his child, and then to infer that the peculiarity was bequeathed.

By this mode of reasoning we might demonstrate any proposition; since in all large fields of inquiry there are a sufficient number of empirical coincidences to make a plausible case in favour of whatever view a man chooses to advocate. But this is not the way in which truth is discovered; and we ought to inquire not only how many instances there are of hereditary talents, etc., but how many instances there are of such qualities not being hereditary.

Until something of this sort is attempted, we can know nothing about the matter inductively; while until physiology and chemistry are much more advanced, we can know nothing about it deductively.

These considerations ought to prevent us from receiving statements (*Taylor's Medical Jurisprudence*, pp. 644, 678, and many other books) which positively affirm the existence of hereditary madness and hereditary suicide; and the same remark applies to hereditary disease (on which see some admirable observations in *Phillips on Scrofula*, pp. 101—120, London, 1846); and with still greater force does it apply to hereditary views and hereditary virtues; inasmuch as ethical phenomena have not been registered as carefully as physiological ones, and therefore our conclusions respecting them are even more precarious.

In this objection, however preposterous it may appear, we find all the qualities of a thoroughly scientific mind—that is, one which receives evidence with caution. Yet it is difficult to see what method Buckle would have us adopt in researches of this kind. Is it the differential method, which consists in comparing the facts of heredity with the exceptions to it, in accounting for the latter, and in showing why they do not come under the law? Possibly this might be done. Or is it the statistical method, which consists in accepting the facts as they present themselves, in grouping, on the one hand, those which have an hereditary character, and on the other those which have not, and in estimating arithmetically the relations of the two groups? We shall see hereafter that this has been attempted.

It must be conceded to Buckle that the question of psychological heredity is by no means one that can be treated with strict scientific rigour; and there are many reasons why this is so. Oftentimes in the course of this present work we have felt the insufficiency of the argument, 'A distinguished father, a distinguished son—therefore talent is hereditary,' whereas we ought to be able to show that to a given mode of mental activity in the progenitor corresponds precisely the same mode in the descendant, or, at least, to say why this is not so. But this is too much to require in the present state of psychology.

This granted, if we revert to the essential point of Buckle's objection, we find that in his view the cases of heredity are simply fortuitous successions, such as are to be found whenever we compare a great mass of facts. If we take from the registers of a lottery the winning numbers through a long series of years, we should probably find that there were occasionally the same succession of numbers, the result of mere chance. In this way, or nearly so, Buckle explains cases of heredity. He reduces the question to a calculation of probabilities. But this singular hypothesis had already been answered by a mathematician.

Maupertuis, after citing a case of sexdigitism which persisted through four generations, adds : 'I presume no one would regard sexdigitism as the effect of mere chance. But suppose we so regard it, let us then see what is the probability that this accidental variation in a parent will not be repeated in the descendants. In the course of an inquiry made by me in a city of 100,000 inhabitants, I found two persons marked by this singular anomaly.

'Suppose—a thing not very easy—that three other cases escaped my observation, and that we have a man with six fingers for each 20,000 souls ; the probability that his son or daughter will not be born with six fingers is as 20,000 to 1, and the probability that his grandson will not have six fingers will be as 20,000 times 20,000 (or 4 millions) to 1. Finally, the probability that sexdigitism will not continue through three successive generations will be as 8000 millions to 1, figures so large that the certainty of things best demonstrated in physics does not approximate to these probabilities.' [1]

---

[1] Maupertuis, *Œuvres*, vol. ii. letter 17.

If we apply Maupertuis' argument to a few cases of psycho-logical heredity, for instance mental disorder, or some special talent (for painting, or music) persisting through three or four generations, it is easy to see what becomes of Buckle's objection.

III.

The greater part of these objections would never have been raised, were it not for the serious error of reasoning only *from the exceptions.* To treat the question fairly, it ought first of all to have been properly stated, that is to say, the fact of heredity should have been considered, not partially, but in its whole extent in the entire domain of life, as we here propose to do.

In order to proceed logically, we should in the first place have to determine what is meant by species. We will not enter into this very difficult question. It will be enough for us to lay down a few very simple, unquestionable and elementary facts, which will be admitted by all.

When we compare together two living beings—that is to say, two sums of attributes—and find that these two beings possess in common a very large number of essential attributes, differing only in those which are secondary, so that the two beings may be regarded as very much alike, we say that they are of the same species. The many essential characteristics possessed by them in common we call specific; the few accidental characters which differentiate them we call individual. Thus, for instance, two individuals of the human species possess in common very many essential characters, being organic, vertebrate mammals, with all that is thereby implied, having senses, physiological or psychological functions, such as sensation, memory, imagination, reason. But they differ from one another in accidental or individual characteristics, as that the muscular system common to both is in the one very well developed, very slightly in the other; that the faculty of memory common to both is weak in the one, and very strong in the other; that the faculty of reason common to both does not in the one go beyond the simplest acts, while in the other it includes the highest abstractions.

Now, by the act of generation, in which heredity has its origin, every creature produces beings like itself. In the lower forms of generation, such as gemmation and fission, this fact is evident. In the higher forms, where the connection of the two sexes is requisite, two contrary forces are brought together, and consequently are antagonistic. The result is, that the product will (though not without exceptions) resemble one or other of the parents, or both at once. This general truth, that the organisms of a given type descend from organisms of the same type, is so well established by countless instances that it has the character of an axiom. 'The tendency of a living being to repeat itself in its progeny,' says a certain naturalist, 'seems to be a sort of necessity. It were difficult to imagine a creature which should not resemble its parents. In fact, so universal is this tendency that it is recognized as one of those fundamental facts which underlie all the natural sciences, and which, with regard to them, take the place held by axioms in the mathematical sciences.'

This being understood, heredity appears in its true light, and the objections brought against it can be appreciated at their value; for the question already stated, 'Are cases of psychical heredity fortuitous, or are they the result of a law?' may plainly be resolved into several parts, each of which easily admits of answer.

1. Are specific characteristics, physical or moral, transmitted by heredity?—They are always transmitted, both in the animal and in man.

2. Are those less general characteristics, which constitute races and varieties, hereditary?—They also are hereditary; a spaniel was never produced by a bull-dog, nor a white man by a negro. And this holds good also of psychical qualities: a given animal possesses not only the general instincts of the species, but also the peculiar instincts of the race. The negro inherits not only the psychological faculties which are common to all men, but also a certain peculiar form of mental constitution, namely, an excess of sensibility and imagination, sensual tendencies, incapacity for abstract thought, etc.

3. Are purely individual characteristics hereditary?—Facts have demonstrated that they are often so, both in physics and in morals.

In conclusion, heredity always governs those broadly general characteristics which determine the species, always those less general characteristics which constitute the variety, and often individual characteristics.   IIence the evident conclusion that heredity is the law, non-heredity the exception.   Suppose a father and mother—both large, strong, healthy, active and intelligent—produce a son and a daughter possessing the opposite qualities. In this instance, wherein heredity seems completely set aside, it still holds good that the differences between parents and children are but slight, as compared with the resemblances.

Let it not be said that we have dwelt too long on points that are self-evident.   They are so clear that we forget them, and argue only from isolated cases, thus changing the state of the question by the way in which it is stated.   But when, on the contrary, we consider the facts as a whole, heredity appears universal, and we are less surprised at finding characteristics that are hereditary, than in finding those which are not.

<hr/>

CHAPTER II.

THE LAWS OF HEREDITY.

THUS, then, heredity presents itself to us as a biological law, that is, inherent in every living thing, having no other limits than those of life itself.   Life under all its forms—vegetal, animal and human, normal and morbid, physical and mental—is governed by this law.   It is, in fact, concerned with the essential and inmost nature of vital activity.   Among the various functions which in their united action constitute life, two are primary—the one, nutrition, which preserves the individual, the other, generation, which perpetuates the species.   Some physiologists even reduce these to one, nutrition being, in their view, only a form of generation, or in the words of Claude Bernard, 'a continuous creation of organized matter by means of the histogenic processes appertaining to the living creature.'   Ultimately, therefore, the vital functions are reduced to generation ; and 'as it is from this that heredity immediately flows, we must conclude that the law of hereditary transmission has its rise in the sources of life itself.

If we accept the foregoing views, the law of heredity would seem to be one of absolute simplicity.   Like produces like : the progenitor is repeated in the descendant.   Thus the primitive types would remain, being continually reproduced, and the world of life would present the spectacle of perfect regularity and supreme monotony. But this is true only in theory. So soon as we come to the facts, we find the law is resolved into secondary laws, or it even appears to vanish in the exceptions. Not to speak of the external causes (chance, influence of circumstances) which interfere with the action of heredity, there are interior causes, inherent in heredity itself, which hinder the law from pursuing the simple course from like to like. A moment's reflection will make this plain.

In the inferior creatures, in which generation takes place without sexual connection, hereditary transmission from the parent to the progeny occurs in a perfectly natural way. This happens in cases of fission, as in Trembley's hydra, or in the Nais, which naturally divide into two or more individuals like themselves ; and also in cases of gemmation, where a bud forms on an animal and is soon itself changed into a new and complete animal.

But in the higher forms of generation sexual connection is indispensable ; as a struggle necessarily arises between the sexes, each parent tends to produce its like. Here hereditary transmission can at best produce only a mixed constitution, holding from both parents. ' Clearly,' says De Quatrefages, ' the mathematical law of heredity would be for the parent creature to reproduce itself completely in its progeny. And perhaps this law, absolute though it be, is to be found underlying all natural phenomena, but in every case it is masked by accessory circumstances, by the conditions amid which heredity acts. But it does not only rest on theoretical considerations, it rests also on facts. Although subject to profound and continual disturbance, still, if we note all the phenomena which show in individuals a tendency to obey the mathematical law, heredity is found to realize in the aggregate of each species the result which it fails to realize in isolated individuals. To use a figurative expression, the true meaning of which cannot fail to be apprehended, while it cannot be verified in the whole, it may be in detail.'

The question is still more complicated when we descend to individual facts. We meet with so many oddities and exceptions, and so many contradictory opinions in explanation of them, that it seems as though, when we pass from theory to practice, all law had vanished. Still these facts, however numerous and varied they may be, may all be brought within the compass of a few formulas, which might be called the empirical laws of heredity. These real laws, which are so many aspects or incomplete expressions of the ideal law, are the following, so far as observation reveals them.

1. *Direct heredity*, which consists in the transmission of paternal and maternal qualities to the children. This form of heredity offers two aspects :

(1.) The child takes after father and mother equally as regards both physical and moral characters, a case, strictly speaking, of very rare occurrence, for the very ideal of the law would then be realized.

Or (2), the child, while taking after both parents, more specially resembles one of them; and here again we must distinguish between two cases.

a. The first of these is when the heredity takes place in the same sex—from father to son, from mother to daughter.

β. The other, which occurs more frequently, is where heredity occurs between different sexes—from father to daughter, from mother to son.

2. *Reversional Heredity*, or atavism, consists in the reproduction in the descendants of the moral or physical qualities of their ancestors. It occurs frequently between grandfather and grandson, grandmother and granddaughter.

3. *Collateral*, or *indirect heredity*, which is of rarer occurrence · than the foregoing, subsists, as indicated by its name, between individuals and their ancestors in the indirect line—uncle, or grand-uncle and nephew, aunt and niece.

4. Finally, to complete the classification, we must mention the heredity of influence, very rare from the physiological point of view, and of which probably no single instance is proved in the moral order. It consists in the reproduction in the children by a second marriage of some peculiarity belonging to a former spouse.

Such are the various formulas under which all the facts of heredity may be classed. We propose to study them in succession. When to this we have added, as the necessary complement, the study of the exceptions to these laws, we shall have passed in review every single case of heredity.

I.

We have first to resort to physiology in order to clear the field, since the laws of physiological heredity have been oftener and far better studied than those of moral heredity; yet so close is the connection between the two orders of facts, that a person can hardly study the one without the other.

In the case of direct heredity, the concurrence of the two sexes in the formation of the product is now admitted by all physiologists. We need, therefore, only refer to the ancient doctrines of the *spermatists* and the *ovists*. The former held that, notwithstanding the apparent concurrence of both sexes in generation, the germ is contained in the male element alone. The latter, who held a doctrine the very reverse of this, but equally exclusive, maintained that the germ exists only in the female element. The first doctrine, which was adopted by Galen, Hartsoeker, Boerhaave, Leeuwenhoek, and the second, which was held by Malpighi, Vallisnieri, Spallanzani, Bonnet, Haller, and even De Blainville, are now equally abandoned. It is admitted that the child is sprung from both father and mother, and embryology demonstrates this. But opinions diverge in regard to the part taken by each of the parents.

If we take a purely theoretic point of view, it is easy enough to formulate the law of direct heredity. According to P. Lucas, it would consist in the 'absolute equilibrium in the physical and moral nature of the infant of the integral resemblances of the two parents.' The procreated individual would be, everywhere and always, nothing but the exact mean of his two parents; the distinct characters of both would be reproduced in their progeny—in every portion of his body, and in every faculty of his mind. But this is only a logical hypothesis, which very rarely becomes a reality in the higher animals; and it is hardly rash to say that the law has never been met with in this ideal form.

And yet we understand that this is the law, that is to say, the only formula broad enough to include all the phenomena; the only rule which flows of necessity from the nature of things, and which expresses the essence of heredity.

It is easy to account for the disagreement between logic and experience. No law of nature is unconditional. They all require certain determinate conditions for their realization; and where these fail, the action of the law rests suspended, or without efficacy. But nowhere are the requisite conditions more numerous or more difficult to fulfil than in the phenomena of generation. For in order to produce in the infant this perfect equilibrium of paternal and maternal qualities, there must evidently be perfect equality of action on the part of both parents; for it will be admitted that in all races, and in all species, the general or partial preponderance in the act of reproduction appertains to that one of the parents in whom the general or partial force of constitution is the greater. A great number of facts, collected by a crowd of writers, show that this rule applies both to the vegetal and the animal world. This preponderance of one of the procreative individuals is very notable in crosses between distinct races or species. It is true that in this case there is a struggle not only between the sexes, but between distinct specific forces. These crosses, however, only exhibit to us, more or less magnified, what takes place in ordinary cases. According to Rursh, marriages between Danes and East Indian women produce children with the physique and the vigour of the European type, while nothing of this kind occurs when these same women marry other Europeans. The intermarriage of Causasians and Mongolians produces, according to Klaproth, half-breeds in whom the Mongolian type is always predominant, whatever may be the sex of the half-breed. From Levaillant's observations (*Voyage en Cafrérie*) on the half-bred children of Europeans and Hottentots, we gather that in them the moral nature is always determined by the race of the father. 'Whenever it happens, which is but rarely, that a white woman has intercourse with a Hottentot, the child has always the good-nature, and the gentle and kindly inclinations, of the father. But the children of white men and Hottentot women, on the other hand, have in themselves the germs of all vices and unruly passions.' Cross breeding in the animal races exhibits also the unquestionable preponderance of one of the parents.

This being admitted, it may be readily shown that among the higher animals the complete conditions necessary for the realization of the ideal law can nowhere be found.

1. There must be first of all a perfect correspondence between the physical and mental constitution of the parents. A moment's reflection will show that each of these two general states—the physical and the mental constitution—is itself the result of many particular states, which, taken together, impress on every individual that distinct and special mark which is in physiology called temperament, in psychology, character.

2. But even if these first conditions are fulfilled, there is something more required. It is not enough that the physical and mental constitution of both parents should be equipoised in a general sense; there are, moreover, particular conditions of age and health, which are indispensable. Disproportion in the ages of the two parents, where it does not produce sterility, gives the preponderance to the younger. Experiments made by Girou de Buzareingues on various animals show that the progeny of an old male and a young female are less like their father, in proportion as he is feeble and the mother vigorous, and that the progeny of an old female and a young male resemble the mother less in proportion as he is vigorous. Nor is the influence of the actual state of health, of vigour, or of cheerfulness in one of the parents less marked in the progeny.

3. Finally, there are sundry other states more accidental and transitory than those named, which influence the act of generation. Positive facts show that these states, all transitory as they are, exert a very powerful influence on the progeny, and ensure the preponderance of one or the other sex. We need only recall the fact that nothing is more common than the intellectual feebleness of children begotten in a state of intoxication; that a popular tradition, adopted by several authors, and to some extent supported by history, represents illegitimate children as cleverer, more handsome, and more healthy than others, because they are 'love-children.' On the other hand, 'when parents,' says Burdach, 'have a dislike to one another, they beget ugly forms, and their children are less lively and vigorous.'

It is easy to see that there are many circumstances of this kind which must influence the act of generation. When we consider how impossible it is to have these general, particular and fortuitous conditions in perfect equilibrium in the two parents, we find it natural that the law already stated should remain in the purely theoretic state.

Hence we have to seek in the facts themselves for some empiric formula, which may be deduced from them. Here arise many opinions, of which the following are the chief.

The simplest is that which holds that there is an invariable connection between the heredity of physical resemblance and the heredity of moral resemblance. That parent who transmits the former, or who influences it most, transmits also the latter, by reason of the strict correlation existing between the two. This doctrine, which has been maintained by Burdach, rests, in principle, on the general relations between the physical and moral natures; and, in fact, on numerous cases furnished by experience. The case of twins is particularly cited, as commonly presenting an extra-ordinary conformity, not only in the external form and in the features of the face, but also in tastes, in faculties, and even in fortune.

Da Gama Machado, author of a *Theory of Resemblances*, which contains a large number of curious facts for the study of physical heredity, holds that the parent who transmits his colour transmits likewise his character. 'In the colonies,' says he, 'the half-breed, called *griffon* or *fusco* (dark), resulting from the union of a mulatto and a negress, is much darker than the mulatto. But this difference of colour is accompanied by a difference in character: the issue of a mulatto and a negress are far more docile than the issue of a negress and a white man. If a wild duck couple with a domestic duck, the duckling resulting from this union, having its father's colour, leaves the barn-yard and returns to the wild life. If the linnet be crossed with the canary or the goldfinch, the transmission of instincts will, according to this author, follow the transmission of colour, and if there is a mixture of colours, there will be also a mixture of instincts.

Girou de Buzareingues, whose experiments on generation are well known, distinguishes two lives in every individual, whatever the sex: The external life, on which depend the nervous system of the animal life and the muscular system, of which motor activity, will, and intelligence are the attributes; and the internal life, which comprises the cellular tissue, the digestive system, the great sympathetic, and the whole nerve-system of the organic life : on this depend internal sensibility and the sentiments.

Each of these two lives would have the faculty of reproduction ; consequently the transmission of the external life would imply the transmission of the intelligence, while the transmission of the internal life would imply that of the sentiments.[1]

Gall and his disciple Spurzheim, rejecting these doctrines, maintained an opinion which results logically from their system—that the analogy in the conformation of the various regions of the cranial arch implies analogous psychological constitution. ' It has been always observed,' says Gall, ' that when brothers and sisters resemble one another, or their father and mother, in the shape of the head, they also resemble each other in psychical and mental qualities.'

We may fairly consider that, since every one of these doctrines is supported by a large number of facts, they all may be esteemed partial generalizations; but since they are all open to many exceptions, none can be accepted as a total generalization. Thus is theory confirmed by experience : reasoning deductively, we arrived at the conclusion that the perfect law of heredity would never be realized ; and now the examination of the facts shows that no empiric formula attains the breadth of a general law.

The only thing that results clearly from this conflict of doctrines is, that in point of fact there is always a preponderance of one of the parents.

In the case of direct heredity, the child is always more specially like either the father or the mother.

This preponderance, moreover, is never exclusive, as will appear hereafter, from some curious facts. In spite of appearances, the heredity of parents to children is never unilateral, but always bilateral. The phenomena of reversionary heredity prove that, although the influence of one of the parents on the child may seem abolished, it never is annihilated, and thus the law of equality of action is as far as possible realized.

The phenomena of cross-breeding confirm what has been said. Anthropologists have drawn up tables wherein the influence of the

---

[1] *De la Génération*, pp. 130, 131.

father and that of the mother, each represented by a fraction, are supposed to be equal in the production of the half-breed. But this hypothesis, as expressed in the following table, is altogether theoretic.

WHITE AND BLACK.

Generations.	Parents.		Offspring.	Blood. White.	Black.
1st	White + Negro		Mulatto	½	½
2nd	Mulatto +	White	Tierceroon	¾	¼
		Negro	Griffo	¼	¾
3rd	Tierceroon +	White	Quadroon	⅞	⅛
		Negro	Ditto	⅛	⅞
4th	Quadroon +	White	Quinteroon	15/16	1/16
		Negro	Ditto	1/16	15/16

But, in fact, cross-breeding does not by any means proceed with such mathematical regularity. Not to speak of the numerous cases in which the union of white and black results in a child entirely black, or entirely white, in half-breeds there is always a preponderance of one or other of the parents. Burmeister, one of the closest observers of the mulattoes of South America and of the West Indian Islands, denies that the mulatto is exactly the mean between his two parents. In the immense majority of cases, his characters are borrowed from both races, but one of them is always predominant, and that usually the negro race. Pruner Bey, who has carefully studied the mulattoes in Egypt and Arabia, passes the same judgment. He observes the marked predominance of the negro type. It is manifest in the curly, woolly hair; in the general form and dimensions of the skull; in the forehead, usually low and slightly receding; in the conformation of the feet, and in a prognathism which scarcely ever disappears in the first generation.

The foregoing observations may be thus summarized: In the case of direct heredity the child derives its qualities from father and mother.

There is always a preponderance of one of these.

It will, perhaps, be asked whether, after having treated the question mainly from the physiological point of view, we ought not now to take it up again from the psychological point of view, and search history for facts in support of this first form of direct heredity—that is, for cases of persons who derived their qualities from both father and mother. Such cases might be found. It might be said that Alexander resembled Philip in some respects, Olympias in others. Nero was the worthy son of Agrippina; but it is not to be forgotten that his father, Domitius Ahenobarbus, was noted for his cruelty : he had one of his freedmen put to death for refusing to drink to excess ; he purposely crushed to death a child on the Appian Way ; and he was wont to say : 'Of me and Agrippina nothing can be born that is not accursed.' Michelet declares that Queen Elizabeth resembled both Henry VIII. and Ann Boleyn. According to the same historian, the Duke de Vendome was most like his mother, Gabrielle d'Estrées ; but in his 'waggish look comes out his Gascon ancestry and the great Béarnais jester.' (Henri IV.) Schopenhauer, who explains the question of heredity according to his metaphysical system, holds that whatever is primary and fundamental in the individual—character, passions, tendencies—is inherited from the father : the intelligence, a secondary and derivative faculty, directly from the mother. He was pleased to imagine that he found in his own person the irrefutable evidence of this doctrine. Intellectual and subtle like his mother, who had literary tastes and lived in Goethe's circle at Weimar, he was, like his father, shy, obstinate, intractable : he was a man of 'scowling mien, and of fantastic judgments.' [1] .

It would not be difficult to multiply instances, but the labour would be wholly useless ; for the question before us now is, not whether the child derives its qualities from both father and mother

---

[1] Schopenhauer, *Die Wdt als Wille und Vorstehung,* vol. i. § 23; vol. ii. book iv. ch. 43.

(about which there can be no doubt), but whether there are cases where it derives them in equal degree from both. If such a case were to occur, we could not show that it did, especially as regards moral resemblances. To that end we must needs have exact processes of measurement, which do not exist; we should have to estimate quantities and not qualities. The foregoing examples, and all the others we might accumulate, could prove only this one thing, that there is always a more or less marked preponderance of one of the two parents. Cases occur where the preponderant action of the father or of the mother is manifested in a singular way, each parent seeming to have, as it were, chosen some particular organ. Thus the father may transmit to the child the brain, and the mother the stomach; one the heart, the other the liver; one the great intestine, the other the pancreas; one the kidneys, the other the bladder. These facts have been established by animal and human anatomy. They give the organic reason for the intercrossing of instincts, which is often so curious, and of the morbid and passionate predispositions of both parents in the child.

Sometimes, too, one of the parents transmits the entire physical, the other the entire moral nature. The most curious and incontestable instance of this is the case of Lislet-Geoffroy, engineer in Mauritius. He was the son of a white man and of a very stupid negress. In physical constitution he was as much a negro as his mother; he had the features, the complexion, the woolly hair, and the peculiar odour of his race. In moral constitution he was so thoroughly a white as regards intellectual development, that he succeeded in vanquishing the prejudices of blood, so strong in the colonies, and in being admitted into the most aristocratic houses. At the time of his death he was Corresponding Member of the Academy of Sciences.

Thus we are brought to the examination of cases of unilateral heredity—the word *unilateral* being here taken, as has been explained, in a restricted sense.

II.

Whenever, then, the strict conditions of intermixture are wanting, the rule is that one of the parents is preponderant. When we study empirically the laws of heredity, we find that this case is of by far the most frequent occurrence. Common language translates this everyday experience into such phrases as these: this child reminds one of his father; or, that child is the image of its mother. But experience also teaches us that this preponderance takes place in two ways, being sometimes direct, sometimes diagonal.

Sometimes the preponderance is manifested in an individual of the one sex on the child of the same sex; in that case the son resembles the father; the daughter the mother.

Again, this preponderance is manifested in the opposite sex; then the daughter resembles the father, and the son the mother.

We will consider the latter case first.

When we study heredity empirically, when, that is, we observe facts and the generalizations which immediately result from it, the formula which includes the largest number of facts and admits of the fewest exceptions is the following: Heredity passes from one sex to the opposite. This assertion may at first appear strange, and even entirely at variance with what has already been said, that like produces like. This will hereafter be explained; but perhaps it will appear less difficult of comprehension if we follow heredity through several generations. It will then be seen to pass from the grandfather to the mother, and then from the mother to the son; or from the grandmother to the father, and from the father to the daughter. Thus it returns to its starting-point.

But not to dwell on this question here, we would remark that the thesis of cross heredity is admitted by several great physiologists, such as Haller, Burdach, Girou de Buzareingues, and Richerand. 'This explains,' says the latter, 'why so many great men have mediocre sons.' Michelet thinks that history justifies him in broadly affirming the existence of cross heredity. 'No other king,' says he, speaking of Louis XVI., 'exemplifies better a law of which history has but few exceptions. The king was a foreigner. Every son takes after his mother. The king was the son of a foreign woman, and had her blood. Succession in such cases has nearly always the effect of an invasion. The evidences of this are numberless. Catherine and Marie de Medicis gave us pure Italians ; in the same way La Farnese may be traced in Carlos II. of Spain ; Louis XVI. was a real Saxon king, and more German than the Germans themselves.'[1]

Dr. P. Lucas, though he does not explicitly accept this law, still does not reject it.

Let us, therefore, look at the facts which support it. These we take at three sources: intermixture of races, mental diseases, and history.

1. From the physiological point of view cases of cross heredity are very numerous under normal conditions, that is, when the parents are healthy and of good constitutions. When one of them presents any anomaly or deformity, we find that cross-heredity is still more common : thus, a curved spine, lameness, rickets, sexdigitism, deaf-muteness, mycrophthalmy—in short, all organic imperfections—pass from the father to the daughters, and from the mother to the sons.[2]

From the psychological point of view, Gall cites the curious case of twins of opposite sexes, where the boy was like the mother, a very stupid woman, and the girl like the father, who was a man of considerable talent.

In cross breeding, this appears very plainly. When a dog is crossed with a wolf-bitch, the males usually inherit the character of the wolf, the females that of the dog. It even appears that this transfer of qualities to the opposite sex takes place more regularly with regard to moral than to physical characters. As will be seen, Buffon, after in vain trying to bring about a crossing of a dog and a she-wolf, abandoned the attempt. But chance brought about that which art could not do. The wolf dropped two cubs ; the one a male which physically resembled the dog, but in character was wild and savage ; the other, a female, physically resembled the wolf, but in disposition was gentle, familiar, and even trouble-somely affectionate. From the crossing of a he-goat and a bitch hound sprang young ones, some of which were like the goat, others like the bitch : the latter had all the habits of their sire.

---

[1] *Histoire de France*, vol. xvii.

[2] Girou has a great number of observations on this point.—*De la Génération,* 276—284.

'A wild tom cat,' says Girou, 'and a domestic cat produced two tom cats which were like their mother, and were gentle and familiar like her, and one she-cat, which resembled the father, and was wild like him, and far more shy than the other two kittens.'

The same author states that hunters have a proverb which says, Dog from bitch and bitch from dog ('*Chien de chienne et chienne de chien*), meaning that the mother's qualities are found in the son, and the father's in the daughter.

The Arabs, who think so much of the genealogy of their horses, show a marked preference for blood on the female side over the male side.

We may also cite decisive facts drawn from the human race. 'P—— was in the habit,' says Girou, 'of going to sleep with the right leg crossed upon the left. One of his daughters came into the world with the same habit; she constantly assumed that posture in the cradle, in spite of the resistance offered by the napkin.

'I know several girls who resemble their fathers, and who from them have inherited peculiar and extraordinary habits, not to be attributed either to imitation or to education; as also of boys who from birth have borne a very striking resemblance, whether physically or morally, to their mothers; but propriety forbids all detail on this subject.

'Here I would observe that the external and the moral resemblance of the son to the mother is far less frequent and less perfect than that of the daughter to the father.'

2. Mental disorders furnish a considerable number of cases in support of cross heredity. These are to be found scattered through the works of writers on insanity. Baillarger, in his *Recherches sur l'Anatomie, la Physiologie, et la Pathologie du Système Nerveux*, has endeavoured to go over the whole ground. In 571 cases observed, he found 246 of cross heredity and 325 of direct. The result, as we see, is not favourable to the thesis which regards cross heredity as of the more frequent occurrence. The author has not failed to draw this conclusion, which will be hereafter examined.

3. We need now to collect some facts from history, restricting ourselves to well-known personages, and eliminating carefully all cases in which hereditary transmission appears questionable.

HEREDITY FROM MOTHER TO SON.

MOTHER.	SON.
Olympias	Alexander the Great
Cornelia	The Gracchi
Livia	Tiberius
Agrippina	Nero
Faustina	Commodus
Sœmias	Heliogabalus
Mammæa	Alexander Severus
Marozia	Pope John XI.
Blanche of Castille . . .	Louis IX.
Berengaria	St. Ferdinand
Charlotte of Savoy . . .	Charles VIII.
Louise of Savoy . . .	Francis I.
Mary Stuart	James I. (?)
Catherine de Medicis . .	Her sons
Jeanne d'Albret . . .	Henri IV.
Marie de Medicis . .	Louis XIII.
Anne-Christine Marlin . .	Buffon
Mdlle. de Tencin . .	D'Alembert
Geneviève de Vassau . .	Mirabeau
Santi Lomaka (Greek) . .	André M.-J. } Chénier
. . . . . .	Goethe
Mrs. Byron (Catherine Gordon)	Byron

Remarks.—Alfonso XI., King of Castille, famed for his religious zeal and his love of warfare against the Moors, was the father of Berengaria, Blanche, and Uraca. The first of these became the mother of St. Ferdinand. The second had four sons, among them St. Louis and Charles of Anjou, both ascetics, who mortified their flesh with iron girdles, scourgings, extreme fastings, etc. The third made her son Sancho take the monastic habit, though called to the throne of Portugal.

Buffon, who held the doctrine of cross heredity, used to say that he himself took after his mother. ' He held it for a principle, says Hérault de Séchelles, ' that children usually inherit intellectual

8

and moral qualities from their mother. And this he applied to his own case, speaking in the highest terms of praise of his mother, who in point of fact was a woman of much ability, extensive knowledge, and of a superior mind.

Mirabeau (Friend of Humanity) was wont to say of his son: ' He possesses all the low qualities of the maternal stock.'

Goethe resembled his father physically, but psychologically he resembled his mother by his strong instinct of self-preservation, his dislike of all strong emotions, and his caustic and biting speech. (For well-known anecdotes on this point, see his *Life* by Henri Blaze, and *Life* by Lewes.)

By his servant maid, whom he married, a woman of inferior intellect, he had several children, one only of them a boy ; they all died young. This son resembled Goethe in bodily vigour, but he was of narrow mind like his mother, and Wieland used to call him the son of the handmaiden (der Sohn der Magd).

HEREDITY FROM FATHER TO DAUGHTER.

FATHER.	DAUGHTER.
Aristippus, the Cyrenaic philosopher	Areta
Theon, the geometrician	Hypatia
Scipio	Cornelia
Cæsar	Julia (Pompey's wife)
Cicero	Tullia
Caligula	Julia Drusilla
Charlemagne	His daughters (?)
Alexander VI.	Lucretia Borgia
Louis XI.	Anne de Beaujeu
Louis XII.	Claude de France
Henry VIII.	Elizabeth / Mary
Henri II.	Marguerite de Valois
Henri IV.	Henrietta of England
Cromwell	His daughters
Gustavus Adolphus	Christina
The Regent	His daughters
Necker	Madame de Staël

Remarks.—Complaint having been made to Caligula that his daughter, two years old, scratched the little children who were her playfellows and even tried to tear out their eyes, he replied with a laugh, 'I see ; she is my daughter.'

'The Regent,' says Michelet, 'took after his mother, a robust, masculine Bavarian woman. She was of an inquiring, active mind, who roamed in all fields of science, and had a liking for general culture, which was in those times rare in France." (*Histoire de France*, tome xiv.) Her son, the Regent, was a fool : her daughters were extremely strange. The eldest, the Duchesse de Berry, a charming woman of unbridled passions, was certainly mad. The second, who possessed her father's versatility, was an encyclopædic whirlwind. The third and fourth were all caprice and folly. They astonished Italy and Spain with such daring scandals that it is impossible not to see madness in all they did.

Lucas, following Carlyle, thus sums up the genealogy of the Cromwells. Robert Cromwell, grandson of the terrible and frenzied instrument of Henry VIII. in his contest with Rome, married Catharine Stuart, a second cousin of Charles I. To Oliver, the only male among the seven children which were the fruit of this strange marriage, passed the enthusiastic and powerful genius of the Cromwells, and it raised him to the highest station. Oliver took to wife Eliza Bouchier, a woman of gentle disposition. His male issue were 'Arcadian Shepherds,' his daughters more fanatical than himself.

III.

We next consider the third form of direct heredity, the preponderance of one parent in the children of the same sex.

This, like the preceding form, is based upon a large number of facts derived from physiology, psychology, and history.

Possibly these are not so numerous as the facts of cross heredity. This, however, is no more than a vague and general impression, in short, a mere hypothesis. Against the questionable arguments derived from the number of facts, the upholders of the contrary opinion might not only cite facts, but might also allege a theoretical consideration in favour of their view, which is not without value; they might say that their thesis is only a special application of a maxim generally admitted with regard to generation, viz. that like produces like. When we treat of reversional heredity, we shall endeavour to show that the conflict between these two opinions is only apparent, and also how they may be harmonized.

Among the physiological facts which exhibit heredity transmitted in the same sex, we may cite the family of Edward Lambert, the human porcupine, in which a peculiar affection was transmitted only to the males. Daltonism, or colour-blindness, manifests itself more frequently, as we have seen, in men than in women; yet it has been transmitted through five generations to twelve persons, all females. Constitution, temperament, fecundity, longevity, idiosyncrasies, or anomalies of every kind, pass as often from father to son as from mother to daughter.

From the psychological point of view, as we have said, Baillarger, resting on the statistical data of mental disease, inclines to the belief that heredity usually occurs between individuals of the same sex. His 671 cases were distributed as follows :—

CASES OF MENTAL DISEASE.

						Total.
In the	father	225	In the mother	346		571
„	sons	128	„	daughters	197	325
„	daughters	97	„	sons	149	246

We now turn to the statistical reports made to the French Government in 1860, of which we have already spoken.

MEN	WOMEN
In 1,000 cases.	In 1,000 cases.
128 inherited from the father	130 inherited from the mother
110 „ „ the mother	100 „ „ the father
26 „ „ both.	26 „ „ both.

It is plain that these two tables lead to the same conclusions.

We hold that the study of mental disease is of great importance for experimental psychology, and well adapted for resolving many problems; yet we would not place over-much confidence in it in the present case.

In the first place, if the author, basing his judgment entirely on the fact of mental alienation, proposes thence to draw a conclusion covering the whole question of heredity, physical as well as moral, he makes so great a mistake in logic that the mere statement is a sufficient condemnation. It would be too arbitrary to rely on a single characteristic, for the heredity of insanity does not include that of the muscular system, of the features, of the complexion, or the apparatus of organic life.

But if, as is probable, he means to speak only of mental heredity, the fault of his reasoning, though less grave, is still very serious. The heredity of mental affections is only one of the forms of psychological heredity, and it is not legitimate to argue from one to all. To derive from parents a morbid predisposition which will hereafter lead to mania, monomania, hallucination, or dementia, by no means necessitates the inheritance of their entire psychological constitution, their character, their genius, their scientific and artistic aptitudes, their memory, passions, or sentiments ; facts prove the contrary. In very many cases the cause of mental disease is altogether physical—a lesion of the brain or of some other organ ; and nothing justifies the assertion, that as these lesions are inherited, therefore the whole mental dynamism is also inherited.

Thus the arguments drawn from mental pathology have not so wide a range as Baillarger assigns to them. But if they are insufficient to prove that heredity in the same sex is more frequent than cross heredity, they do, however, prove that it is of frequent occurrence.

We now cite from history some well-established instances of this form of heredity.

HEREDITY FROM FATHER TO SON.

FATHER.	SON.
Nicomachos	Aristotle
Scipio (Publius Cornelius)	Scipio (Africanus major)
Vespasian	Titus
Verus (Ælius)	Verus (Lucianus)
Pepin d'Heristal	Charles Martel
Charles Martel	Pepin the Short

HEREDITY FROM FATHER TO SON (*continued*).

FATHER.	SON.
Pepin the Short . . .	Charlemagne
Hamilcar . . .	{ Hannibal Hasdrubal Mago
Seneca (Marcus) . . .	{ Seneca Gallio
Artevelt (Jaques van) .	Artevelt (Philip van)
Guise (François) . .	Guise (Henri)
Nassau (William of) . .	Nassau (Maurice of)
Scaliger (Julius Cæsar) .	Scaliger (Joseph)
Casaubon (Isaac) . .	Casaubon (Méric)
Tasso (Bernardo) . .	Tasso (Torquato)
Sanzio (Giovanni) . .	Rafaelle (Sanzio)
Bellíni (Jacopo) . . .	Bellini (Giovanni)
Teniers (David) . .	Teniers (David)
Miéris (F.)	{ Guillaume-Miéris Jean
Van der Velde (William) .	Van der Velde (William)
Racine (Jean) . . .	Racine (Louis)
Mozart (Johann George) .	Mozart (Johann)
Beethoven (Johann) . .	Beethoven (Ludwig)
Niebuhr	Niebuhr (Carsten)
Buckland (W.) . . .	Buckland (F.)
Herschell (W.) . .	Herschell (J.)
Ampère (André) . . .	Ampère (J.-J.)
Geoffroy St.-Hilaire (Étienne)	Geoffroy St.-Hilaire (Isidore)
De Candolle (A. Pyrame) .	De Candolle (Alphonse)
Arago (François) . .	Arago (Emmanuel)
Pitt (Lord Chatham) . .	Pitt (W.)
D'Israeli (Isaac) . .	D'Israeli (Benjamin)
Mill (James) . . .	Mill (J. Stuart)
Schopenhauer . . .	Schopenhauer (Arthur)

Remarks.—In many families the transmission from father to son has continued for several generations, as has been already noticed in the family of Charlemagne; among artists it is frequent (Beethoven, Mozart, Van der Velde, etc.).

L. Verus, colleague of Marcus Aurelius, is commonly known, but not so his father, Ælius Verus. Yet a knowledge of his character would serve to explain that of his son. In Spartianus (*Historia Augusta*) are some curious details as to his beds of roses carefully picked and prepared, etc., showing his extreme effeminacy.

HEREDITY FROM MOTHER TO DAUGHTER.

It is not surprising that there are not many instances under this head. Probably any one who will tax his memory a little will recollect instances of this kind occurring in ordinary families. In history, science, literature, this is more difficult. Women have there acted but an inconsiderable part, and it is therefore natural that cases of heredity between famous mothers and famous daughters should be rare. Still here are a few.

The Emperor Augustus, who was several times married, had by his wife Scribonia his celebrated daughter Julia. She became the wife of Agrippa and had a daughter, another Julia. Both of them caused much grief to Augustus by their infamous conduct, 'Julias, filiam et neptem,' says Suetonius (c. 65), omnibus probris contaminatus relegavit.'

We may remark in passing that according to the same historian Cæsar had by Cleopatra a son, 'similem Cæsaris formâ et incessû.' He was called Cæsarion, and died very young.

Agrippina, the wife of Germanicus, 'Mother of the camps,' was a strong-willed, heroic woman, 'pervicax iræ,' says Tacitus. Being Agrippa's daughter, she had in her character some of her father's sternness. 'My daughter,' said Tiberius to her, 'you are always complaining because you do not reign.' She was the mother of the famous Agrippina, who made Claudius her slave, and raised Nero to the imperial throne.

We have already mentioned Marozia, mother of Pope John XI. This woman, who was famous in the tenth century for her wealth, her influence, and her misconduct, had her vices from her mother, Theodora, and transmitted them to her son.

Michelet points out the resemblance between Marie Leczinska

and her daughter Adelaide. 'The queen, before her marriage, had a tendency to epileptic fits. Even after her marriage, being agitated with causeless fears, she would rise from her bed at night and walk about. Madame Adelaide appears to have inherited much of this excitability. She was brave, with the courage of her race, with some childish fears, as for instance of thunder. . . . . The queen loved her father (Stanislas), and was very much beloved by him, which aroused her mother's jealousy. This, too, Adelaide inherited from her mother, and she loved her father beyond all bounds of reason.' (*Histoire de France,* tome xvi.)

To sum up all that we have said about direct heredity: it is certain that the child inherits from both parents. It never happens that either parent exercises an exclusive influence. The action of one is always preponderant, this preponderance takes place in two ways, either within the same sex or from one sex to the other. As we have seen, both of these are of very frequent occurrence. The only question is, which is the more frequent?

An answer is impossible, and even if it were possible, it would be to no purpose. To make it perfectly exact we should have to bring together all the cases of direct heredity and range them in two groups: on the one hand, cross heredity, and on the other heredity in the same sex, and then compare the totals. Yet all this labour, even if possible, would lead to nothing. Between these totals there would probably be so small a difference that no one could say which expressed the law and which the exceptions. Whenever a case of this kind arises, we may say that both sides are right and both wrong; that each possesses only a fragment of the law, thinking he possesses the whole, and that there is some higher point of view which will reconcile the two. With regard to heredity, we seek that law of which fragments only have so far been given to us by our empiric generalizations. But we must first study the phenomena of atavism.

SECTION II.—ATAVISM.

Whenever a child, instead of resembling his immediate parents, resembles one of his grandparents, or some still remoter ancestor, or even some distant member of a collateral branch of the family— a circumstance which must be attributed to the descent of all its members from a common ancestor—this is called a case of atavism. This is called reversional heredity (Lucas); reversion, or in the more expressive German term, *Rückschlag* and *Rückschritt.*

The fact was known to the ancients; Aristotle, Galen, and Pliny speak of it. Plutarch mentions a Greek woman who gave birth to a negro child, and was brought to trial for adultery, but it transpired that she was descended in the fourth degree from an Ethiopian. Montaigne expresses his astonishment at this, 'Is it not marvellous,' says he, 'that this drop of seed from which we are produced should bear the impression, not only of the bodily form, but even of the thoughts and the inclinations of our fathers? Where does this drop of water keep this infinite number of forms? and how does it bear these likenesses through a progress so haphazard and so irregular that the great-grandson shall resemble the great-grandfather, the nephew the uncle?'

In the first part of this work are recounted a large number of cases of atavism; here it will suffice to call attention to some curious facts which will serve to show the tendency of heredity.

The phenomenon of reversion is of very frequent occurrence in vegetal and animal races. Dr. Broca gives a curious example, the result of an experiment he made with a view to study the formation of races by methodical selection. He took the seeds of cornflower which he gathered promiscuously in the fields, and sowed them. This produced blue and red cornflowers. He then sowed the seed of the red cornflowers only, and obtained about a hundred flowers, two thirds of which were blue, the remainder varying from violet to rose colour. If again the seed of the rose cornflower be sown, the result will be a few blue flowers, many red, rose, and even white. It would thus be possible to create a white species, but only by a constant struggle against the phenomena of reversion which persistently reproduce the primitive type.[1]

Girou de Buzareingues gives at length the history of a strain of dogs, a cross between the pointer and the spaniel, which is briefly as follows. In the first generation the product is a spaniel; this, being crossed with a pure pointer, the result is a mongrel male with all the external characters of the pointer. By coupling this mongrel

---

[1] *Bulletins de la Société d'Anthropologie,* 2ᵉ série, tome iv. See Darwin, *Variation, etc.,* ch. xiii., for several instances of reversion in plants and animals.

with a pure pointer bitch, pointers were produced, outwardly resembling the pure pointer.   Here, then, we have the phenomena
of heredity, alternating with atavism, revealing themselves from one
generation to another in the mixed nature of the mongrel.

Facts of the same kind occur in many other domesticated races.
P. Lucas tells of a half-bred Arab mare which gave no sign of her
noble origin: covered by a stallion of inferior breed, she produced a colt possessing a strong likeness to its maternal ancestors.
The contrary often takes place, and breeders often find instances
of the inferior type reappear after a long time in stock that has
been improved by crossing.   Atavism presents itself in the silk-
worm, after more than a hundred generations.

In man it is a common fact that certain affections, such as
rheumatism, and especially gout, pass from grandfather to grandson.   In the portrait galleries of old families, and in the monu-
mental bronzes of the neighbouring churches, types of feature
are often seen which still are repeated from time to time in the
members of those families.[1]

It is common to find children with their father's or mother's
nose or mouth.   The nose is, perhaps, of all the features of the
face, the one which is best preserved by heredity.   The Bourbon
nose is well known.   P. Lucas tells us that in the beginning of
this century Dr. Gregory, while visiting at a country house in
England, the residence of a lady of high family, was struck with
the resemblance between the nose of his hostess and that of the
Chancellor of Scotland in the reign of Charles I.   He was, therefore, not surprised to learn that the lady was the great-granddaughter of that personage, who died two centuries before; nor
is this all.   As Dr. Gregory walked in the neighbourhood he
noticed the same form of nose in several labourers, and he
learned from the steward that these were also descended from
the Chancellor, but in illegitimate line.   Moreover, the re-appear-
ance of features is so frequent an occurrence that it has become
a popular belief.   Marryat has turned it to account in his novel,
Japhet in Search of a Father.   'From Dr. Parsons,' says
Quatrefages,[2] 'I borrow a case which is doubly interesting, as it

[1] Herbert Spencer, *Principles of Biology*, § 83.
[2] *Unité de l'Éspèce Humaine.*

is officially vouched for, and as it shows, in the case of a pair of negroes, a very singular hereditary disposition.

'Two negro slaves, living on the same Virginian plantation, were married. The wife gave birth to a daughter who was perfectly white. On seeing the colour of the child she was seized with alarm, and while protesting that she never had intercourse with a white man, she tried to hide the infant, and put out the light, lest the father should see it. He soon came in, complained of the unusual darkness of the room, and asked to see the babe; the mother's fears were increased when she saw the father approach with a light, but when he saw the child he appeared pleased. A few days afterwards he said to his wife : " You were afraid of me because my child was white, but I love her all the more on that account. My own father was white, although my grandfather and grandmother were as black as you and I. Although we are come from a country where white men were never seen, still there has always been one white child in families related to ours." This girl was sold to Admiral Ward when she was fifteen years old, was brought by him to London, and exhibited before the Royal Society.

'It appears that phenomena of this nature have occurred even in Africa, and Admiral Fleuriot Delangle lately told me of an analogous case.'

Reversional heredity in insanity is well established, as we have seen. It is not unusual to find persons descended from insane ancestors living to the age of thirty or forty with every sign of judgment and reason, who then became insane without any assignable cause. Gintrac records that a man who had become insane had sons, men of ability, filling public offices with distinction. Their children were at first sane, but at the age of twenty gave signs of insanity. Facts like these are recounted by all writers on insanity.

As regards the reversional heredity of talents, character, aptitudes, and passions, it is of as frequent occurrence as purely organic heredity. In the following table we give some instances of this, which have been already treated of in detail in the First Part.

REVERSIONAL HEREDITY.

1st Generation.	2nd Generation.	3rd Generation.	4th Generation.
Theodosius	Arcadius	Pulcheria	...
Scipio	Cornelia	The Gracchi	...
Charles Martel	Pepin the Short	Charlemagne	...
Henry I. of		Henry II. of	...
England	Matilda	England	...
Philippe le Bel	Isabelle	Edward III.	...
Charles VI. of		Henry VI. of	...
France	Catherine	England	...
Charles d'Or-		Marguérite de	
léans	...	Valois	...
Joanna	Charles V.	...	Don Carlos
Gustavus Vasa	...	...	Gustavus Adolphus
Van der Velde	Van der Velde	Van der Velde	
Mendelssohn,		Mendelssohn,	
(philosopher)	...	(musician)	...
Mozart, J.	Mozart, J.	Mozart	...
Beethoven, J.	Beethoven, J.	Beethoven, L.	...
Lord Chatham	...	Lady Hester Stanhope	...
Darwin, Eras-		Darwin,	
mus	...	Charles	...

Remarks.—All the names in the second column held in a latent condition the characteristics of the first generation, and transmitted them to the third.

The case of Charles VI. of France is peculiarly remarkable. This mad king gave his daughter Catherine in marriage to his conqueror, Henry V. of England. The fruit of that union was the weak and unfortunate Henry VI., the sad victim of the wars of the Roses.

SECTION III.—INDIRECT HEREDITY.

Indirect heredity is 'the representation of collaterals in the physical and moral character of the progeny.' We often observe between distant relatives out of the direct line of descent—between uncle and nephew, aunt and niece; granduncle and grandnephew, and cousins, even in the remoter degrees—striking resemblances of conformation, face, inclinations, passions, character, deformity, and disease.

But while the two forms of heredity, hitherto considered direct heredity and atavism, are generally admitted, that now to be discussed has been received with considerable distrust and doubt. In the last century, Wollaston,[1] in *The Religion of Nature Delineated*, after having shown that a child often more closely resembles an uncle, an aunt, or a cousin, than it does either of its parents, adds: ' Neither uncle, nor aunt, nor cousin have anything to do with generation in this instance ; therefore the resemblance does not proceed from the act of generation.' In this century indirect heredity has been often denied, or doubted. Piorry, in his *Traité sur l'Hérédité des Maladies* (1840), views it with suspicion. Baillarger, in the work already quoted, brings together one hundred and forty-seven cases of mental disease traceable to collateral heredity ; but he judged it best to omit them from his calculations, for the reason that ' heredity, under this indirect form, although in most cases quite probable, still does not appear to be unquestionable.'

To explain these facts, which are so well established that it is impossible to deny them, these authors have recourse to various hypotheses. Some speak of the force of circumstances ; others of accident ; others see in them nothing more than coincidence. They all agree in finding here, in the last analysis, only the result of chance.

We have already seen, while considering Buckle's objection, what is the value of such an explanation as this, how improbable and inaccurate it really is. But the doctrine which insists on collateral heredity has something better to offer than these negative reasons. To show that it is correct, we need only remark that indirect heredity is only a form of atavism—a form which is rarer and less easy of apprehension than direct atavism, but differing from it only in appearance. The nephew resembles the uncle, the

---

[1] Quoted by Lucas.

cousin resembles the cousin, because each of them hold some characteristic from a common ancestor, who transmitted it to the intermediate generations, in whom it has been latent. The researches made into the subject of generation during the past fifty years, and the discovery of alternate generations, have greatly enlarged our view of heredity, and this transmission in collateral line has in it nothing wonderful. Hence this form of heredity, which was admitted by Burdach and proved by Lucas, no longer meets with opposition. We now regard it as nothing more or less than a somewhat complicated case of atavism. We treat it here under a special heading, merely for the sake of making the whole subject plain: in fact, we are but continuing our study of reversional heredity. However, a few facts will show the identity of direct atavism with collateral heredity.

'I am acquainted,' says Quatrefages, 'with a family into which married a grand-niece of the illustrious Bailli de Suffren Saint-Tropez, the last French commander in the great Indian wars against the English, with Hyder Ali for his ally. This lady had two sons, the younger of whom, judging from a very fine portrait, bore a very striking resemblance to his great-great-uncle, but was not at all like his father or mother. The celebrated sailor, therefore, and his great-great-nephew reproduced, with an interval of four generations between them, the features of a common ancestor. Plainly, atavism acted here in both branches, for in this case there is no direct heredity.'

A well-formed man had two relatives affected with hare-lip; by his first wife he had eleven children, two of them hare-lipped, and by his second wife, two who possessed the same deformity. —A woman in whose family were several members hard of hearing gave birth to two deaf and dumb boys.—A man whose brother and whose aunt were deaf-mutes had five children, one of them deaf and dumb. There are many similar cases of deaf-muteness on record. A still more singular case is that of a woman come of a family in which there had been several cases of hypospadia, and who gave birth to two boys affected with that anomaly.[1]

[1] Lucas, ii. p. 36.

COLLATERAL HEREDITY.

Ancestors.	Descendants.	Degree of Kinship.
Cæsar	Octavius	Grandnephew (His mother was Cæsar's niece)
Seneca	Lucan	Nephew
Pliny the Elder	Pliny the Younger	Nephew (sister's son)
Alexander the Great	Pyrrhus	Grandnephew
Doria (Andrea)	Doria (Felipó)	Nephew (brother's son)
Montmorency	Coligni	Nephew
Nassau (Maurice of)	Turenne	Nephew
Mazarin	Prince Eugène	Grandnephew
Gustavus Adolphus	Charles XII.	Grandnephew
Marlborough	Berwick	Grandnephew
Corneille	Fontenelle	Nephew (sister's son)
Murillo { Juan Agustin Antonio	Murillo, Esteban	Nephew and cousin on mother's side
Caracci, Agostino Caracci, Annibale	Caracci, Luigi	First cousins
Bernouilli, Jacques		Several nephews and grand nephews, named already in the genealogy of this family
Jussieu, Bernard	Jussieu, Laurent	Nephew (see genealogy)
Bentham, Jeremy	Bentham, George	Nephew, celebrated botanist

Some authors reckon among cases of collateral heredity those where two or more illustrious brothers are found in the same family, *e.g.* Æschylus and Cynegirus, the two Boileaus, the two Corneilles, the two Van Eycks, the two Van Ostades, the Schlegels, the two Cuviers, the two Humboldts, Charles Lamb and his sister, Napoleon and his brothers, etc. We do not regard as strictly collateral heredity anything save that heredity which passes from an ancestor to a descendant. In all the cases just cited, and in others like them, it seems to us very probable that this talent common to several brothers springs from one common source—from some kinsman whose merits lie unnoticed, for merit does not belong exclusively to history : or else it is the result of some quiet work of nature, for who can tell how and through what metamorphoses she produces talent? We know not, and doubtless we should be profoundly surprised if we could understand it. But as we wished in the foregoing table to state only incontestable facts, we have carefully narrowed our ground.

SECTION IV.—THE HEREDITY OF INFLUENCE.

We admit that, from the psychological point of view, we are sceptical in regard to this form of heredity, especially as regards man. It consists in the influence of a former alliance on the children born of a subsequent marriage.

The fact seems to be perfectly out of the order of things. Atavism, though it may appear strange at first view, is explained by the community of blood and of origin ; if the father and mother seem to bear absolutely no resemblance to their child ; if they are merely the channels of some quality or some feature of the ancestors, at least there exists between these and the descendants a continuous chain which accounts for the transmission. Here is nothing of the kind : a child resembles a person who has nothing in common with him, save that the person was once its mother's husband.

Still, among the lower and even the higher animals there are facts to show that heredity of influence frequently occurs.

We would mention in the first place Bonnet's well known experiments on the aphis. He took a young aphis just after it was hatched, isolated it completely, and saw it, in that state of undoubted virginity, produce, after twenty-one days, ninety-five young ones. The aphides thus produced were able themselves to produce others. Bonnet placed one apart, and obtained from it five successive generations without the aid of a male. An aphis of the fifth generation produced young under the same conditions, and Bonnet saw this fecundity prolonged through over ten generations. This viviparous condition ceased in the autumn, when the males begin to appear; then the aphis becomes oviparous.

This is a curious example of the influence of the male on a whole series of generations, fecundated as it appears by one single act. Facts of a like nature occur in certain caterpillars, and in some species of molluscæ.

Among the higher animals it is still more easy to study the heredity of influence. Burdach [1] gives the following examples.

When a mare is crossed by an ass and produces a mule, if she be afterwards put to a stallion, the colt she then drops will have some points of resemblance to the ass.

An English mare which in 1815 was once covered by a quagga gave birth to a mule marked with spots; she never saw the quagga again. In 1817, 1818, and 1823, she was covered successively by three Arab stallions, and produced three brown colts with bands like those of the quagga.

A sow which had had by a wild boar a litter in which the brown colour of the sire was predominant, was put, long after his death, to boars of domestic breeds; among the pigs of the second and third litters were several having patches of the colour of the wild boar.

If a bitch be once put to a dog of another race, every litter of puppies afterwards will include one belonging to that other breed, except the first time she be put only to dogs of her own breed.

'It is the same with the human species,' says this physiologist. 'We sometimes find the children of a second marriage resembling the former husband, who may be long since dead, and showing a closer relation to him, even from the moral point of view, than to their true father.'

Burdach is content with affirming this without citing any instance.

---

[1] *Traité de Physiologie,* ii. 243.

Lucas does the same. He prudently confines himself to observing that the fact that children begotten in adultery resemble their putative father does not prove the case, as the putative father may also be the real father; and that only in case of the husband's death or prolonged absence could the fact be absolutely conclusive. I find in Michelet, and repeat with all reserve, an assertion which, if admitted, would be a true case of the heredity of influence, from the psychological point of view, but it is the only case I know. 'Madame de Montespau,' says Michelet, 'had already had a son by M. de Montespau. The first child she had by the king—the Duc de Maine—resembled only her husband : he had his Gascon disposition, his buffoonery. He might have passed for the grandson of Zamet, the buffoon.' [1].

When this question of the heredity of influence was discussed before the French Anthropological Society, most of the members took the negative side. While admitting that cases of it are frequent among animals, they doubted whether a widow could have children resembling her first husband. [2]

We can only repeat what we have already said, and while we do not deny a fact which is not at all impossible, and which could perhaps be explained, we may consider it so rare, so difficult to establish psychologically, that it is useless to insist on it in a study of mental heredity.

We will now endeavour to get a general view of what has been said on heredity, and to appreciate the results.

We first reduced the facts to a few empiric formulas, which include them all, viz. direct cross heredity, direct heredity in one sex, reversional heredity and collateral heredity. These we hold to be so many fragments, as it were, of a single law, of which we are sensible, though we do not understand it. We now have to find this law. We do not speak here of the theoretical and ideal law of heredity, which we have already given, but only of an empirical law, a more general formula, which includes and explains all the others. If we succeed in finding all the ties which bind these various formulas together, this simplification of the work will render it easier to understand the nature of heredity.

---

[1] *Histoire de France*, tome xiii.
[2] *Bulletins de la Société d'Anthropologie*, tome i. p. 291.

We remark, in the first place, that the empiric formulas given above are capable of being simplified and reduced under two chief heads : immediate and mediate heredity. When we find a child resembling its father or mother, the fact appears perfectly simple, either because it is so common, or because we judge it to be quite natural that like should produce like. But when we see the great-grandchild resembling the great-grandfather, or the great nephew resembling the great uncle, and this without any intermediate stage to explain the resemblance, this case of heredity appears to us so strange that many have rejected it. It would then be a great point if we could show that this mediate heredity resolves itself into the other form. To do this we must make a brief digression.

All naturalists are agreed that no studies are of more advantage for them than those of comparative anatomy and comparative physiology ; that the knowledge of rudimentary organisms has given them a better understanding of organs and functions, and that these results have been specially remarkable as regards generation. The study of the lower forms of this function has greatly enlarged their views, and even entirely modified the ideas of scientific men on that subject. Among these discoveries, that of alternate generations appears to us, of all others, the best fitted to throw light on the subject which now engages our attention.

In 1818 Chamisso's studies on certain molluscs called biphoræ, or salpæ, led him to the discovery that these animals are alternately free and aggregated. In the first generation strings of biphoræ are found, the product of gemmation ; in the second, solitary biphoræ produced from spores ; in the third, the strings reappear: so that the young never resemble the parent, but always the grand-parent.

1st generation	Aggregated salpæ	Grandfather
2nd „	Free „	Father
3rd „	Aggregated „	Son

The researches of Saars, Steenstrup, Owen, and Van Beneden, show that in some animals the cycle is not limited to three generations, but that often it is more extended, and that the resemblance, instead of passing from the grandfather to the grandson, passes from the great-grandfather to the great-grandson. In those species which propagate by alternate generation, the process is this : an ovum produces a simple organism, and this propagates by gemmation ; the creatures thus produced resemble neither the parent nor the original organism ; next the primitive type reappears, and with it the attributes of the two sexes, and propagation by ova. Thus, in the medusa, between two perfect types we find three, as follows :—

1st generation	Medusa	Great-grandfather
2nd „	Ciliated larva	Grandfather
3rd „	Polyp	Father
4th „	Strobila	Son
5th „	Medusa	Great-grandson

It is not here, as in cases of metamorphoses, the same individual which passes from the larval to the nymph state, and then becomes a perfect adult : here we have several individuals totally different from one another.

The conclusion to be drawn from these facts is, that we ordinarily understand heredity in too narrow a sense, looking at it only under its immediate form—from one generation to the next. But, as we see, it may embrace a much larger cycle. It is true that these phenomena are met with only in the lower species, and there are no instances of alternate generation among vertebrates : but still they show how strong, tenacious, and, so to speak, unlimited is heredity. At the same time it gives us a better understanding of atavism. The two facts, indeed, are not identical, and we do not at all mean to say that atavism is a form of alternate generation, yet the mind readily perceives an analogy between them. Reversional heredity in man seems less singular to us when we compare it with these orderly cycles ; and on witnessing these indisputable facts we can better understand how great is the force of heredity.

At a time when alternate generation was yet unknown, Burdach and Girou de Buzareingues were led by their researches to admit that there are stronger resemblances between grandfather and grandson, grandmother and granddaughter, than between father and son, mother and daughter. This is expressed in the following table. (Burdach, *Physiologie*, ii. 269) :—

	Paternal Line		Maternal Line	
First Generation	Grandfather	Grandmother	Grandfather	Grandmother
Second Generation		father	mother	
Third Generation	son	daughter	son	daughter

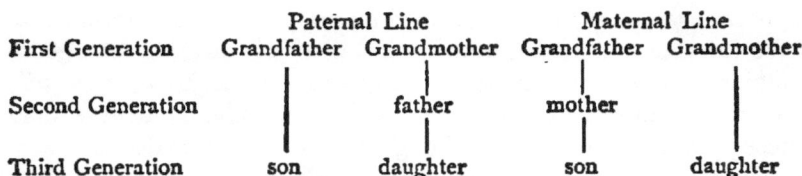

If we compare this table with that given above for the salpæ, it is impossible not to be struck with the resemblance.

But a difficulty still remains. In cases of reversional heredity where the grandson resembles the grandfather, the grandnephew the granduncle—the intermediate stages being totally unlike either —how is this resemblance to be explained? Above all, how can it be said, as we have done, that these cases are to be referred to immediate heredity? The reply to this question is to be found in one of two hypotheses; either these resemblances are fortuitous. or else they have been preserved in the latent state by the intermediate generations, and thus what appears to be mediate heredity is really immediate. The first hypothesis cannot be accepted, therefore we must hold the second. And this leads us to ask what is meant by 'latent characters.'

One of the best examples of these, says Darwin, is afforded by secondary sexual characters. In every female all the secondary male characters, and in every male all the secondary female characters exist in a latent state, ready to be evolved under certain conditions. It is well-known that a large number of female birds when old or diseased, or when operated on, partly assume the secondary male characters of their species. Waterton gives a curious case of a hen which had ceased laying, and had assumed the plumage, voice, spurs, and warlike disposition of the cock; when opposed to an enemy she would erect her huckles and show fight. Thus every character, even to the instinct and manner of fighting, must have lain dormant in this hen as long as her ovaria continued to act. We see something of an analogous nature in the human species.

On the other hand, with male animals, it is notorious that the secondary sexual characters are more or less lost when they are subjected to castration, as in the case of capons.

Thus the secondary characters of each sex lie dormant in the opposite sex, ready to be evolved under peculiar circumstances. 'We can thus understand how, for instance, it is possible for a good milking cow to transmit her good qualities through her male off- spring to future generations, for we may confidently believe that these qualities are present, though latent, in the males of each generation. So it is with the game-cock, who can transmit his superiority in courage and vigour through his female to his male offspring.'[1]

As Darwin remarks, these facts oblige us to admit that certain characters, aptitudes, and instincts may remain in the latent state in an individual, and even in a series of individuals, while yet we are unable to find any trace of their presence; and on this hypo- thesis the transmission of a characteristic from grandfather to grand- child, with the apparent omission in the intermediate parent of the opposite sex, becomes very plain.

What has now been said respecting latent characteristics applies to a form of heredity of which we have not yet treated specifically, heredity occurring at corresponding periods. This, it appears to us, may be explained on the hypothesis of latent characteristics contained in the individual in the germ state, and which come to light only under definite conditions, and at some particular point of his development, and this particular moment corresponding with a similar moment in the progenitors. Hereditary diseases are a good instance of heredity at corresponding periods. Thus, chorea, which usually makes its appearance in childhood, con- sumption in middle age, gout in old age, are naturally hereditary in the same periods.

Blindness furnishes still more striking instances. In one family it was hereditary for three generations, and thirty-seven children and grandchildren became blind between their seventeenth and eighteenth year. In another instance, a father and his four children were all attacked with blindness at the age of twenty-one. It is the same with deafness. Two brothers, their father, their paternal grandfather, all became deaf at the age of forty.[2] Esquirol

[1] *Variation, etc.,* ii.
[2] Dr. Sedgwick, *British and Foreign Medical and Chirurgical Review,* 1861, p. 485. See also Lucas ii. 739, and Darwin *Variation, etc.,* ii. 80

cites some instances of insanity which made its appearance at the same age in several generations. One of these cases is that of a grandfather, father, and son, who all committed suicide at about the age of fifty; another is that of a family all of whose members became insane at the age of forty.

Such facts as these—and they are numerous—are a strong argument in favour of the hypothesis of latent characteristics, and this in turn does much to throw light upon many singular features of heredity, as we can show by passing in review all the cases we have cited.

When the child takes equally after father and mother, the case needs no explanation, it being the realization of the ideal law, as far as that is possible.

When the child resembles one of its parents to the exclusion of the other, this exclusion does not really take place. That parent whose influence appears destroyed may reappear in the next generation, or later.

It will be observed that the question already debated, 'whether heredity is more frequent in one sex or between the two sexes,' loses much of its importance when we regard heredity as a cycle. When we see the father reappear in the daughter, and finally in the grandson, the mother in the son, and finally in the grand-daughter, we have no difficulty in believing that each sex reasserts its rights, though it does not receive them at first.

Finally, the hypothesis of latent characteristics gives a plausible and simple explanation of all the phenomena of reversion, whether in direct or collateral line.

Still it is evident that these formulas cannot pretend to give a complete explanation of a fact so abstruse and so complex as hereditary transmission. Our only purpose is to show that the term is taken in too narrow a sense when it is restricted to two generations, and that the facts seem less strange so soon as we grasp them as a whole. We desired also to exhibit the wonderful tenacity of heredity. Its law is absolute transmission; and, in spite of all the obstacles which tend to weaken or destroy it, it struggles on without truce or pause, losing much of its strength as it advances, dissipating itself, so to speak, so as to appear no longer to exist. And yet, when we see the same characters reappear, sometimes after a hundred generations, here is indeed matter for reflection. It may be said that heredity verifies in its own way the axiom, Nothing is lost. With its character of unconquerable firmness, of obstinate persistency, it appears to us as one of those many inflexible bonds by which omnipotent nature imprisons us in necessity.

We have now to see what attempt has been made to subject the facts of heredity to the control of numbers.

CHAPTER III.

ESSAYS IN STATISTICS.

I.

It is rightly said that there is no perfect ideal science except that which is exact, that is to say, submitted to the control of number, weight, and measure; but it is not correct to say that there is no science save that which is exact. Yet distinguished and even eminent thinkers have maintained this paradox. If we are to believe Herschel, 'no branch of human knowledge can be considered as having left the state of infancy, if it does not base its theories and correct them practically by means of numbers.' If this be true, the domain of science at the present day would be somewhat narrow. We should have to exclude from it a large number of studies which rightly count as scientific, and even to despair of ever bringing them under the conditions of science. Admitting, what is probable, that certain branches of physics and chemistry, at present refractory, may be subjected to all the strictness of mathematical formulas, it is very doubtful whether the facts of biology, and still more those of psychology and sociology, can ever be so subjected. But it is not therefore necessary to exclude them permanently from the domain of science.

When we compare scientific knowledge with ordinary knowledge, such as serves the ordinary needs of life, and when we consider the nature of both, we find that they differ only in degree, that science is not a mode of knowledge apart and *sui generis*, employing processes exclusively its own, but that it springs from ordinary knowledge by a natural evolution, tending always towards more and more complex and more and more exact previsions, until finally they attain to a close relation or identity, the most perfect end which they can reach. In this process of evolution there are, as it seems to us, two principal stages : the first of these, which constitutes science properly so called, consists in the employment of verification ; the second constitutes exact and ideal science, and it consists in quantification, or, to avoid neologism, quantitative determination.

This we will try to show.

When we are aware of a large number of phenomena which are analogous, that is, at once like and unlike, we endeavour to seize the fixed basis in the production of these phenomena—their law. But whether this law result from an intuition of genius, or from a slow and minute comparison of facts, followed by induction, must be submitted to the process of verification, for it has to explain all the facts, or at least most of them ; and it alone must explain them, otherwise it remains an hypothesis.

Thus every science, in order to become science, passes through three stages, the facts, the law, and the verification. First, the phenomena are collected and observed, scrutinized, turned over and over, placed on the rack of experiment, then from them is drawn their generic constant element ; finally, the law thus discovered is anew tested by application to facts, just as a seal is verified when applied to its impression. This last process—verification—is essential.

Without verification there is no science, because this process alone can give to our theories an objective value. It is a complete mistake to suppose that what is not true can be scientifically established. There are a hundred ways of looking at facts, of interpreting, and of generalizing them. Of course, these are not all correct, but who is to decide between them? In such case science gets only the individual, personal opinion of one man, his special mode of understanding and accounting for the facts. But this is an entirely subjective doctrine, which may indeed be science, but if so is science only by accident, nor have we any means of knowing that it is science, or any grounds for affirming that it is.

It may be said, parenthetically, that this is what distinguishes metaphysics from science.

9

When in the works of one of the great philosophers, Aristotle, Leibnitz, or Hegel, we read the scheme of some grand doctrine, the argument, especially to a novice in such studies, is attractive and convincing. The grandeur of the views, the breadth of the method, the fruitfulness in results, are all alike charming. On reflection some difficulties present themselves : these are the usual processes of science, the inductions are legitimate, the deductions exact, and yet we are dissatisfied—some infirmity of mind hinders an entire assent. The mind is undecided, hesitates between two opinions. Yet, for the most part, no cause can be assigned for this indecision, although the true reason is that to these doctrines verification is wanting, which alone gives perfection to science and produces an absolute conviction. When Aristotle reduces everything in nature to the opposition between the possible and the actual ; when Leibnitz reduces all to forces, and Hegel to the evolution of ideas, their doctrine is irreproachable for logical strength and precision. Yet we dare not assert that these doctrines are true, since verification is impossible. When, in the last century, the doctrine of the pre-existence of germs in embryogeny was taught, it was acceptable, was logically deduced, perhaps true. Experiment alone could decide : and experiment showed it to be false by proving epigenesis to be true; and this last theory has been therefore adopted by science.

Thus, of the three stages to be travelled, metaphysics traverse the first two, the facts and the laws, but never reach the third, strict verification by the differential method, and not that arbitrary and hasty verification which explains some facts without concern for those which it overlooks. Thus metaphysics remain beyond and above verification, beyond and above science, confined for ever to what is subjective.

But, as has been already said, verification is but the first degree in science. The second degree, that which completes the work, is quantitative determination. That is the ideal to which all sciences aspire, but to which but few attain.

It is clear that, as the domain of quantity is that of number, weight, and measure, every process from the qualitative to the quantitative conducts us to more and more precise determinations. But how does this transformation of quality into quantity take place. and under what conditions?

Hegel somewhere says: 'Quantity is quality suppressed'—a somewhat obscure way of saying that quantity is the canvas on which quality is embroidered. To understand this, let us observe, in the first place, that what we call quality comes to us originally by sensation and feeling, that is to say, under an agreeable or disagreeable form, which is consequently subjective. If I feel any sensation—that, for instance, of heat—it has the property of affecting me in a certain way; but, further, I notice that it may increase, or diminish, or vary indefinitely. There is, then, in it a greater and a less, a something measurable, or quantity. It is the same with all sensations. If, then, in any quality I suppress, by the power of thought, all that is agreeable or disagreeable—all that is simply *affective*, all that depends on the constitution of our organs—there remains a possibility of indefinite variation to greater or less; in other words, what belongs specially to quality having been suppressed, there remains what belongs to quantity.

Thus under all quality lies quantity. The category of quantity is the more general, consequently the more simple, and so the more measurable. If, then, we can transform quality into quantity, we make quality measurable; and this transformation is sometimes possible. If it be found that some variations of quality in a class of phenomena correspond regularly to variations of quantity, then every mathematical formula that is applicable to the variable quantities may be applied to the corresponding qualities. Thus it has been proved by experiment that every variety of sound corresponds to a distinct and determinable variety of motion. Thus the physicist, in regard to light and heat, can eliminate all that is purely qualitative, and see only a movement of vibration subject to mechanical laws. Thus, too, mechanics, hydrostatics, optics, acoustics, and thermology, have gradually become mathematical. But this transformation grows, as is natural, more and more difficult in proportion as we ascend from simple qualities to complex existences. In the world of life and thought number is as yet powerless, and there is no reason to suppose that it can hold dominion there for some time to come.

We now apply what has been said to the special question of heredity.

We began by collecting a large number of facts belonging to the

domain of physiology, to mental maladies, to animal and human
psychology and history—facts of various kinds, and adapted for
showing all the varieties of hereditary transmission. We next
endeavoured to disengage what is constant in the production of
these phenomena, and proposed heredity as a biological law, the
exceptions being, as we shall see, only the results of disturbing
causes; and we examined the various forms of this law. We
believe that this theory may be verified, that it has a scientific
value.

The facts which have served to establish the law will serve also
to verify it, for it is nothing more than a simple generalization.
Of course it were puerile to suppose that, in the present state of
physiology, and yet more of psychology, any theory of heredity
could be final. Nevertheless, we persist in the conviction that the
laws already · recited, being only the expression of facts, are no
merely subjective view : and this is the important point.

But it may be possible to go even beyond this, and to submit
the laws of heredity to a quantitative test. In a recent work,
entitled *Hereditary Genius,* the statistical method has been applied
to this subject. Before giving our opinion on the question, we
will briefly state the results obtained by this author.

II.

Mr. Galton's book possesses merits and defects somewhat common
in English works : many figures, a sufficiency of facts, very little
generalization. His method is purely statistical. His investigations
have for their object not heredity in general, nor even psychological
heredity, but simply this question : Is genius hereditary, and to what
extent? Given an illustrious or eminent man,[1] what are the chances
of his having had an illustrious or eminent father, grandfather, son,
grandson, brother, etc.? To answer this question, the author has

[1] 'There are,' says he, 'in the British Isles, two millions of male persons
above the age of fifty. Among these I find 850 that are illustrious, and 500
eminent. In one million men, therefore, there will be 425 *illustrious* and 250
eminent.' The author declares that he has got these same figures by various
methods, viz. by consulting the *Dictionary of Contemporaries,* the necrological
notices in the *Times,* etc. This will give an idea of Mr. Galton's method, and
of his taste for exact research.

searched the biographies of great men, drawn out their genealogies, traced their relationships, compared the results, struck averages, and the following are his conclusions.

He first entered this field with a work on *English Judges from 1660 to 1865.* These judges, always eight in number, constitute the highest magistracy in England, and are, as he assures us, universally admitted to be exceptional men. Their biography is known, as are also their family connections. Here, then, is a fair number of facts, which may be grouped together in order to examine the results.

In the course of 205 years there were 286 judges, and among these the author has found 112 who had one or more illustrious kinsmen. Hence, the probability that a judge has in his family one or more illustrious members exceeds the ratio of 1:3—in itself a striking result.

Passing now from these general results to details, it may be shown how this probability diminishes as we pass from relations of the first degree (father, son, brother), to relations of the second degree (grandfather, uncle, nephew, grandson), and those of the third degree (great-grandfather, granduncle, cousin, grandnephew).

Suppose 100 families of judges, and let N stand for the most eminent man in each of them, the number of their illustrious kinsmen will on the average be distributed as follows:—Father, 26; brother, 35; son, 36; grandfather, 15; uncle, 18; nephew, 19; grandson, 19; great-grandfather, 2; granduncle, 4; first-cousin, 11; grandnephew, 17. This statement will be more readily understood from the following table :—

TABLE I.

2 great-grandfathers		
15 grandfathers	4 granduncles	
26 fathers		18 uncles
100 N	35 brothers	11 cousins-german
36 sons	19 nephews	
19 grandsons	17 grandnephews	
6 great-grandsons		

If now we pass from thi partial work on the judges to broader researches, we meet with results of very much the same kind.

Mr. Galton distributes into seven groups the remarkable men who have been the objects of his investigations—statesmen, generals, men of letters, men of science, artists, poets, and divines. He pursues the method already indicated. He sets out from the hypothesis of 100 families studied, modifying his results according to circumstances; for example, when his researches have extended to only twenty, twenty-five, or· fifty families, he multiplies his results by five, four, or two. Thus he is enabled to institute a direct comparison between the various groups. These results are given in the following table, with the addition of the group already considered, that of the judges :—

TABLE II.

	Judges.	Statesmen.	Generals.	Men of letters.	Scientific men.	Poets.	Artists.	Divines.	Averages.
Father	26	33	47	48	26	20	32	28	31
Brother	35	39	50	42	47	40	50	36	41
Son	36	49	31	54	60	45	89	40	48
Grandfather . . .	15·	28	16	24	14	5	7	20	17
Uncle	18.	18	8	24	16	5	14	40	18
Nephew	19	18	35	24	23	50	18	4	22
Grandson	19	10	12	9	9	5	18	16	14
Great-grandfather . .	2	8	8	3	0	0	0	4	3
Granduncle	4	5	8	6	5	5	7	4	5
First-cousin . . .	11	21	20	18	16	0	1	8	13
Grandnephew . . .	17	5	8	6	16	10	0	0	10
Great-grandson . . .	6	0	0	3	7	0	0	0	3

We will not follow our author through the extended observations he makes on each column and on each of its figures, nor through the remarks, often ingenious, often very problematical, which he makes with a view to explain whatever differs overmuch from the average. There is no question but that, if we omit columns six and seven (poets and artists), which present some singular deviations, we cannot fail to be struck with the resemblance between the figures here compared. The impression made by the table will be still more striking if we compare the first column, that of the judges—of the men whose kinships the author has studied most closely—with the last column, that which gives the averages, that is, with the column which purports to express the law in numerical terms.

The number of families that has served as the basis of the work is about 300, and includes nearly 1000 men of note, of whom 415 are illustrious. The author thinks that, if there is a law, so great a mass of facts ought to bring it to light. This law is given in the last column of Table II. The probability that a man of mark would have remarkable kinsmen is, for his father, thirty-one per cent.; brothers, forty-one per cent.; sons, forty-eight per cent., etc. (See Table II., column 9.)

If we estimate the probability of the kinsmen of illustrious men rising to be eminent—and the author shows that eminent men are in general less numerous by one half than illustrious men—it will be found to be as follows :—

In the first degree, for the father as one to six ; for each brother as one to seven ; for each son as one to four. In the second degree, for each of the grandfathers, as one to twenty-five ; uncle, one to forty ; nephew, one to forty ; grandson, one to twenty-nine ; In the third degree, for each cousin-german, one to one hundred ; each of the other relatives one to two hundred.

Before we dismiss statistics we must clear up one point. In Table II. the word 'father' stands for 'mother,' as well, and 'brother' includes 'sister'; in a word, the male and female relatives are indicated by one term. We have now to determine the respective positions of the males and females in the eight groups of one hundred families each.

TABLE III.

	Judges.	Statesmen.	Generals.	Litterateurs.	Savants.	Poets.	Artists.	Divines.	Average.
Male Line . .	74	64	68	74	71	94	85	27	70
Female Line .	26	36	32	26	29	6	15	73	30
Total . .	100	100	100	100	100	100	100	100	100

On comparing the two averages, seventy for males, thirty for females, we cannot fail to be struck by the great difference between the two, and the marked preponderance of the male line. The author has inquired into the cause of this, but without arriving, as he himself admits, at any very satisfactory conclusion. He allows but little weight to the hypothesis that in the biographies of great men, if their mothers are mentioned, but little is said with regard to their other female relations ; for in the case of statesmen and great commanders, whose genealogy is well known, the female line is likewise very much inferior to the male, as is shown in columns two and three of Table III. The author thinks that a more satisfactory solution would be to admit that the aunts, sisters, and daughters of illustrious men, being accustomed at home to an intellectual and moral atmosphere above the common, do not, on an average, marry as much as other women ; and he is of opinion that his hypothesis would bear the test of facts, though he confesses that it is impossible to apply the test.

III.

We have now given in a few pages the results of a thick volume filled with facts and figures. While regretting again the absence of larger views, we must bestow high praise on this taste for exact research, this constant aiming at precision, this fear of elevating to the rank of objective truths merely subjective impressions. But the work does not give what it promises to give.

It will be noticed in the first place that Mr. Galton's method, being chiefly quantitative, differs totally from our own, which is chiefly qualitative. In the foregoing chapters we have striven to show that by comparison of facts we arrive at a great biological, universal law—heredity ; a law that is necessary, invariable, and without exception, provided secondary causes do not intervene. In the next place, descending from the more to the less general, we have examined the various aspects of this law, and have shown how the facts of heredity fall under three formulas, or four at the most. The laws have been in our view only the simple generalization of facts.

Mr. Galton proceeds differently ; facts are for him only a matter of calculation, he groups them with a view of arriving not at laws but only at averages. We do not find in his book anything like an analytical research into the general formulas of heredity. His method is statistical. And here the question arises, What is the value of this method, applied to moral facts?

Statistics, according to the definition of its professors, is ' the science of social facts expressed in numerical terms.' Its object is to collect and group methodically all moral or social phenomena which are susceptible of numerical valuation. Its method consists in exposition and induction. The method of exposition, which is the simple and the more certain, consists in the calculation of averages, and is based on this undoubted truth, that ' in an indefinitely protracted series of events, the action of regular and constant causes must in the long run outweigh that of irregular causes.' (Laplace). The inductive method, which is less certain, consists in obtaining numerical expressions for social facts, by means of arithmetical or algebraic processes applied to a small number of observations, and in admitting, on the ground of analogy or probability, results not directly established. Mr. Galton employs both methods, but chiefly the second. He feels, therefore, confident in regard to his method.

In spite of all the attacks and jokes levelled against it, I hold that statistics is a genuine science, and that it is of high importance. But its mistake, in my opinion, is to suppose that it furnishes a quantitative determination. As we have seen, science has two chief phases : the one where it takes its rise in becoming objective; the other where it attains its perfect form in becoming quantitative. Statistics halts at the first, while thinking to reach the second.

To see that this is so, in spite of appearances, in spite of columns of figures and the imposing array of calculations, we will take a moral and social fact of high importance—human liberty. An attempt has been made to study it by means of statistical data. Quelelet in his *Physique Sociale*, and after him Buckle in his *History of Civilization*, have used these with great ability. They have shown that the amount of crime in general, and of each species of crime in particular, varies much less than is supposed ; that in the beginning of each year, supposing the circumstances to remain the same, we might almost predict with certainty the number of crimes that will be committed in each country during the year. If we look into the French criminal reports and compare several years, we shall be surprised to find that various crimes and offences, classed under a score of heads, oscillate within very restricted limits. The number of suicides, too, is much the same for each year; in five years it varied in London between two hundred and thirteen and two hundred and sixty-six. Nay, even occurrences which might appear to be governed entirely by chance, and to result from pure stupidity, are not without regularity. It has been shown that in London and in Paris about the same number of letters without an address are posted every year.

I have no wish to discuss here whether or no we are free agents, nor whether that problem can be resolved by the present method. My object is only to inquire whether it can lead to quantitative determination—that is, to absolute certitude. It is plain that it cannot do so. When we are told that the statistical method enables us to predict the number of murders, larcenies, suicides, marriages, etc., the meaning is that they are foreseen in the gross and approximatively; but in true quantitative knowledge nothing is determined in the gross or approximatively. Given a great man in a family, does any one imagine that by means of Galton's averages we can determine how many illustrious brothers, sons, or nephews he will have, with as much certainty as we can calculate the day and the hour of an eclipse?

It is, therefore, a mistake to fancy that because mathematical processes are employed we can arrive at mathematical certainty. The real service rendered by figures is this : there is a multitude of scattered facts, which have no visible connection, and appear to be perfectly fortuitous. The statistician compares these together, and discovers in them uniformities, or, in other words, laws. And as from uniformity of effects we may infer uniformity of causes; as from moral and social facts we can ascend to the psychological states from which they result, the consequence is that statistics can be of service in the study of morals and even of psychology. By grouping together certain phenomena of social life it gives us a means by which we can verify and check our conclusions; it gives to the purely subjective views of the mind the means of acquiring an objective value, and so of passing from the conjectural to the scientific state. It supplies the psychologist and the moralist with materials—with observations and experiments. But this is only the beginning of science, not its perfection.

And, indeed, how could it be expected, in the present state of the moral sciences, that figures could solve every problem? The philosophers of the present century have shown (and the positivist school have performed a fair proportion of the work) that the sciences are not isolated systems of doctrine, each detached from each, but that there exists among them an hierarchical subordination, so that the more complex rest on the more simple, and presuppose them. The mathematical, physical, biological, moral, and social sciences represent so many phases of a continuous process, which advances from the simple to the complex. Social phenomena presuppose thought and sensation; these presuppose life; life presupposes physical and chemical conditions; physical and chemical facts presuppose mathematical conditions, time, space, and quantity, which are simply the most vague and general conditions of existence. In this series of an increasing complexity, and of a decreasing comprehensiveness, it would be folly to imagine that the superior science could exist before the inferior science were constituted. But quantitative determination exists only in mathematics, and to some extent in physics; it has not yet penetrated into biology; how, then, could it have attained to the moral and social sciences? It is, perhaps, doubtful if it will ever reach them. Number is an instrument at once too coarse to unravel the delicate texture of these phenomena, and too fragile to penetrate deeply into their complicated and multiple nature. With all its apparent precision it stops at the surface of things, for it can give us only quantity, which is a very unimportant thing as compared with quality.

In short, this statistical research into heredity fails to do what it promised. Yet, by comparing facts and grouping figures, it arrives at the same result as ourselves, but by another route : it establishes psychological heredity, and the objective reality of its laws.

CHAPTER IV.

EXCEPTIONS TO THE LAW OF HEREDITY.

I.

THE study of the laws of heredity would not be complete without an examination of the exceptions. Nothing gives a clearer notion of the nature of a law, than a knowledge of its anomalies.

Here, especially, this is indispensable, for the infractions of hereditary transmission are so numerous and so striking, that from time to time we ask with hesitation if the law exists at all beneath the phenomena which conceal it. On considering these difficulties, we shall understand why the author of the most famous work upon this subject should have set up over against heredity an equal and contrary law, that of innateness, which as he considers explains all the exceptions.

Before discussing this hypothesis, and showing how heredity may explain the exceptions no less than the regular cases, we will, as usual, begin by a statement of facts.

In the physiological world, these exceptions are readily shown in the internal or external structure, the physiognomy, the stature, constitution or temperament.

Though, generally, brothers and sisters have a family likeness, it is not rare that there is between them such a diversity of feature and countenance that no external sign would indicate their common blood. This difference is sometimes seen even in twins. Sinibaldi asks 'how it comes that at Rome ugly boors and women from the dregs of the people, with hideous features, produce sons and daughters of surprising beauty, and of such perfect form that their equals are not to be found in the palaces of nobles, or in the courts of princes.' [1]

Fathers and mothers of erect form, none of whose families have ever been misshapen, produce children hunchbacked and deformed. Deformed parents have had perfectly straight children. Parents of middle height sometimes beget tall children, while other

---

[1] Might not this be a fact of atavism?

parents, of good station, in good health, and belonging to families of good constitution, beget children of very low stature. A man had by his wife eight children, of whom four were dwarfs. Bébé, the famous dwarf of King Stanislas, and whose height was thirty-three inches, was born in the Vosges of well-formed, vigorous, healthy parents. The celebrated Polish gentleman, Borwslaski, whose height was twenty-eight inches, had a brother and sister, dwarfs like himself, and three other brothers, each five feet six inches in stature.[1]

Such idiosyncrasies as the predominance of some one organ, one of a viscus, or even of an entire system of organs, likewise present curious instances of spontaneity. Family constitutions, as P. Lucas remarks, very often begin with individuals, and the most rooted constitutions, those that are most general in families, are yet not those of all the members.

We may quote especially, as remarkable facts of spontaneity, those called by Zimmermann exceptions in temperament. He has gathered several examples; as, for instance, of a man who suffered extreme agonies when his nails were clipped ; another when his face was washed with a sponge. For some persons coffee is an emetic, jalap a constipant. Hachn could not eat more than seven or eight strawberries without falling into convulsions, and Tissot could not swallow sugar without vomiting.

But there is no need to cite a large number of such facts, if the reader will bear in mind that peculiarities of organization—congenital or natural varieties—are necessarily exceptions to the law of heredity. Thus polydactylism, ectrodactylism, harelip, and all deformities of a similar nature, begin by a deviation from the specific type. The celebrated case of Edward Lambert, 'the man-porcupine,' may be remembered, whose parents were healthy and well formed, but he transmitted his singular carapace to his children. Thus we see from facts that heredity imposes its law even on its own exceptions.

Among animals all races which are not due to intercrossing, but which spring from spontaneous variation, are at once the result of innateness and heredity : of the former for their origin, of the latter

---

[1] Lucas, i. 108 ; Burdach, ii. 427.

for their continuance. Thus it is with the hornless bulls, or *mochos*, of the Argentine Republic, with rumpless fowls, bantams, etc.

If we pass from the physiological to the psychological order we shall find no less striking instances of spontaneity.

Phrenologists have accumulated facts to show that among animals, where we see only uniformity of habits, characters, and physical aptitudes, there exist between members of the same family individual differences, which, as they do not result from education, are due to spontaneity. In a litter of wolf cubs taken from their dam, says Gall, and which were all brought up in the same way, one became tame and gentle like a dog, while the others preserved their natural savagery.

In twins there sometimes occur extreme contrasts of tastes, propensities, and ideas. This was observed by the ancients :

> Castor gaudet equis, ovo prognatus eodem
> Pugnis.

What is still more curious is, that double monsters, when they survive, may possess different psychical constitutions. Serres observed this in the case of Ritta and Christina, the female twins of Presburg, who were united by the inferior lumbar vertebræ. They differed completely in character. One was handsome, gentle, sedate, with sensuous character little marked ; the other ugly, ill-conditioned, quarrelsome, and of strong passions. Her outbursts of rage against her sister, and their disputes became so frequent, that in the convent where Cardinal von Saxe-Zeits had placed them, the inmates were compelled to give them in charge of a watcher, who never left them alone. Notwithstanding these quarrels, they lived to the age of twenty-two.

It has been said that the law of spontaneity cannot be disputed, since we see the sons of great men unworthy of them. By what singular freak of nature did two fools like Paxalos and Xantippos, and a maniac like Clinias, spring from Pericles ? or from the upright Aristippos, the infamous Lysimachos? from the grave Thucydides, a silly Milesias or a stupid Stephanos? from the temperate Phocion, the dissolute Phocus? from Sophocles, Aristarchos, Socrates, and Themistocles unworthy sons? And the like differences are to be found in Roman history : Cicero and his son, Germanicus and Caligula, Vespasian and Domitian, Marcus

Aurelius and Commodus. In modern history, 'it is enough to mention the sons of Henri IV.,' says Lucas, 'of Louis XIV., of Cromwell, of Peter the Great; as also those of La Fontaine, Crébillon, Goethe, and Napoleon.'[1]

We do not, however, accept these cases as facts conclusive of spontaneity. The greater part of them are doubtful, and many of them are false. It is not enough to say, Such an illustrious man has mediocre sons, in order to conclude that therefore heredity is at fault. A son who does not inherit from his father, may perfectly do so from his mother. As we have already seen, this case is so frequent that some authors have regarded it as a rule.

Among the examples cited by Lucas, there are some in which the maternal heredity is clear, as Commodus, Louis XIII., Goethe, Napoleon. And it is probable in the case of others in the list, especially those taken from Greek history, that if we had precise data regarding the wives of those great men, or their immediate ancestors, it would be easy to show that these obscure or dissolute personages have inherited from their mothers, or of their grand-parents. Thus heredity would recover a large number of facts which have been wrongfully removed from its domain.

However, we would not deny that there are exceptions, and very important exceptions. But the conclusive way to establish them is, not to show that a great man has mediocre children, which proves nothing, but that a great man has sprung suddenly from an obscure family. Nor is this case rare. 'Often,' says Burdach, 'the parents possess very limited intellectual faculties, while all their children display abilities of the first order. From simple parents often spring those superior men, those minds whose influence is felt for thousands of years, and whose presence was a need for humanity at the moment when they entered life. The greatest men have belonged to lowly, poor, or obscure families.'

In the negro race, whose lack of capacity is recognized, anthropologists have noted individuals possessed of remarkable faculties. Toussaint L'Ouverture was certainly no ordinary politician. According to Pritchard, even the stupid Esquimaux and Greenlanders can produce men of intelligence.

---

[1] i. 153.

A peculiar conformation of certain organs of sense, or a total lack of them, are facts at once both of physiological and psychological spontaneity. There are some persons whose eyes are unable to discern some given colour—blue, red, yellow, etc. Others are born blind of parents possessed of perfect vision. Deaf-muteness in many cases cannot be explained by anything in the parents. Physicians cite many examples of families where the parents both hear and speak very well, while their children are all born deaf and dumb. Finally, the taste and the smell are sometimes struck with anæsthesia, or complete insensibility, which cannot be explained by hereditary transmission.

We will, in conclusion, glance at psychological idiosyncrasies, and exceptional mental facts. Psychology, even as physiology, has its rare cases, but unfortunately not so much pains have been taken to note and describe them. Not to speak of insanity, idiocy, or hallucination, which may occur, apparently at least, without visible antecedent in the progenitors, there are some purely moral states which are met with in a certain class of criminals—murderers, robbers, and incendiaries—which, if we renounce all prejudices and preconceived opinions, can only be regarded as psychological accidents, more painful and not less incurable than those of deaf-muteness and blindness. We have given sundry instances of these anomalies, and of their heredity; but they also frequently occur in the shape of isolated and nontransmitted cases of moral monstrosity. These creatures, as Dr. Lucas says, partake only of the form of man; there is in their blood somewhat of the tiger and of the brute : they are innocently criminal, and sometimes are capable of every crime.[1]

II.

Having shown by facts of every kind that there exist grave exceptions to the law of heredity, we have now to explain them. As we have seen, it is perfectly clear and unquestionable that heredity is the law; that this cannot be doubted; and that even in those cases which we qualify as exceptions, the exception is

---

[1] See several instances of moral monstrosity in the work of Dr. Despine already quoted, vols. ii. and iii.

never more than partial : for even where heredity does not transmit
the individual characters, it at least transmits the specific characters.
The question, therefore, is not to ascertain whether heredity is a
biological law, but whether that law is absolute.   As the exceptions are no less unquestionable than the law, and as they must
necessarily have a cause, there can be but two hypotheses.

α. We may hold that there is in nature an essential, permanent
cause, of which the phenomena of spontaneity are the effects—in
other words, that the biologic fact of generation is governed by
two laws, one of spontaneity, the other of heredity, the law being
only the expression of what is constant in the production of
phenomena—the invariable relation between cause and effect.
This is the thesis maintained by Dr. Lucas.

β. Or we may say that the causes of spontaneity are only acci-
der.tal ; that it is never more than a chance, the result of the
fortuitous play and concurrence of natural laws ; but that it is not
the effect of any distinct and special law.   On this theory there
would be one law of heredity with its exceptions, not two laws, the
one of heredity, the other of spontaneity.   This second thesis is
our own.   But before demonstrating it we must consider the opposite opinion.

Of this Dr. Lucas has given a full exposition, applying to it
philosophic principles.   He holds that every living being, considered in its origin—that is, in its generation—is the product of
two laws, which he places both on one plane and on the same
level.   One is the law of spontaneity, by which nature ever
creates and invents.   The other is the law of heredity, by which
nature ever imitates and repeats herself.   The former is the
principle of diversity, the latter of resemblance.   If the former
stood alone, there would be in the world of life nothing but
differences infinite in number ; if the latter stood alone, we
should have nothing but absolute resemblances.   But taken
together, these two principles explain how all living things of the
same species may at the same time resemble one another in their
specific characteristics, and differ in their individual characteristics.

If we regard the question here proposed from a metaphysical
point of view, it cannot be denied that a difficult, and probably an
insoluble, problem arises.   In the middle ages, it was hotly

debated under the singular titles of 'the problem of individuation,' of 'hoccity,' and of 'hæccity.' This barbarous jargon has
been ridiculed, but yet, if we turn from words to things, we cannot deny that this problem pressed upon the schoolmen, and
was of paramount importance. Modern philosophy, as it seems
to us, has been far more concerned with what is general—laws,
genera, species—than with what is individual. ˙ Now, if we are
hence led to consider what is general as the true reality, the
logical conclusion is that the individual is only a momentary
phenomenon, of no importance, the ephemeral result of laws
which intersect and combine in a thousand ways during the endless evolution of the universe. To use the words of Dr. Lucas, we
should have to affirm resemblance by rejecting diversity : heredity
would be the law, spontaneity the exception. If, on the other
hand, we regard the individual as a reality, as a sort of nomad,
governed and hemmed in on all sides by the laws of nature,
but whose essential, impenetrable being is never modified, then
we set diversity above resemblance, and sacrifice heredity to
spontaneity.

We have here undertaken only a study of experimental psychology, and hence we need not discuss this difficult metaphysical
problem. We may note, in passing, that if we descend to the
ground of experience, it is impossible to deny absolutely the existence of diversity, for it is demonstrated by facts. There are in
nature no two beings alike. When we see a large flock of sheep
we may regard most of them as copies of one another, but the
practised eye of the shepherd can distinguish each one. The
courtiers of Alfonso X. sought in vain for two leaves like each
other. But though diversity exists, we do not believe that it is
only explicable by a special law.

If we consider the act of generation under the simplest possible
conditions, as a single being engendering another, without the
intervention of any disturbing cause, it is absolutely impossible to
conceive how the product could differ from the producer ; for
there is no reason for admitting one deviation rather than another,
such deviation would be an effect without a cause. Linnæus'
aphorism, like produces like, strikes us therefore with all the
evidence of an axiom. But in reality the process does not take

place with such ideal simplicity. In the first place, there are ordinarily in the act of generation two sexes, and consequently two antagonistic heredities; this is the first cause of diversity. There are, furthermore, accidental causes which are in action at the very moment of generation; and this is another cause of diversity. Finally, there are external and internal influences subsequent to conception.

It is clear, says M. Quatrefages, that in every procreation the parents import influences which may be ranged in the following three orders of facts: their characters may be similar, or opposite, or different. In the first case there will be a persistence or an augmentation of the characters transmitted; in the second a diminution of them, or a reciprocal neutralization. Suppose two parents, one of them presbyopic and the other myopic; the child will have the chance of good sight, in consequence of the conflict of opposite influences. In the third case, if the characters are simply different, the product is the resultant of the father and mother; that is to say, a new character appears, differing from the other two, though due to heredity. Thus, among animals, when the parents are of uniform different colours, the progeny very often have the skin mottled, parti-coloured, or striped, and consequently very different from that of the father and mother.

Thus heredity, in virtue of its fundamental law, may play the part of this force of spontaneity devised by Lucas. We hold that there are cases of spontaneity which result from natural causes; we do not admit a law of spontaneity. Indeed Lucas's hypothesis is contradictory. To understand how little spontaneity possesses the character of a law, we need but observe that a law is identical with the phenomena it governs, since it is only the expression of what in them is permanent and essential, so that it enables us to fore-tell them. If the law of heredity may be supposed to be alone in operation, without disturbing influences, it may be predicted that the product will resemble one of the parents, or both. But suppose a law of spontaneity, no prediction or provision is any longer possible, since anything whatever may occur where diversity is the rule. This is permanent disorder. But it is impossible from this to deduce a law. A law is declared by a process of abstraction and generalization, which cannot be applied to cases which are

totally diverse, since the very object is to find resemblances and
to eliminate differences.   All scattered facts, all diversities which
cannot be grouped together, are called anomalies, or facts without
laws.   We may, therefore, speak of facts of spontaneity ; but a law
of spontaneity is a contradiction in terms.   Where, *ex hypothesi*,
there are no two facts which resemble each other, we may in
strictness admit the arbitrary intervention of a creative power,
but in no degree the regular and constant action of a law.

It is therefore impossible to recognize two antagonistic laws, the
one heredity, the other spontaneity.   And we may add that
theories of our own day concerning the origin of species and their
evolution, do not admit of anything like a law of spontaneity.
Besides selection and heredity, which are the chief factors in this
transformation, they do, indeed, presuppose what Wallace calls 'the
tendency of varieties to depart indefinitely from the original type;'
but this tendency, which is the prime source of all variation, is
owing to the action of surrounding conditions—that is to say, of
accidental and fortuitous causes—but by no means to an unintelligible entity such as the hypothetical law of P. Lucas.

III.

If, then, there is no law of spontaneity, we have only to recognize
in the foregoing facts exceptions to the law of heredity.   We can
only explain these by attributing them, not to a single cause, but to
causes.   No doubt it is far simpler to say, whenever heredity is at
fault, This is the result of spontaneity ; spontaneity causes the
sudden appearance of such a great man—of such a great criminal
—in a given family; but the simplicity of the explanation is of little
account, if it is imaginary.   In truth, there is no problem more
difficult and more complex than that of accounting for these
exceptions, and of pointing out how heredity may be so transformed as to become unrecognizable.   In the present state of
physiology and psychology it is impossible to explain these exceptional cases in a complete and satisfactory manner.   We get but
an indistinct view of the explanation.

The doctrine which regards heredity as the absolute rule, beyond
which are only anomalies, is very ancient.   Aristotle taught it in
its strictest form.   ' He who does not resemble his parents,' says

he, 'is a sort of monster, for in him nature departs from her specific form ; this is the first step in degeneration.' The authors who in modern times have adopted this opinion, attribute these exceptions to various causes, which may be ranged under three heads, according as they act after birth, before birth, or at the moment of conception.

1. We are inclined to assign but little importance to causes acting after birth, such as diet, climate, circumstances, education, physical and moral influences. They often produce serious effects, but it is not possible for them to produce the radical transformations we are now considering. This proposition, upheld by Bossuet, Helvetius, and by the writers of the eighteenth century, resulted from the philosophy of that period. But there is now no need to prove that spontaneity is not to be explained by external and late-acting causes, and we no longer believe with Helvetius that we can manufacture great men by means of education.

2. The causes anterior to birth, but subsequent to conception, are all the physical and moral disturbances of uterine existence— all those influences which can act through the mother upon the fœtus during the period of gestation ; impressions, emotions, defective nutrition, effects of imagination. These causes are very real, despite the objections of Lucas, who attacks them in order to establish his law of spontaneity. We shall see from examples that between inconsiderable causes and their effects there exists an amazing disproportion.

3. Finally, there are causes anterior to intra and extra-uterine life, which act at the instant of conception. These depend less upon the physical and moral natures of the parents than on the particular state in which they are at the moment of procreation. 'One fact which fully proves the universality of the law of heredity,' says M. de Quatrefages, 'is the frequent transmission from parent to child of the actual and momentary state of the former at the instant of conception. This fact had attracted the attention of physicians and philosophers, but it had been exaggerated. They went so far as to assert that the past history of the parents was as nothing in the constitution of the child, who, according to them, depends altogether on the state of the parents at the moment of procreation. On the other hand, modern writers had lost sight of

this class of phenomena, and P. Lucas did well in calling fresh attention to the matter, and citing facts in its favour.

'It has been long remarked that children begotten in a fit of intoxication often present for ever after the characteristic signs of that state : obtuse senses, and the almost total absence of the intellectual faculties. I had occasion at Toulouse, during my brief medical career, to observe a fact of this kind. A couple of artisans, man and wife, belonging to families all of whose members were of sound mind and body, had four children. The first two of these were quiet and intelligent, the third was half-idiotic and nearly deaf, and the fourth was like the elder two. From details communicated to me by the mother, who was much afflicted by the mental state of her child, I learned that it had been conceived when the father was brutalized by drink. By itself, this fact would have little or no significance, but when added to those collected by Lucas, Morel, and others, it is of very great importance.'[1] In fact, it enables us to understand that those transitory states which exist at the moment of conception may exert a decisive influence on the nature of the being procreated, so that often, where now we see only spontaneity, a more perfect knowledge of the causes at work would show us heredity.

But it may be said that the causes classed under the foregoing heads explain the exceptions very insufficiently. It may be said : We have no hesitation in admitting that heredity, like every other law, is subject to conditions; that since these conditions are numerous and delicate it is impossible to realize them perfectly, and that consequently hereditary transmission always falls far beneath its ideal. But is it not going too far to pretend, as you do, that transitory, accidental causes can produce in the beings that are procreated radical metamorphoses? We can understand how from parents of but mediocre intellect should spring a child more intelligent than they; but could a man of genius? How could a consummate scoundrel descend from honourable and honest parents? And there is a multitude of such cases.

Without pretending to give a conclusive answer, we propose to set before the reader a certain number of facts and reflections

---

[1] Quatrefages, *Unité de l'Éspèce Humaine.*

which appear to bring under the law of heredity the most refractory cases, the most formidable exceptions. By penetrating farther into the vital and mental dynamism of man, we shall probably have a glimpse of that mysterious elaboration whereby unity produces diversity, and causes give rise to effects very dissimilar to themselves. We shall then see how heredity seems to disappear, when it cannot be grasped.

These obscure causes of deviations from heredity may be reduced under two heads :—

1. Disproportion of effects to causes.
2. Transformations of heredity.

IV.

If we take up any engine of simple structure, such as a winnowing machine, a plough, or a scarifier, and some slight injury befalls it, it is probable that it will not be less serviceable : a trifling cause produces only trifling effects ; effect and cause are mutually equivalent, and there is in their relation nothing surprising. But if the one in question is a complicated engine, such as a locomotive, or a factory engine, the case is very different ; here an insignificant cause may produce terrible effects : the engine may run off the rails, an explosion or a fire may take place. Between causes and effects there is a disproportion which experience alone reveals. If now we consider, instead of a mechanism constructed by the hand of man, those natural mechanisms called organisms, where wheelwork and arrangement extend to even the minutest details, then the disproportion between effects and causes will become enormous ; a drop of prussic acid or the puncture of a carbuncle will throw the machine out of order in a few hours. Finally, in that mental mechanism—which is still more complicated, and where the impulses, tendencies, forces, conscious and unconscious processes, do but attain that momentary equilibrium which we call the actual state of consciousness—the disproportion between causes and effects transcends all assignable limits. A rush of a little alcoholized blood to the brain, the fumes of opium or hasheesh may produce the most surprising results in the mental machine. A few drops of belladonna or of henbane give rise to fearful visions. A little pus accumulated in the brain, a lesion so slight that the microscope can scarce detect it, gives rise to mental disorganizations called delirium, insanity, monomania. In short, we may lay it down as a general truth, solidly based on experience, that the more complicated the mechanism, the greater the disproportion between accidental causes and their effects.

The study of anomalies, and the artificial production of monstrosities, afford us convincing proofs of this truth. The researches of Geoffroy Saint-Hilaire and of Dareste have shown that it is possible to produce monsters at will, and that these deviations from the type are brought about by trifling causes. Hens' eggs when set on end, or in any way disarranged, produce monstrous chickens. And the same thing occurs if the eggs be shaken, or perforated, or partially coated with varnish. Isidore Geoffroy Saint-Hilaire shows that women of the poorer class who are obliged to work hard during pregnancy, as also unmarried women who are forced to conceal their pregnancy, far more frequently than other women give birth to monsters. ' Certain monstrosities,' he writes, ' are often caused by lesions which happen to the embryo in the uterus or in the ovum. Yet it would seem that complex monstrosities are more often determined at a later period than at the beginning of embryonic life. This may in part result from the fact that a point which suffered injury in the origin of the phenomenon, afterwards by its anomalous growth, affects the other points of the organism which have afterwards to be developed.' His *Histoire des Anomalies*, to which we would refer the reader, is full of curious facts, well fitted to stimulate thought. It will be seen that insignificant causes are sufficient to effect either a fusion of homologous parts, or inequalities of development—checks to growth 'which make anomalous beings, in some respects, permanent embryos, in which nature has halted half-way.'

In presence of such facts, it is not possible to accept futile explanations which have only an appearance of simplicity : for instance, ' As is the effect, so is the cause ; there must exist in the cause at least as much as in the effect.' Such explanations are available only in very simple cases, or at best in complicated cases of a purely mechanical kind. According to a profound remark of John Stuart Mill, whenever an effect is the result of sundry causes (and nothing is more frequent in nature), we can have two cases :

either the effect is produced by mechanical laws or by chemical laws. In the case of mechanical laws each cause is found in the complex effect, precisely in the same way as though it alone had acted : the effect of concurrent causes is exactly the sum of the separate effects of each. On the other hand, the chemical combination of two substances produces a third, the properties of which are entirely different from each of the other two, whether taken separately or together : thus, a knowledge of the properties of sulphur and oxygen does not imply a knowledge of the properties of sulphuric acid.[1] But psychological laws are analogous, now to mechanical, now to chemical laws. It is even probable that the greater number of them are chemical. Hence it is impossible to proceed by deduction from causes to effects. Here experience alone can guide us. It is curious to notice that prior to the discoveries of modern chemistry the idea of a total dissimilarity between causes and effects, and, what is still more striking, between the composite and its component parts, seems to have been unknown to science, except perhaps the dreams of alchemists about the transmutation of metals. It would surely have been a surprise for the scientific men of that epoch had they been told, Here is oxygen, a gas without colour or odour, combustible, and the active agent of all combustion ; and here is hydrogen, another and a very different gas. Combine the two in definite proportions, and you will get a liquid which may be either the water you drink, or the mist on which is painted the rainbow. The chemistry of life, by showing us how inorganic matter is transformed into the plant, the plant into the animal ; how in the animal the organic matter returns by death to the inorganic world to recommence its course, has revealed to us metamorphoses far more astounding than those whose explication we seek.

We may, then, regard it as certain that in the domain of life (including thought) a disproportion often exists between cause and effect which cannot be foreseen by reasoning, which is given us only by experience, and that it is a wholly gratuitous assertion to say, There is too much difference between such a fact and such another—between the simplicity of the one and the com-

---

[1] Mill's *Logic*, book vi., iv., and book iii., vi.

10

plexity of the other—to allow of the one being the cause and the other the effect.

This would be the place to consider the famous theory of the relations between genius and idiocy and insanity (Moreau of Tours, Lelut). In it we should find many arguments for our thesis on the disproportion between effects and causes in the physical world. But not to dwell on this point, we confess that most of the criticisms which have been made on this doctrine do not appear very conclusive. If the authors had maintained the identity of insanity and genius, as regards the facts which manifest them—as, for example, that the lucubrations of a madman are of equal value with the works of Newton, or of Goethe—the assertion would be so monstrous that we could only regard it as a joke. But what have they maintained? That the secondary causes, the organic conditions of genius and insanity, seem to be almost identical ; so that it is only by reason of accessory circumstances that a certain nervous organization produces grand, artistic, or scientific creations instead of expending itself on the dreams of a madman.

• Plainly, in order to reach a conclusion on this point we need a large number of well-attested, well-interpreted, and well-verified facts. But the only arguments that have been b.ought against this thesis are sentimental ones, which possibly are only prejudices ; and it is probable that if we knew clearly and scientifically the conditions on which genius is produced, we should find much to surprise us.

In our opinion, what has excited most hostility against this doctrine is that unconscious materialism which leads us to attach so much importance to the organic conditions of phenomena. But, even though from the point of view of physiological experience there existed between the causes of insanity and those of genius only insignificant differences, would there be any less difference between the two from the standpoint of psychological and social experience? The analogy between the causes would in no degree change the enormous difference between the effects. Even were genius the result of a certain state of the cerebral mass, it would, nevertheless, still be the most exalted thing in the world. The diamond has not lost its value since it has been discovered that it is carbon. As John Stuart Mill well says, ' It is only for low minds that a great and beautiful object loses its charm by losing somewhat of its mystery, and discovering a part of the secret process whereby nature has given it birth.'

If we reflect on the preceding facts, we shall, I think, agree that the exceptions to heredity, great as they may be, are less embarrassing than at first they seemed. Suppose two children as different as possible in psychical constitution: it is probable that if we could ascend to the causes of these differences, we should find them very simple. But unfortunately there is no mental chemistry by which we can transform these probabilities into certainty.

v.

We will now examine another cause of deviation from hereditary type, another source of diversity in the act of generation—the metamorphoses or transformations of heredity. This case is more simple than the preceding, to which, indeed, it may be referred as a species to its genus. Here we can trace the course of heredity, because the transition is not now from contrary to contrary, but from like to like; no longer from genius to idiocy, from virtuous father to debauched son; but from epilepsy to paralysis, from eccentricity to insanity. We might say that in the present case there are partial exceptions, and in the preceding case total exceptions, were it not that we are anxious always to keep in view the important truth that there is never a total exception to heredity, the exceptions to it never going beyond the individual characteristics.

The study of the transformations of heredity has been made in detail by Dr. Moreau, of Tours, in his *Psychologie Morbide.* To that work we refer the reader for particulars, and here extract from it only the facts of most interest for psychology.[1]

'It shows an incorrect conception of the law of heredity,' says he, 'to look for a return of identical phenomena in each new generation. There are some who have refused to subject mental faculties to heredity, because they would have the character and intelligence of the descendants exactly the same as those of the progenitors; they would have one generation the copy of the other that went before it, the father and son presenting the spec-

---

[1] *Physiologie Morbide,* pp. 108—193.

tacle of one being—having two births, and each time leading the same life, under the same conditions. But it is not in the identity of functions, or of organic or intellectual facts that we must seek the application of the law of heredity, but at the very fountain-head of the organism, in its inmost constitution. A family whose head has died insane or epileptic, does not of necessity consist of lunatics and epileptics ; but the children may be idiots, paralytics, or scrofulous. What the father transmits to the children is not insanity, but a vicious constitution which will manifest itself under various forms, in epilepsy, hysteria, scrofula, rickets. Thus it is that we are to understand hereditary transmission.'

Dr. Morel, in his *Traité des Dégénérescences*, published at about the same time, says in much the same terms :—

We do not mean exclusively by heredity the very complaint of the parents transmitted to the children, with the identical symptoms, both physical and moral, observed in the progenitors. By the term heredity we understand the transmission of organic dispositions from parents to children. Mad doctors have, perhaps, more frequent occasion than others for observing this hereditary transmission, as also the various transformations which are exhibited in the descendants. They are aware that a simple neuropathic state of the parents may produce in the children an organic disposition which will result in mania or melancholy—nervous affections which in turn may give rise to more serious degeneracy, and terminate in the idiocy or imbecility of those who form the last links in the chain of hereditary transmission.'

Speaking of the young inmates of houses of correction, Dr. Legrand du Saulle calls attention to an entire category among them of ' creatures who are whimsical, irritable, violent, with little intelligence, refractory, ungovernable and incorrigible.' These are the children ' sometimes of old men, blood relations, drunkards, epileptics, or lunatics. Sometimes, and this is the more frequent case, their father is unknown, and their mother is scrofulous, rickety, hysterical, a prostitute, or a lunatic.' [1]

In the *Psychologie Morbide* will be found several cases of the transformation of heredity, taken from pathology and from history.

---

[1] *Gazette des Hôpitaux*, 6 Oct. 1867.

Many of the biographical facts there given are not beyond criticism, but the following are a few of the most conclusive :—

Frederick William of Prussia was the victim of a sort of insanity. He was an excessive drunkard, eccentric, brutal ; he several times attempted to strangle himself, and at last fell into a profound hypochondria. He was the father of Frederick the Great.

' We should seek in vain,' says Dr. Moreau, ' for a more striking proof of the relations subsisting between the neuropathic state and certain intellectual and affectional states, than in the family of Peter the Great. Genius of the highest order, imbecility, virtues and vices carried to extremes ; excessive ferocity, ungovernable maniacal outbursts, followed by remorse ; habits of debauch, premature deaths, epileptic attacks—all these are found united in the Czar Peter, or in his family.'

The Condés offer an analogous example. Talent, eccentricity, originality of character, moral perversity, rickets, and insanity, stand side by side, or succeed one another in the most unexpected way.

We may recall what has been already said of the Pitt family Lady Hester Stanhope, the Sibyl of the Lebanon, her father Lord Stanhope, her grandfather Lord Chatham, her cousin Lord Camelford, and Pitt her uncle, were all remarkable for their genius, their eccentricities, or their extravagances.

Tacitus had an idiot son. The gloomy Louis XI. was grandson of Charles VI., a lunatic. Hoffmann, author of fantastic stories, had lunatics in his family, and was himself subject to hallucinations.

If now we quit the ranks of illustrious men,[1] and consider those of common stamp, we shall find in writers on insanity a great many cases of transformations of heredity, in all that concerns the psychical faculties. The lypemania of parents is seen to become a tendency to suicide in the children ; insanity becomes convulsions or epilepsy, scrofula is replaced by rickets, and *vice versâ*.

Fixed ideas in the progenitors may become in the descendants melancholy, taste for meditation, aptitude for the exact sciences, energy of will, etc. The mania of progenitors may be changed in the descendants into aptitude for the arts, liveliness of imagination,

---

[1] For further details see *Psychologie Morbide*, 3ᵉ partie.

quickness of mind, inconstancy in desires, sudden and variable will. Just as real insanity, says Moreau of Tours, may be hereditarily reproduced only under the form of eccentricity, may be transmitted from progenitors to descendants only in modified form, and in more or less mitigated character, so a state of simple eccentricity in the parents—a state which is no more than a peculiarity or a strangeness of character—may in the children be the origin of true insanity. Thus, in these transformations of heredity we sometimes have the germ attaining its maximum intensity ; and, again, a maximum of activity may revert to the minimum.

We cannot say what are the causes of these metamorphoses, by what mysterious transmutation nature thus extracts better from worse and worse from better ; for the question is beyond the present range of science. We cannot tell why a given mode of psychic activity is transformed in process of transmission, nor why it assumes one form rather than another. Were the solution of the problem attainable, it would doubtless reveal some singular mysteries. Thus many physiologists have thought that when both parents present the same characteristics, heredity may acquire such power as to destroy itself. Sedgwick thinks that in this way the fact may be explained that two deaf-mute parents oftentimes give birth to children that can hear. In truth, we can only ascertain the facts : but this is quite enough, since the facts show by what concurrence of fortuitous circumstances and accidental causes nature produces diversity.

But these metamorphoses, occurring between generation and generation, will cause us less surprise if we bear in mind that they are also frequent in the same individual. There is no doubt as to this point ; pathology supplies countless instances of it. To restrict ourselves to mental diseases : ' Madness,' says Esquirol, ' may affect all forms, either successively or alternatively. Monomania, mania, and dementia, alternately replace one another in the same individual.' Thus a lunatic will pass three months in lypemania, the following three months in mania, four months in dementia, and so on in succession, now in regular order, anon with great variations. A lady, fifty-four years old, is one year lypemaniac, and the next year maniacal and hysterical. Often, in the same subject convulsions are seen to pass into epilepsy, epilepsy into hysteria, and *vice versâ;* or lypemania will take the place of pulmonary consumption, hysteria, hypochondria, epilepsy.

To sum up briefly what has been said : M. Lemoine, in his study on *Morbid Psychology,* has made a very just criticism on this resort to two laws, the one of spontaneity and the other of heredity, both reciprocally supplying each other's defects. 'When the one is at fault,' says he, 'and puts the system in danger of failure, the other is hastily adduced, and everything is set right with a word. A madman's son is a madman : the law of heredity is invoked to explain his insanity. An idiot is born of parents and descends from ancestors who are all of sound body and mind : spontaneity is invoked to account for the fact.' We hold, with Lemoine, that spontaneity thus understood is an occult quality, an explanation that explains nothing, like the *Quia est in eo virtus dormitiva.*

But M. Lemoine, speaking of the reduction of spontaneity to heredity, adds : 'The reduction of these two laws to one is rather ingenious than legitimate, for it appears to me that the law of spontaneity should rather absorb the law of heredity. If we ascend from generation to generation, we certainly do not always find lunatics the children of lunatics, or idiots the children of epileptics. But at length we shall be more fortunate ; probably in the distant past, not so far back as the deluge, we shall find a lunatic, or epileptic, or idiot, who is the child of parents and ancestors, sound of mind and body—in short, an idiosyncrasy. This idiosyncrasy, whatever it may be, is the starting-point, is the pattern after which nature has fashioned all the descending gen-- erations. In creating this first case of disease, whensoever it appeared, nature acted freely. On the contrary, when she transmits disease as a heritage from fathers to children, she does but imitate herself, and copy her own model. The law of spontaneity explains the law of heredity, instead of being explained by it, if, indeed, it explains anything.'

To our mind there is here a confusion of two questions, which it is important for us to notice : a metaphysical question regarding the first cause, and a scientific question concerning secondary causes.

If we take metaphysical and transcendental ground—which we

do not here propose to do—spontaneity undoubtedly takes precedence of heredity, since it is clear that the derivative presupposes the primitive, and the imitation presupposes the model.

But if, as now, we take our stand on the ground of science and experiment, heredity becomes the only law; for it alone has a character of constancy, fixedness; and because it alone is reducible to formulas. Whether we admit with Lamarck the spontaneity of a single type, or with Darwin of three or four types, or of a very great number with Cuvier, so soon as we quit that region of origins and enter the domain of experience we see that nothing subsists except by heredity.

We have, therefore, to return to our starting-point. Heredity is the law. It is no *à priori* conception, any more than the axiom, like produces like. It is the accumulated and generalized result of an innumerable mass of experiences. Facts prove that between the *partus* and the *parens* there is never anything more than individual differences, and that the immense majority of characteristics is always inherited. Thus, according to the standpoint which we take, it is equally true to say that the law of heredity is always realized, and that it is never realized. The heredity of the greater share of the characteristics is a thing of universal occurrence; but the heredity of the sum of all the characteristics is never found. So that heredity, while it is the law, is always the exception. But no argument can be drawn from this; for it is a logical necessity that where the conditions of a law are not completely realized the law cannot attain its ideal.

PART THIRD.

THE CAUSES.

Die Materialisten bemühen sich zu zeigen dass alle Phœnomene, auch die geistigen, physisch sind : mit Recht ; nur sehen sie nicht ein, dass alles Physiche andererseits zugleich ein Metaphysisches ist.—*Schopenhauer.*

CHAPTER I.

I.

To inquire into causes we must hazard hypotheses. This cannot be avoided; for though science begins with the investigation of laws, it is perfected only in the determination of causes. Here, too, as in every experimental study, we have only to deal with secondary and immediate causes, or, in plainer terms, with invariable antecedents. As far as our purpose is concerned, to explain physiological heredity means to define an aggregate of conditions, of such a nature that if these conditions are present heredity necessarily follows, and when they are wanting heredity is invariably wanting. In what follows, therefore, there is no question of ultimate causes; and, without inquiring here whether they are accessible or inaccessible to the human mind, we shall never speak of them except with the admission that we are entering on hypotheses.

Heredity is only a special case of the great problem of the relations between physics and morals, as will more clearly appear in the course of this work. We can, however, note in advance, in a more precise way, the position of our question, by observing that every inquiry into the relations between physics and morals necessarily comprises two parts, the influence of the moral on the physical, and the influence of the physical on the moral. The problem of heredity is concerned only with the latter. The influence of physics on morals manifests itself in many ways, of which we here consider one only, heredity. With this explanation we can now indicate the line of inquiry we shall follow in our study of causes.

We shall, in the first place, examine in a very general way the relations between the physical and the moral, as the problem in its most general form necessarily governs all the particular cases.

Then, passing from the abstract to the concrete, from theory to
experience, we shall strive to show that every mental state implies
a corresponding physical state.

Thence we shall draw the conclusion that an habitual mental
state, such as psychological heredity, must have as its condition
an habitual physical state, such as physiological heredity.

In the seventeenth century, the question of the 'union of soul
and body' was put in a form which rendered it insoluble.   It was
a problem of metaphysics.   There were held to be two substances,
body and mind; between the two an abyss.   All their characteristics were opposed; then, as was to have been expected, it was
found impossible to join together again what had been so
thoroughly sundered.

Since the time when the progress of physiology showed that the
nervous system is the physical condition of moral phenomena, and
that every variation in the one is coupled with a variation in the
other, researches into the correlation of the physical and the
moral have had a firm basis, for the reason that it has been
possible to rest them on a something which is the body, even
while it is the instrument of the soul.   Thus is explained the
invasion, ever widening since the seventeenth century, of neurology
into psychology.

Nor is this all.   A further step in progress, which now appears
to have been made by all partisans of experimental inquiry,
consists in substituting for the metaphysical the experimental
point of view, and for the antithesis of two substances the antithesis of two groups of phenomena.   Hence the problem is no
longer the relations between body and soul, but the relations
between a group of phenomena pertaining to the unit which we
call life, and the group pertaining to the unit called the *ego*.   It is
true that this way of putting the question simplifies it only by
making it insoluble; for when we restrict ourselves to experience,
we renounce in advance all ultimate and absolute reason.   But as
the experimental sciences are strictly speaking made up of two
things—facts and hypotheses—and as the human mind has an invincible tendency always to sacrifice the facts to the hypotheses,
we, if we resist this tendency, run the risk of throwing away
the booty for its shadow.

For us, who desire as far as possible to adhere to facts, it is clear that we can examine the general relations of the physical and moral only under the experimental form. But when we try to state the question without any of the prejudices of the average mind, which render it equivocal, or of metaphysics, which render it insoluble, the only tolerably precise formula we get is this : We distinguish in ourselves two groups of phenomena or operations ; those in one group are conceived as external, unconscious, subject to the twofold condition of space and time ; those in the other as conscious, internal, and successive. The correlation which we discern between the two groups consists in this, that certain modes of existence in one group are the habitual antecedents of certain modes of existence in the other ; for example, that sum of states of consciousness which we call a pain is accompanied by certain states of the organism, motion, play of the physiognomy, states of the viscera, and *vice versâ*. A little belladonna, opium, or even alcohol, introduced into the circulation, produces certain determinate states of consciousness ; in a word, we observe between the two groups of phenomena relations, whether of invariable co-existence or of invariable succession. It appears to us that this is the only clear and unambiguous way of putting the question with which we are now occupied. Finally, when we strive to get a nearer view of the opposition between the two groups, we find that the higher or psychological group has for its fundamental character consciousness ; and thus the antithesis of physical and moral may without too great inaccuracy be regarded as the antithesis of the conscious and the unconscious. If, therefore, we should succeed in showing that this attribute of consciousness which characterizes one of the groups, and which consequently differentiates the two groups, does not belong to the higher group so essentially or so exclusively as it seems ; if we succeed in showing that operations which are considered specially psychological, such as feeling, enjoying, suffering, loving, judging, reasoning, willing can in some cases be either absolutely or relatively unconscious, then the antithesis of physical and moral instead of being absolute would become relative, and the problem would present itself under a new aspect. With a view to resolve it, we will endeavour to penetrate into the mysterious region of the unconscious.

II.

The psychological study of unconscious phenomena dates from scarcely half a century back, and is yet in its first stages. The school of Descartes and that of Locke—that is to say, the whole seventeenth and eighteenth centuries—expressly held that psychology has the same limits as consciousness, and ends with it. What lies without consciousness is remanded to physiology, and between the two sciences the line of demarcation is absolute. Consequently, all those penumbral phenomena which form the transition from clear consciousness to perfect unconsciousness were forgotten, and not without injurious consequences, for hence came superficial explanations, and insufficient and incomplete views. The nature of things cannot be violated with impunity ; and as everything in nature forms series, continuity, insensible transitions, our sharp divisions are always false. If we did not lose sight of the fact that our subdivisions of universal science into particular sciences, however useful and even indispensable, are always artificial and arbitrary on one side or another, we should be saved much idle discussion. Thus, as regards the unconscious phenomena which pertain at once to physiology and psychology, it makes very little difference which of these two sciences is occupied with them, provided only that they be studied, and studied well.

Leibnitz alone in the seventeenth century saw the importance of this. Less was not to be expected of the inventor of the infinitesimal calculus, the apologist of the *Lex continui in natura*, the man who in the highest degree possessed the faculty of insight. By his distinction between perception (conscious) and apperception (unconscious), he opened up a road on which in our times most physiologists and psychologists have somewhat tardily entered. There is, however, as yet no comprehensive work on this question,[1] and the undertaking would be no light one ; for a psychology of

---

[1] The completest and most recent work on this subject is Hartmann's *Philosophy of the Unconscious* (*Philosophie des Unbewussten, Versuch einer Welt-anschauung*, Berlin, 1869). The author takes a metaphysical point of view close to that of Schelling and Schopenhauer ; but he gives a good number of facts, some of which will be hereafter quoted.

the unconscious would have the same limits, and the same extent as ordinary psychology. It would be necessary to show—at least, as we view the matter—that most, if not all, of the operations of the soul may be produced under a twofold form ; that there are in us two parallel modes of activity, the one conscious, and the other unconscious. This study would require a volume. For our purpose it will suffice here to show by some positive facts what this unconscious activity is, and in what degree it can explain the correlation of the physical and the moral.

Passing from the simple to the composite, from reflex action to unconscious cerebration, we will address our study of the unconscious to the nerve-centres in the following order, viz. spinal cord, rachidian bulb, annular protuberance, cerebellum, cerebral hemispheres.

1. The spinal cord is regarded by physiologists under a twofold aspect: as a conducting cord it transmits sensations to the brain, and brings back thence motor excitations ; as nerve-centre it is the seat of reflex action. Simple reflex action, which we may define to be a simple excitation followed by a simple contraction, is the first act of automatism, or of unconsciousness, that presents itself to us. Reflex action consists essentially in movement in a part of the body, called forth by an excitation coming from that part, and acting through the intermediary of some nerve-centre other than the brain. Proschaska, who was the first to study these movements, called them 'phenomena of reflection of sensitive impressions in motor impressions.'

If we examine here, from our own point of view, the reflex actions whereof the spinal cord is the centre, we shall find that their distinctive character is that they are automatic, unconscious, and, what concerns us far more closely, co-ordinated. ' In those purely reflex reactions,' says Luys, ' which, owing to their automatism, possess that determined and necessary character which is peculiar to the mechanical contrivances of human industry, everything betrays a sort of predestined *consensus* between the centripetal impression and the centrifugal action which it calls forth, so essential to them is it to be regular and co-ordinate.'[1] A few facts will place this in

---

[1] *Recherches sur le Système Nerveux*, p. 280.

clearer light. If, after having cut off the head of a frog, we pinch any part of its skin, the animal at once begins to move away, with the same regularity as though the brain had not been removed. Flourens took guinea-pigs, deprived them of the cerebral lobes, and then irritated their skin : the animals immediately walked, leaped, and trotted about, but when the irritation was discontinued they ceased to move. Headless birds, under excitation, can still perform with their wings the rhythmic movements of flying. But here are some facts more curious still, and more difficult of explanation. If we take a frog, or a strong and healthy triton, and subject it to various experiments; if we touch, pinch, or burn it with acetic acid ; and if then, after decapitating the animal, we subject it again to the same experiments, it will be seen that the reactions are exactly the same ; it will strive to be free of the pain, to shake off the acetic acid that is burning it ; it will bring its foot up to the part of its body that is irritated, and this movement of the member will follow the irritation wherever it may be produced.[1] We can hardly say that here the movements are co-ordinated like those of a machine ; the acts of the animal are adapted to a special end; we find in them the characters of intelligence and will, a knowledge and choice of means, since they are as variable as the cause which provokes them.

If, then, these and similar acts were such that both the impressions which produce them and the acts themselves were perceived by the animal, would they not be called psychological? Is there not in them all that constitutes an intelligent act, adaptation of means to ends, not a general and vague adaptation, but a determinate adaptation to a determinate end? In the reflex action we find all that constitutes, in some sort, the very groundwork of an intelligent act—that is to say, the same series of stages, in the same order, with the same relations between them. We have thus in the reflex action all that constitutes the psychologic act except consciousness. The reflex act, which is physiological, differs in nothing from the psychological act, save only in this, that it is without consciousness.

---

[1] For further details see Vulpian, *Physiologie du Système Nerveux*, pp. 417—428 ; it will there be seen that headless animals act precisely as though they had heads. See also Despine, *Psychologie Naturelle*, tome i. ch. vii.

On this obscure problem some say that 'where there can be no consciousness, because the brain is wanting, there is, in spite of appearances, only mechanism.' Others say that 'where there is clearly selection, reflection, psychical action, there must also be consciousness, in spite of appearances.' For the present, we will not join in this discussion. A German physiologist, however, quoted by Wundt, holds that he has by the following experiment proved the absence of all consciousness in the spinal cord. He takes two frogs, the one blinded, in order to diminish the number of impressions from without, and the other without its head. He places them in a vessel containing water at 20° Cent. of temperature; the two frogs remain perfectly quiet in their warm bath, But he gradually heats the water in the vessel, and then the scene changes. The non-decapitated frog appears to be ill at ease, changes its place, breathes with difficulty, and its sufferings become greater as the temperature rises. At 30° it makes all possible efforts to escape; finally, at 33° it dies of tetanic convulsions. In the mean time, the headless frog remains quietly in its place; 'the spinal cord slumbers, it does not perceive the danger.' The temperature goes on rising, the other frog is now dead, and still the headless one continues motionless. Finally at 45° its carcase rises to the surface, 'it is as stiff as a board.'

Yet, perhaps, as Wundt observes, this experiment is not decisive; first, because other experiments have given the opposite results. Moreover, the development of consciousness must necessarily depend on the entire organization, and it is quite possible that if a headless animal could live a sufficient length of time there would be formed in it a consciousness like that of the lower species, which would consist merely of the faculty of apprehending the external world. It would not be correct to say that the amphioxus, the only one among fishes and vertebrata which has a spinal cord without a brain, has no consciousness because it has no brain; and if it be admitted that the little ganglia of the invertebrata can form a consciousness, the same may hold good for the spinal cord.

But not to insist on a point which cannot here be profitably discussed, we go on with our study of the phenomena of unconsciousness.

2. The grey substance of the medulla oblongata has higher and more intelligent functions than those of the spinal cord. It governs certain muscular co-ordinated contractions which do not depend on the will, and which are often unconscious ; these acts are respiration, deglutition, simple exclamation, sneezing, coughing, yawning, and those muscular contractions which constitute the play of the physiognomy.

If to the spinal cord and the medulla oblongata we add the annular protuberance, removing all the rest of the encephalon, the automatic acts produced are still more remarkable. Animals thus treated utter, when pinched, plaintive cries, having the true expression of pain. A rat with the cerebral hemispheres removed makes a sudden jump when one comes near him, and imitates the 'spitting' of an angry cat. Dogs and cats with the cerebral lobes removed will, if a decoction of colocynth be poured down their throats, make grimaces with their lips as though they would free themselves from a disagreeable sensation. Thus, then, the nerve-centres we have enumerated produce, in the absence of the brain, unconscious sensations of pleasure and of pain, of hearing and of taste.

If to these we add the tubercula quadrigemina we shall have unconscious visual sensations. A pigeon with the cerebral hemispheres removed makes a movement of the head as though to avoid a danger that threatens, when the fist is suddenly brought close to it. An experiment first made by Longet shows that the pigeon follows with its head the motions given to a lighted candle.

All these phenomena are of the same nature as those which depend on the spinal cord, and suggest the same reflections. They are intelligent—that is to say, adapted to an end. At bottom they are identical with physiological acts, and differ from them only by this one character, that they are unconscious, or reputed as such.

3. The same remark also applies to the automatic phenomena dependent on the cerebellum. The function of that organ seems to consist in co-ordinating the muscular contractions which produce the various movements—'a co-ordination which requires infinite science, that is utterly ignored by the mind.' 'I have often,' says Despine,[1] 'admired this automatic science, when seeing a dog follow his master's carriage, leaping in front of the horse, passing between the wheels, while they are revolving at every rate of speed; and all this without ever being touched either by the wheels or by the horse's feet. What mathematical precision there must be in the action of the numerous muscles which concur to execute all these movements! It all occurs without the volition of the animal, nor does he know how he performs it. In man this automatic science strikes us as more wonderful still. Instrumentalists whose cerebellum is imperfect never can perform a piece of music as they think it ought to be performed. Some highly intelligent men are very awkward, while other men of very moderate intelligence are possessed of very remarkable dexterity; in point of address some inferior races may equal superior ones. To be a good horseman, a good juggler, a good rope-dancer, a good shot, the commonest grade of intelligence suffices; but there is need of very perfect automatic organs. It is not the shape of the hand that gives dexterity; some hands that are very well formed are yet very unskilful, while some ill-shaped hands perform prodigies of dexterity. The hand and the fingers are only the instrument that operates.'

To all these facts, which appear to denote an unconscious intelligence seated in the organism, and which we have referred to distinct nerve-centres, we might add others no less curious; such as the tendency by which the living thing attains its typical form, or, in case of lesions, restores and completes it. Some physiologists, Burdach for instance, see in this an unconscious instinct of individual conservation; but most authors simply state these facts without explanation. We will not insist upon them, so that we may the sooner arrive at the unconscious operations of the brain.

4. Automatism was long considered as appertaining exclusively to the spinal cord and to the secondary nerve-centres. In England, it has been chiefly the researches of Carpenter and Laycock which have proved that the brain also possesses an automatic activity of its own, which they have called 'unconscious

---

[1] *Psychologie Naturelle*, vol. i. p. 485.

cerebration,' or, ' the soul's preconscious activity.' Here we touch the quick of our subject, since the brain, or at least the ganglionic matter spread over the surface of the hemispheres, is the seat of the highest and most complex psychological operations. But, as we have already remarked, there is no mode of mental activity which may not be produced under its unconscious form. Facts will prove this.

But how are we to study these phenomena if they are withdrawn from our direct observation? if, on the one hand, they are cognizable only by the consciousness, and if, on the other, they lie outside of consciousness? We do not profess here to sketch a method whose processes vary, of necessity, according to the cases. Most commonly we reach them by induction, advancing from the known to the unknown. We arrive at the unconscious by ascertaining the influence it may have on conscious life, just as we discover an invisible planet by the perturbations it produces. We infer the unconscious from its well-ascertained conscious results. If I am a somnambulist, and rise from my bed at night, dress myself, and sit me down at a table to write verses, I must, when I wake next day, admit that I am the author, because I see them in my own handwriting, though I may have no recollection of what has occurred; in other words, I infer, from the material result before my eyes, that my mind must have performed, in a certain interval of time, a certain number of very complicated operations which differ from ordinary psychological work in only one point, viz. that they are effected without consciousness.

On entering upon the study of the facts, we meet with a group of morbid states, comprising natural and artificial somnambulism, ecstasy, catalepsy—all facts so common that there is no need to describe them. ' There are well-authenticated cases in which automatic action of this kind has not only produced results perfect of themselves, but has produced them by a shorter and more direct process than would have been thought possible in the waking state. The absence of every distracting influence seems to favour the uninterrupted action of the mental mechanism, if the phrase is permissible.' (Carpenter.) A thing not so well known is, that in a certain form of epilepsy the patient often goes on doing automatically, though consciousness is abolished, what he was doing at the instant of the attack. Schrœder van der Kolk knew a woman who went on eating, drinking, or working, and who, on coming to her senses, had no recollection of what she had done. Trousseau[1] speaks of a young musician subject to epileptic vertigo, attacks of which lasted from ten to fifteen minutes, and who, during that interval, would continue playing the violin unconsciously. An architect who had long been subject to epilepsy was not afraid to mount the highest scaffoldings, though he had often had attacks when walking on narrow planks at great heights. No accident ever befell him ; when the attack came on he ran swiftly along the scaffolds, shouting his own name at the top of his voice. A few seconds later he would come to himself, and would then give his orders to the workmen. He would have had no idea of the strange way in which he had acted, had he not been told of it.

If now we pass from the morbid to the normal state, and review all the forms of mental activity, distinguishing each after the manner of analytical psychology, we shall see that for every conscious form there is a corresponding unconscious one.

The first forms of unconscious life must be sought for in the fœtal life—a subject full of obscurity, and very little studied from the psychological point of view. We may hold, with Bichat and Cabanis, that though the external senses are in the fœtus in a state of torpor, and though in the constant temperature of the amniotic fluid the general sensibility of the fœtus is almost null, still its brain has already exercised perception and will, as seems to be evidenced by the movements of the fœtus during the last months of pregnancy.

But to take simply the adult man or animal. We shall first find, at the common frontiers of physiology and psychology, a notable group, that of the instincts, which of themselves alone constitute the psychological life of a great number of animals. If we consider these as composite reflex actions, the instincts form, as we have seen, the transition from simple reflex action to memory.

With instinct we may couple habit, which resembles it in many respects, and is no less wonderful. Habit constitutes a true return

---

[1] Trousseau, *Leçons Cliniques*, i. 59,—in vol. ii. are cases no less curious.

to automatism, and it is never perfect unless when it is entirely unconscious.

These facts have long been recognized ; but here are some that have received less attention. In the group of the phenomena of sensibility we discern, both from their effects and directly, the existence of unconscious pleasure and pain, whence come our causeless joy and sadness. The instincts peculiar to man, such as modesty and shame, maternal love, presentiments, secret sympathies and antipathies, only become conscious exceptionally and incidentally ; yet we feel that all these instincts spring from the depths of our being, from the dim region of the unconscious. Nowhere is this fact more striking than in the sexual instinct, which, both in man and in animals, takes its rise prior to all experience. This instinct, which perhaps even determines individual selection, where it takes place, caused Schopenhauer to maintain ingeniously that love is the tendency of specific conservation, and that we must recognize ' in this dæmon a certain unconscious idea of species.' In a word, are not the intellectual sentiments (those of the true and the false) an unconscious, half-perceived cognition? Every cognition is in its origin instinctive. The experimental method was instinctively anticipated by the alchemists before it was clearly perceived by Galileo and Bacon. What in medicine and the sciences is denominated diagnosis is an unconscious cognition.

If we pass from phenomena of sensibility to intellectual operations, we shall see that every mode of intelligence has its unconscious form. In the first place, the difference between conscious perception and unconscious (or rather semi-conscious) impression is well known ; the sensorial nerve-centres can receive and preserve impressions which either never attain the state of consciousness or do so only after a time. Perception can exist only by the aid of two principal *forms*, space and time, and by certain processes which ultimately determine the position of the object in a certain point in space; and thus the unconscious serves as support and condition for conscious perception. We need say nothing of memory, which is altogether a form of unconsciousness, recollection being nothing but the transition from unconsciousness to consciousness. The latent association of ideas is a phenomenon of the same kind. The mind goes through a series of operations of which consciousness holds only the two extremities. Finally, the highest creations of the imagination spring from the unconscious. Every great inventor, artist, man of science, artificer, feels within him an inspiration, an involuntary invasion, as it were, coming out of the depths of his being, but which is, as has been said, impersonal. All that comes under consciousness is results and not processes. The difference between talent and genius is the difference between the conscious and the unconscious. Artists, prophets, martyrs, mystics, all those who in any degree have felt the *furor poeticus*, have ever acknowledged their subjection to a higher power than their own *ego*, and this power is the unconscious overlapping the submerged consciousness.

The mystics of every country and of every age put faith only in their unconscious knowledge, and it is not to be denied that they have brought back from the world of unconsciousness high and entrancing visions.

The logical operations of the intellect, namely, judgment and ratiocination, may also be performed without consciousness. It is a known fact that after a night's rest the mind finds the materials of its work classed with an order that we should never have been able to give them, with all our industry and all our dexterity. Men of science of the first rank commonly foresee results by quick intuition—a thing which can only come from unconscious ratiocination. 'The art of divining, without which it is almost impossible to advance' (Leibnitz), is nothing but this. Every man, however mediocre the quality of his mind, is unconsciously guided by a hidden logic. A proper study of the unconscious would throw some light on the question of 'innate' ideas, and on those fundamental truths which we do not hesitate to admit under the unconscious form; and would, in particular, explain the induction which presupposes a belief more or less vague in the uniformity of the laws of nature. Probably the difference between deduction and induction is only the difference between the conscious and the unconscious, so that, outside consciousness, the two processes would constitute only one, and that one would be deductive.

As for the will, it derives ultimately from character, and the root of character is in the unconscious. And, to our mind, it is this that makes the question of the freedom of the will insoluble, consciousness being incapable of giving us all the elements of the problem. We know motives and acts ; but that which causes the possible to become the actual is unconscious.

'Languages,' says Turgot, 'are not the work of self-conscious reason.' If his age had understood this as he did, it would have discussed the origin of language less; above all, it would not have seen in it a conscious creation. The source of language is in the unconscious. 'Without language it is impossible to conceive the philosophic consciousness, or even human consciousness, and hence it is that it has never been possible that the foundations of language should be laid in a conscious manner. Still, the more we analyze language, the more clearly we perceive that it exceeds in depth the most conscious productions of the mind. It is with language as with all organic beings. We fancy that these beings come into existence, being produced by a blind force, and yet we cannot deny the intentional wisdom that presides over the forma-tion of each one of them.'[1] Many philosophers of our day have in other terms pronounced the same opinion as to the unconscious origin of language.

In fact, we meet with a final manifestation of the unconscious in sociological phenomena, in history. A people arrives at conscious-ness only as it becomes civilized ; perhaps it was only in the last century that that ideal state was reached wherein the human race has clear consciousness of itself and of its history. Among primi-tive peoples, however, societies are formed, and a certain division of political powers and of vocations is made, though without any definite consciousness of the end or of the means. From this the consciousness of the species afterwards springs by degrees. The process of development is the same in the species as in the indi-vidual ; compare Homer with Aristotle ; Gregory of Tours with Montesquieu. Here, as everywhere, consciousness springs from the unconscious and presupposes it.

We have now, in the compass of a few pages, given a sketch of a question which would require a volume; but, brief as it is, it is enough for our purpose. To sum up, we have seen that there is no psychological phenomenon, simple or complex, high or low,

---

[1] Schelling, *Einleitung in die Philosophie der Mythologie.*

normal or morbid, which may not occur under an unconscious form. In a word, we find in ourselves or in others, and we conclude that there exists in animals, a great number of acts, often complex, which, as a rule, are willed, deliberated upon, conceived, felt—in short, accompanied by consciousness ; that is, by a more or less clear knowledge (1) of the means, and (2) of the end. In some cases the consciousness of the end to be attained, and of the means to be employed disappears : yet we know that the end has been attained, though we know it only through the effect produced. Such acts are unconscious.

Two hypotheses only are possible to interpret these facts.

1. It may be said that consciousness is the habitual, though not indispensable, accompaniment of mental life ; that the intellect is by nature unconscious: that its essence consists in the co-ordination of means, and its progress in a more and more complex, a more and more perfect, co-ordination ; but that consciousness is only a secondary phenomenon, though of the highest importance ; somewhat as the brain, which is the noblest of all the organs, is nevertheless only a complementary organ, superadded to the rest, though it is the noblest of all. This thesis has even been applied to physiology, when it has been said that the unconscious phenomena presuppose only nerve-currents terminating in the secondary centres (rachidian bulb, annular protuberance, tubercula quadrigemina, etc.), while the conscious phenomena presuppose a second series of currents terminating in the ganglionic substance of the brain. In this way consciousness would be a fact of a higher order, but not indispensable to psychological life, which could subsist without it under all its forms. Consciousness would be like the intermittent flashes from the furnace of an engine, which allow us to see glimpses of a marvellous mechanism, but which do not constitute the mechanism.

2. On the other hand, consciousness may be regarded as being pre-eminently the psychological fact. The operation which constitutes consciousness (*Bewusstwerden*), never being identical with itself through two consecutive moments, possesses every possible degree of clearness and of intensity ; consciousness increases and diminishes, but in its progressive decrease it never reaches zero : what we call the unconscious is only a minimum of consciousness.

11

The brain is the seat and the condition of clear consciousness; but every secondary nerve-centre and every ganglion is conscious after its own fashion. This view, which is also based on physiology, holds that, inasmuch as sensibility is a histological, not a morphological property, wherever there is a nerve-substance there must also be a more or less vague consciousness, and that the general consciousness of the creature is composed of these infinitesimal quantities, which are lost in it even while they constitute it.

We need not decide between these two hypotheses, nor are we competent to do so. We would merely show that, as far as they touch upon our subject, they both lead to the same conclusion.

We have already said that the antithesis of the physical and the moral, considered in the phenomenal order, resolves itself into the contrast of the conscious with the unconscious, and we now see that, as we bring both groups together, the one encroaches on the other, so that it is impossible to say where the conscious ends and where the unconscious begins. For the present, we only observe that it would be premature to draw a conclusion before we have studied the purely psychological—that is, the conscious—phenomenon. This we now proceed to do.

III.

We therefore now pass from phenomena of a mixed nature—half-physiological and half-psychological — to those which properly constitute intellectual life. But we must not forget that here we are concerned only with phenomena; we know not what the mind is in itself, nor need we discuss that question here. We have merely to inquire whether psychological life may not in the last analysis be brought down to a few irreducible elements, given, or at least suggested, by experience, and whether there is any relation between the primordial facts of mental life and the primordial facts of physical life. Leaving, therefore, all questions as to the substance of the mind, which concern metaphysics, and all details as to its faculties and phenomena, which concern descriptive psychology, let us see to what ultimate form we may reduce the fact of conscience, or thought, considered as a phenomenon.

It may be said generally, that to think is to unify and to diversify; to reduce phenomenal plurality to the unity of the subject, and to realize the unity of the subject in a phenomenal plurality. Every act of thinking is definitely reducible to a perception of either differences or resemblances, that is to say, it resolves one into many, or reduces many into one. This double process of analysis and synthesis can be infinitely repeated and complicated, but it underlies all our intellectual operations, whatever they may be. Contemporary psychologists have well shown that on comparing the phenomena of intelligence we find a true unity of composition, and that this essential unity of all intellectual phenomena consists in this, that always and everywhere we are integrating or disintegrating something. Their studies, which we need not detail here, enable us to pass from these rather vague considerations to a more precise knowledge of the fact of consciousness in its ultimate form.

Since in every act of thinking there are necessarily two elements, plurality and unity, we will examine these in order that we may see to what they are ultimately reducible.

1. We will begin with the dividing element of thought. Every one will readily admit that if we start from some very composite mental state—for instance, from the idea of a certain social system, or of a certain form of government—and then proceed by continuous analysis, constantly passing from the more to the less complex, from the less complex to the simple, from the simple to the most simple, we must, in traversing this descending series, finally arrive at primitive elements. Thus we are able to resolve our system into a sum of ratiocinations and relations, each ratiocination into a sum of judgments and relations, each judgment into a sum of ideas and relations, each idea into a number of images or of concrete forms from which it is drawn, and each image and concrete form into internal or external, subjective or objective, sensations. Sensation, therefore, would appear to be the primitive element upon which all rests, the molecule to which this complicated diversity may be reduced.

The researches of physicists and of physiologists, however, have led some psychologists to ask whether sensation is indeed, as it appears to be, an irreducible phenomenon, and the reply has been in the negative. When treating of the so-called simple sensations of sound, colour, taste, smell, they found themselves in the same condition as chemistry once was when dealing with bodies supposed to be simple. Analysis has shown that the so-called primitive sensations are themselves composite. For the analysis of these sensations we refer the reader to recent treatises on psychology, giving here only a single example.

We take some sensation usually esteemed irreducible; for instance, that of a musical note. It is known that if we cause a body to vibrate, and that the vibrations do not exceed sixteen in the second, we perceive a regular succession of identical sensations, of which each is a separate and distinct sound. But if the vibrations grow more rapid, these sounds, instead of being each apprehended as a separate state of consciousness, blend into one continuous consciousness, and that is the musical note. If the rapidity of the vibrations be increased, the quality of the sound varies, becoming sharper; and if the rapidity goes on steadily increasing, it becomes at length so sharp that soon it becomes inappreciable as sound. Nor is this all ; the researches of Helmholtz have shown that the differences of tone between instruments (as the violin, the horn, and the flute) are owing to the fact that different harmonies are added to the fundamental note. These differences of sensations, known as differences of tone, are therefore due to the simultaneous integration of other series, having other degrees of integration, with the original series. In plainer terms, the fusion of these primary noises in a single state of consciousness produces the sensation of a musical note ; and this fusion, combined with the principal note of other less intense vibrations, produces differences of tone.

This analysis, summary and insufficient as it is, will enable us to understand how illusory is the apparent simplicity of the phenomenon we call sensation. The same is to be said of colours, tastes, odours, and in general of all sensations, though with some of them the analysis could not be carried so far.[1] If, then, sensation is a composite phenomenon, it may, perhaps, be possible to discover its primary element.

The most recent work written on this subject is Herbert

---

[1] For details, see Helmholtz' *Physiological Optics (Lehre von der Tonempfindung)* ; Herbert Spencer, *Principles of Psychology*, § 60.

Spencer's *Psychology.* Pushing his analysis beyond the very limits of consciousness to a final element, which is rather felt than seen, he finds 'the unit of consciousness' in what he terms a 'nervous shock.' If we examine our various sensations, we shall see that in spite of their specific differences they possess one thing in common—the nervous shock which constitutes the basis of them all, and to which they all appear to be reducible. It is not possible to say precisely wherein consists this ultimate element, though a few examples may help us to form an approximate idea of it. Thus, the effect produced in us by a crash which has no appreciable duration is a nervous shock. An electrical discharge traversing the body, and a flash of lightning striking the eye, resemble a nervous shock. The state of consciousness thus produced is in quality like that produced by a blow (leaving out of consideration the consequent pain), so that this may be taken for the primitive and typical form of a nervous shock. 'It is possible—may we not even say probable—' writes Herbert Spencer, 'that something of the same order as that which we call nervous shock is the ultimate unit of consciousness ; and that all the unlikelinesses among our feelings result from unlike modes of integration of the ultimate unit.' [1]

We would observe, with the same author, that there is a perfect agreement between this view and the well-known character of nervous action. Experience shows that the nerve-current is intermittent, that it consists of undulations. The external stimulus does not act continuously on the sensitive centre, but sends up to it, as it were, a series of pulsations, so that, objectively, this phenomenon may be said to resemble what is subjectively called a nervous shock.

It does not seem possible, in the analysis of consciousness, to push any farther the reduction of what we have called diversity, for the nervous shock is hardly a state of consciousness. From the synthesis of these shocks would come states of consciousness properly so-called—that is to say, sensations and sentiments ; and then by syntheses of sensations and sentiments, and by associations of images, ideas, and relations, is built the whole edifice of our cognitions.

---

[1] Herbert Spencer, *Psychology*, ib.

2. In the whole of the foregoing we have constantly spoken of synthesis, integration, fusion, association. How is this operation performed which reduces diversity to unity? Does it result from the elements themselves? Are these syntheses formed after the manner of chemical combinations, and according to laws dependent on the quantity and the quality of the combined elements? Must we deduce the unity of the facts of consciousness from the unity of the vital phenomena, and look for the cause of mental synthesis in organic synthesis? This would scarcely help us, for we know how difficult it is to explain physiological unity in the living being.

The unity of the fact of consciousness is indisputable, and, to our mind, inexplicable, so long as we do not go beyond phenomena—that is to say, beyond the sphere of science. But, though we here treat of the composition of the mind, we desire in no respect to go beyond the phenomenology of the mind. We will, then, examine the different aspects of the question from the point of view of experience.

The question which arises with regard to the unity of life arises again with regard to the unity of consciousness : whether it be an effect or a cause. We have seen that some physiologists, instead of regarding life as a cause on which the functions depend, place, on the contrary, all the reality in the functions of which vital unity is only a resultant or composite effect. The same hypothesis has been introduced into psychology, and it is upheld by the following arguments.

In psychology the idea of personality is fundamental, as in biology is the idea of individuality. But the person, the *ego*, the thinking subject, assumed as a perfect unity, is but a theoretic conception. It is an ideal which the individual approaches as he rises in the scale of being, but to which he never attains. Our personality breaks up into an infinity of sensations, sentiments, images and ideas, past or future; it is only a synthesis, an aggregate, a sum that is ever undergoing addition and subtraction, but of which the whole reality is in the concrete events which compose it.

If we scan the whole biologic scale, we shall see that at the lowest grade, where there is simply life, the phenomena and the functions have for their characteristic the fact that they are simultaneous: digestion, circulation, respiration, the secretions, etc., with all their subdivisions, take place at the same time, and depend on one another. But if we pass from plants to the lower animals, and from them to the higher, we find added to the vital actions other actions which have a tendency to range themselves in simple succession, to be produced under the form of a series. These actions we call psychical. In the radiata, the mollusca, and the articulata, the psychical life has for its centres ganglia dispersed through the animal; the actions of these are very imperfectly co-ordinated, so that there is rather simultaneousness than succession: hence their mental inferiority. This dispersion of psychical life explains the fact that if we cut in two or more pieces an earthworm, a centipede, or a praying mantis, each piece of the insect moves and acts on its own account. But in proportion as we ascend in the animal series, the nervous system grows more and more perfect, and the centres are co-ordinated with a view to a higher unity; simultaneous action gives place to a more and more perfect succession, without however attaining it. This fusion of simultaneousness with succession can never be complete; and thus the tendency of psychical actions to take the form of a simple series is ever approaching this ideal, but never absolutely attains it.

We can also attack this problem of the unity of consciousness in another way. We have just seen that it necessarily occurs under the form of a series, a succession—that is to say, under condition of time. But time is measurable; and since to study is to measure, and as accurate science consists of measurement, it follows that consciousness in some degree comes under the cognizance of exact science.

The experiments made on this subject are of recent date. Towards the close of the last century the Greenwich astronomers remarked that the various observers did not observe in the same way the coming of a star to the meridian. The variations sometimes amounted to half a second. Bessel, of Königsberg, was the first to suppose that this difference was owing to psychological causes, and he set himself to determine this error, or personal equation. From observations made by astronomers, it resulted that some time elapses between the instant when an act is performed and the instant when an attentive observer signals his perception of it. Though the velocity of thought seemed to defy all measurement, still it has been determined by Helmholtz, Donders, Hirsch, and Marey, by means of ingenious experiments.

From these experiments it results that the velocity of impressions varies according to the individuals, and even for the same individual according to the temperature : at a low temperature the velocity of the nervous agent is less. Impressions travel from the periphery to the nerve-centres, and volitions from the nerve-centres to the periphery, with an average velocity of thirty metres per second. Between visual, auditory, and tactile impressions and the reaction of the hand showing that the perception has been perceived, there elapses one-fifth of a second in the case of visual impressions ; one-sixth in case of auditory impressions ; and one-seventh in case of tactile impressions. But, as Donders remarked, this case is itself complex, and is resolvable into two psychical stages : (1) impression travelling from periphery to centre ; (2) volition travelling from the centre to the hand. By some curious experiments he thinks he can prove that the simplest act of thought, the solution of a very easy dilemma, requires one-fifteenth of a second. Wundt, from experiments of his own, finds that the most rapid act of thought requires one-tenth of a second.[1]

The velocity of thought, and consequently the number of states of consciousness, vary considerably. In some dreams, and in the mental state produced by opium and hasheesh, this velocity is such that phenomena of consciousness which can have lasted only a few seconds appear, by an illusion that is easily explained, to have lasted several minutes or several hours. The well-known opium eater, De Quincey, had dreams which appeared to ' last ten, twenty, fifty, or seventy years, or even transcended the limits of all possible experience.' The reason of this is, that we measure the length of time by the number of our states of consciousness. Retrospectively, a space of time during which we have been active seems much longer than one in which we have been idle. A week spent in travel seems longer than one spent in the habitual mono-

---

[1] For a study of this subject in its psychological relations, see Wundt, *Menschen und Thierseele*, Lectures 4 and 23.

tony and routine of life. Under the enormous and sudden afflux of sensations and ideas, space, like time, expands beyond all measure in the consciousness. 'The buildings, the mountains,' says De Quincey, 'loomed up in proportions too grand to be taken in by the eye. The plain stretched out, and was lost in immensity.'

Thus these facts, chosen from among many others, show that the succession which constitutes consciousness is ever varying in velocity and complexity, and consequently we appear to be far enough removed from that *ego*—that simple, invariable, unchangeable unit—which some have imagined.

These researches into the measurement of the phenomena of consciousness as to their duration will doubtless sooner or later lead to important conclusions; for the present we think we may draw a few of these provisionally.

1. The inner sense, like all the other senses, has its limits, beyond which it perceives nothing. There is a psychical minimum, just as there is a visual, or an auditory minimum. Suppose one-eighth of a second to be the briefest state of consciousness, then a cerebral phenomenon lasting one-fifteenth or one-twentieth of a second will lie outside of consciousness.

2. In consciousness, simultaneousness is only apparent. If certain states of consciousness seem to be simultaneous (and Hamilton supposed that we could entertain seven ideas at once) it is simply because their succession is so rapid that we cannot note their want of continuity. If consciousness could have its microscope, as the eye has, we should see succession where now we see simultaneousness; for instance, in the perception of a complex object, as a house.

3. The greater part of our internal states can never enter the consciousness. Our total life is made up of sundry particular lives, and the life of each organ has its echo in the various ganglia and nerve-centres scattered throughout the body. But as all these internal states are simultaneous, while consciousness is a succession, the result is that the majority of them remain in the unconscious state. There exists between them a real 'struggle for life,' a strife to attain consciousness—a strife which has place, now between phenomena of the same class, as between sensation and sensation, image and image, idea and idea; again, between phe-

nomena of different classes—a sensation and an image, a sentiment and an idea.

Every analysis, therefore, of whatever kind, issues in this : that consciousness conveys to me only a small part of what passes within me. My personality is complex; my unity is that of a regiment, rather than that of a mathematical point. For, without attempting the long and delicate task of analysing our personality, we may say that it comprises at least four essential elements : (1) We have as a basis for all the others, the general sense of the existence of our body, of the play of its functions, of its normal or morbid state. (2) The knowledge of our perceptions or actual ideas. (3) The knowledge of our previous states. (4) The sense of our activity—that is to say, the faculty of knowing how we act upon the outer world, and how we are acted on by it.

But the same question constantly presents itself. How does all this attain unity? We are brought back again to this unavoidable difficulty. Is the unity, without which there is no consciousness, a reality or an abstraction? There is here, we take it, an insoluble antinomy.

On the one hand, if we suppose the unit, the *ego*, the person, to have any reality beyond the phenomena, we attribute real existence to an abstraction. For if, *ex hypothesi*, I abstract from my *ego* all the phenomenal plurality which manifests it—my sensations, sentiments, ideas, resolutions, etc.—the subject so denuded is a mere possibility ; that is to say, the poorest, emptiest, hollowest of abstractions.

On the other hand, if we suppose that the phenomena alone are real, and that the unit, the *ego*, the person, is but a sum, a resultant—that is to say, an abstraction—we enunciate an unintelligible proposition ; for these phenomena which constitute *me* possess the twofold character of being given to me as phenomena, and of being given to me as *mine*. My sensations, sentiments, ideas—in short, all my states of consciousness—imply a synthetic judgment, in virtue of which they are referred to my personality and integrated therewith. Without this synthetic judgment, all those phenomena which are most intimate to me would be as foreign to me as those which take place beyond Herschel's nebulæ. Scattered pearls do not make a necklace, there is need of a string to connect them ; if we cut an apple into twenty pieces, and scatter them to the winds from the summit of a tower, these scattered fragments no longer make up an apple. The same would be the case with that phenomenal, disintegrated, and unconnected plurality, which nothing can reduce to unity. But, like the *ego* and the non-*ego*, the internal and the external are correlative terms, and the one cannot be assumed without the other ; if I cannot know myself, I cannot know anything ; and thus, if there is no unity of consciousness there is no cognition, whether internal or external, nor is there in the universe any such thing as thought. To suppose, as some appear to have done, that the unity of the *ego* is nothing but the continuity of the consciousness, is an illusion, for consciousness being, as we have seen, discontinuous, could produce only an intermittent unity.

Thus, then, we find it impossible to reach a conclusion, or rather, we find ourselves forced to conclude that here science ends and metaphysics begins. We are face to face with the unknowable ; it is within us, in the profoundest depths of our being. We are equally unable to suppress the two terms of our antinomy and to reconcile them ; equally unable to say whether our unity is real or only apparent. The fact is, that the study of the ultimate conditions of consciousness withstands analysis. The analytical method is the only one possible, and here the analytical method is illusory. We think we have explained a complex fact, when, by successive simplifications, we have reduced it to its constituent elements. And this is generally true ; but in the biological and psychological order, the synthesis made after analysis is not identical with the synthesis that existed prior to analysis. Here the whole is not equal to the sum of the parts. Chemistry, by its synthesis and analysis, enables us to understand this apparent paradox. It shows that if two or more simple bodies, each having special properties, combine, the resulting whole usually possesses physical, chemical, and physiological characteristics altogether different from those of its constituent parts ; thus, sulphuric acid resembles neither sulphur nor oxygen. In the mental order there are analogous combinations, and possibly our *ego* is one which is made and unmade every moment. But we cannot know this.

We must, then, be on our guard against supposing that we have explained all when we have analysed all. In pyschology, analysis is of service in making us acquainted with the emphatic conditions of phenomena, which is nearly the whole extent of our science; but our science is not everything.

IV.

We can now arrive at a summary view of the general relations of the physical and the moral. In the first place, all the foregoing discussions and expositions are reducible to two essential propositions :—

1. The phenomena which constitute physical and mental life, taken in their totality, seem to form a continuous series of such a nature that at the one extremity of the series all is unconscious and purely physiological, and at the other end all is conscious and purely psychological; and that the transition from the one extreme to the other is performed by insensible gradations, whether it be that the unconscious rises to the conscious, or that the conscious returns to unconsciousness.

2. The purely physiological phenomena appear to be reduced in the last analysis to motion, and purely psychological phenomena to sensation; and thus we have the problem of the relations between the physical and the moral brought down to this question : What is the relation between a nerve-vibration and a sensation ?

Some, taking their stand in metaphysics, think the problem to be resolvable; others, holding to experience, regard it as unsolvable.

If we examine the tendencies of contemporary metaphysics on this point, we shall find two currents of doctrine quite distinct, and both equally logical. Either we may regard motion as the only reality, all else being but a modification of it, thought being the maximum of motion; or we may regard thought as the only reality, of which all the rest is only a modification, motion being the minimum of thought. The former hypothesis might be called mechanism, or, by a somewhat antiquated term, materialism. The second hypothesis is idealism. It is enough for our purpose to show briefly that neither of these hypotheses can be scientifically established.

1. The mechanical theory is very simple—it starts from motion,

to which it affirms that everything can be reduced. So long as it holds to the inorganic world it is not easily assailable; to motion, in fact, the properties of brute matter may be reduced—heat, light, cohesion, sound, and, probably, also the phenomena of electro-magnetism. It is even known with exactitude what numerical ratio subsists between a given quantity of motion and a given quantity of heat. As regards chemical action, its reduction to motion is less clear; but suppose that all this should one day be explained, the inorganic would be reduced to simple bodies and motion. According to the mechanical hypothesis, the world of life is reducible to the same terms. In the first place, since the researches of Wöhler, chemical synthesis has effaced every line of demarcation between organic and inorganic chemistry. The ternary and quarternary compounds which constitute organic matter are chiefly confined to oxygen, hydrogen, carbon and nitrogen. Their elements, therefore, are not bodies of a peculiar kind. Living substance possesses no properties due to any imaginary 'vital principle.' Life, together with the play of the functions which compose it, is but a very complicated chemistry and mechanism. But if we were to admit that this mechanical conception of life is confirmed in all its details (which is not the case), it would still have to explain what is most essential in living beings, their unity. To say, as has been said, that living matter is endowed with the peculiar property of 'adapting itself to ends,' explains nothing. We thus attribute to it an unconscious intelligence, but in so doing we go beyond the bounds of mechanism. This unity, this *consensus*, is so important in the living creature that Auguste Comte himself admits that here 'we must substitute for analytic study synthetic considerations'—that is to say, instead of passing from the lower to the higher, from the components to the resultant, we must descend from the higher to the lower, from the end to the subordinated means.[1] But if we suppose that mechanism explains life, and endeavour, with its assistance, to

---

[1] In his *Rapport sur la Physiologie Générale*, Claude Bernard thinks that we are justified in reducing life to the laws of inorganic nature, but that we have no right to say that the processes are identical. Life has processes of its own See also some excellent observations in Renouvier, *Critique Générale*, tome iii. p. 90, *et seq.*

arrive at an understanding of thought, we have first to explain how the nervous system is constituted, which is the indispensable condition of all thought. As we are aware, it is only a complementary apparatus : certain infusoria, whose bodies are only an amorphous mass, entirely void of muscles and nerves, have yet a relative life. Relying on the law of evolution, on the passage from the simple to the complex, and on the physiological division of labour, some have endeavoured to explain the genesis of the nervous system. The most curious essays in this direction have been made by one who in other respects rejects the mechanical hypothesis. Mr. Herbert Spencer, in his *Biology* (§ 302), and more particularly in his *Psychology* (Part 5), strives to show how a nerve might be produced in an extremely simple primitive organism by the laws of motion ; and how, from this beginning, more and more complicated nervous systems might be developed. If this bold genesis were beyond question, it would be a great victory for the mechanical theory, but still the necessity would remain of explaining how nerve-vibration becomes a fact of consciousness. We are utterly incapable of understanding how motion becomes thought. The hypothesis is indemonstrable in theory, and inconceivable in fact. If it be said that, subjectively, heat and light are as different from motion as the fact of consciousness is different from nerve-vibration, we must observe that the comparison is not exact. For a motion to become light there is need of an optical apparatus and consciousness ; for a motion to become sound there is need of an acoustic apparatus and consciousness. But for a nerve-vibration to become consciousness—which as yet has no existence—what is needed? How shall we explain this metamorphosis ?

Such, briefly, is the mechanical hypothesis, which it would require a volume to set forth in its details. According to it, phenomena differ in nothing from one another save in this, that the higher are produced by a concentration, and the lower by a dispersion of force. A unit of thought would be equivalent to several units of life, and a unit of life to several units of purely mechanical force. At least, such would seem to be the tenour of the observations made by one of its most recent exponents, Dr. Maudsley, in his *Physiology of Mind.* ' All ascending transformations of matter and force are, so to speak, concentrations of the same within a less space. One equivalent of chemical force corresponds to several equivalents of a lower force, and one equivalent of vital force to several equivalents of chemical. The same holds good for the various tissues. . . If we suppose a higher tissue to undergo a decomposition, or a retrograde metamorphosis, which shall necessarily coincide with the resolution of its energies into lower modes, we may say that a simple monad of the higher tissue, or one equivalent of its force, is equal to several monads of the lower kind of tissue, or to several equivalents of its force. The characteristic of living matter is that it is a complexity of combinations, and a variety of elements so brought together in a small space that we cannot trace them; and in nervous structure this concentration and this complication are carried to the utmost degree. . . The highest energy of nature is, in fact, the most dependent. The reason of the powerful influence it is capable of exerting on the lower forces which serve in its evolution is, that it implicitly contains the essence of all lower kinds of energy. As the man of genius implicitly comprises humanity, so the nervous element implicitly comprises nature.' In another place, the author adds the following remark, which can hardly be reconciled with mechanism : 'What is this progress, this *nisus*, which is so evident when we take all nature into account? Is it not a striving of nature to attain consciousness, to attain the possession of itself? In the series of manifold productions, man, says Goethe, was the first wherein nature held converse with God.'

We shall not attempt, in this place, the discussion of the mechanical theory. We shall hereafter submit both it and its opposite, idealism, to criticism. We would only remark for the present that, from the standpoint of experience, we may object to it that it is an excessive abuse of hypothesis, which it exalts to reality.[1] While

---

[1] Those who occupy the metaphysical point of view refute mechanism by saying that from the less it deduces the greater.

Taken by itself, this axiom is incontestable, for it is only another form of the plain truth that the whole is greater than a part, but we must here be careful. The terms greater and less are quantitative expressions, and hence they have no value except in the domain of the measurable, the homogeneous, the mathematical. To employ them aright, the two terms must be comparable and

among these hypotheses there are some which share in the present imperfection of the sciences, but which may be accepted in advance, there are others which so far transcend all possible experience that there is no rashness in rejecting them.

2. Idealism is not so easily set forth as the opposite theory : not that it is less simple, or that it does not hang so well together, but because it conversely follows the scientific order, proceeding always from the end to the subordinated means, descending step by step the series which mechanism ascends step by step. The starting-point of mechanism is very definite, if it is not very certain; idealism at the outset takes up its position in the absolute, which is the only point of view from which the universe can be surveyed, ' For God serves to explain the soul, and the soul to explain nature.' We are here beyond the reach of experience, and consequently of science. Yet we must attain to science, must pass from the absolute to the relative, from ourselves to phenomena. But how, by what mysterious operation is this done ? Idealism answers only in metaphors—which is inevitable, since the finite and the infinite are incommensurable, and, *ex hypothesi*, there is no possible ratio between the first and the second term. If we suppose this first difficulty solved, we are then on the ground of experience, in possession of a reality derived from the absolute, which will serve ultimately to measure and explain everything. This reality is thought.

According to Schopenhauer and his school, thought would occupy only the second place, intelligence would be only 'the physics of the mind' imprisoned in the subjective forms of time,

---

consequently of the same nature. To say that mind is the greater and matter the less, is to be the dupe of words ; it is to apply to quality what is true only of quantity. The relation of mind to matter is not a relation of greater and less, but of object to object.

It is also said that the mechanical theory subordinates the higher to the lower. This refutation, for which we are indebted to A. Comte, is more exact, because it substitutes the qualitative point of view for the quantitative. For my own part, I certainly consider the psychological order superior to the vital order, and the latter to the inorganic world. But these ideas of higher and lower may well possess only a subjective value, and be only a mere human way of considering things, so that this refutation, however true in fact, has no logical cogency or true scientific value.

space, and causality. The supreme reality would be will, which alone springs not from intellectual experience, and which alone is directly conceived. Yet will thus posed, without and above all consciousness, all idea, is only in name like that will of which we have consciousness, or of that which enters into the texture of the effects and causes which constitute experience. We cannot define this absolute will because, *ex hypothesi*, it is not knowable, and because nothing exists for us, except so far as we know it. But not to dwell on these inner discordances of idealism, let us admit that thought, in its broad sense, is the principle of all things. Astonishing and paradoxical as this thesis might at first appear to the average mind, it is in many respects true, incontestable, even in the eyes of the partisan of pure experience. By an un-scientific illusion, we imagine that were man and, in general, every thinking and sensing brain to disappear, the universe would still sub-sist with its light, its colours, its forms, its harmonies, its æsthetics. But this is not so, since the universe, at least for us, is only a sum of states of consciousness. Resistance, form, colour—in short, all the attributes of matter—exists for us only on this condition. The order of these phenomena, their existences, or their uniform suc-cessions—that is to say, their laws—exist for us only on this condi-tion. ' And this world,' says Schopenhauer, 'would no longer exist if human brains were not unceasingly multiplied, springing up like mushrooms, to take in the universe, which is ready to founder in nothingness, and to toss between them like a ball this great image identical in all, of which they express the identity by the word object.'

Without accepting this absolute idealism, which is hypothetical, experience alone compels us to admit that for us all real or possible existence is bounded by the limits of our real or pos-sible thought. If, then, we place thought at the summit of all things—as well in the absolute as in the experience, since it is thought which, in revealing itself, reveals all things—it follows that, for idealism, in proportion as we descend from pure thought to sensation, from sensation to the vital phenomena, and from the vital phenomena to chemical and mechanical action, the universe grows obscure and mean ; there is constant diminution of reality, of being. Sensation and sense-impressions are intelligible, but life is an unconscious thought enclosed in matter; 'the body is a mind of a moment's duration.' In the inorganic world, at the lowest grade of the scale, the phenomena of shock or of the communication of motion, the clearest of all for mechanism, is in fact the most obscure, because there the effort, the will, which constitutes all thought, is more widely separated than elsewhere from its effect: there thought is *aliena a se.* Further, the phenomenon of shock includes that which some would have it replace, viz. spontaneity. 'Inertia, with the elasticity which results from it, is to the body what is to the soul the innate tendency to preserve the action that constitutes its essence, and to restore it when it is deranged.' Inertia is analogous to and derived from will, and all motion is in its essence an aiming at something. Thus everything is explained by thought, all that is intelligible; and, as Berkeley says, 'In all that exists is life, in all that lives is sensation, and in all that has sensation is thought.'

Such is the idealistic system—a system that hangs well together, even if it be not conclusive. We do not accuse it of depending on an hypothesis, such as: 'Thought is the only reality,' for this it shares in common with metaphysics, and, indeed, with all human science. All our scientific knowledge, however coherent, however solid and fruitful in results, is like a gold chain, of which we do not see the first link. As we are alike incapable of transcending experience and of being content with experience, and as science has the same limits as experience, the only way of transcending these limits is hypothesis. Every system of thought employs hypothesis more or less; idealism more frankly than any other system. A graver defect, as we view it, is, that even though the hypothesis be admitted, the system nevertheless still contains an insuperable difficulty. How does thought, which is the only reality, become something else for itself, something so different that it no longer recognizes itself? What is the cause of this continuous and ever-increasing lapse of thought? It evidently cannot be any external cause, for by the hypothesis there is nothing beyond thought. What, then, is the internal cause? Nature, it will be said, is 'an exterioration of the mind' —a proposition that relatively is incontestable, but absolutely doubtful, for experience shows that we are as incapable of sup posing matter without mind as mind without matter; subject and object, external and internal, are correlative terms.   If the object is in the last analysis reduced to states of consciousness which come from within, states of consciousness are reduced in the last analysis to sensations which come from without.   The object is constituted by the aid of elements derived from the subject, and the subject is constituted by the aid of elements derived from the object.   From this alternative there is no escape.

Moreover, the radical weakness of these two rival doctrines, mechanism and idealism, has been so well demonstrated in a recent work by Herbert Spencer, that we cannot do better than to give that author's remarks in his own words.

'Here, indeed, we arrive at the barrier which needs to be perpetually pointed out, alike to those who seek materialistic explanations of mental phenomena, and to those who are alarmed lest such explanations may be found.   The last class prove by their fear almost as much as the first prove by their hope, that they believe that mind may possibly be interpreted in terms of matter; whereas many whom they vituperate as materialists are profoundly convinced that there is not the remotest possibility of so interpreting them.   For those who, not deterred by foregone conclusions, have pushed their analysis to the uttermost, see very clearly that the concept we form to ourselves as matter, is but the symbol of some form of power absolutely and for ever unknown to us; and a symbol which we cannot suppose to be like the reality without involving ourselves in contradictions.   They also see that the representation of all objective activities in the terms of motion is but a representation of them, and not a knowledge of them; and that we are immediately brought to alternative absurdities if we assume the power manifested to us as motion to be in itself that which we conceive as motion.   When, with these conclusions that matter and motion, as we think them, are but symbolic of unknowable forms of existence, we join the conclusion, lately reached, that mind also is unknowable, and that the simplest form under which we can think of its substance is but a symbol of something that can never be rendered into thought; we see that the whole question is at last nothing more than the question whether these symbols should be expressed in terms of those, or those in terms of these—a question scarcely worth deciding, since either answer leaves us as completely outside of the reality as we were at first.

'Nevertheless, it may be as well to say here, once for all, that were we compelled to choose between the alternative of translating mental phenomena into physical phenomena, or of translating physical phenomena into mental phenomena, the latter alternative would seem the more acceptable of the two. Mind, as known to the possessor of it, is a circumscribed aggregate of activities; and the cohesion of these activities one with another, throughout the aggregate, compels the postulation of a something of which they are the activities. But the same experiences which make him aware of this coherent aggregate of mental faculties, simultaneously make him aware of activities that are not included in it—outlying activities which become known by their effects on this aggregate, but which are experimentally proved to be not coherent with it, and to be coherent with one another. As, by the definition of them, these external activities cannot be brought within the aggregate of activities distinguished as those of mind, they must for ever remain to him nothing more than the unknown correlatives of their effects on this aggregate, and can be thought of only in terms furnished by this aggregate. Hence, if he regards his conceptions of these activities lying beyond mind, as constituting knowledge of them, he is deluding himself; he is but representing these activities in terms of mind, and can never do otherwise. Eventually, he is obliged to admit that his ideas of matter and motion, merely symbolic of unknowable realities, are complex states of consciousness built out of units of feeling. But if, after admitting this, he persists in asking whether units of feeling are of the same nature as the units of force distinguished as external, or whether the units of force distinguished as external are of the same nature as units of feeling; then the reply, still substantially the same, is, that we may go further towards conceiving units of external force to be identical with units of feeling, than we can towards conceiving units of feeling to be identical with units of external force. Clearly, if units of external force are regarded as absolutely unknown and unknowable, then to translate units of force into them is to translate the known into the unknown, which is absurd. And if they are what they are supposed to be by those who identify them with their symbols, then the difficulty of translating units of feeling into them is insurmountable ; if force, as it objectively exists, is absolutely alien in nature from that which exists subjectively as feeling, then the transformation of force into feeling is unthinkable. Either way, therefore, it is impossible to interpret inner existence in terms of outer existence. But if, on the other hand, units of force, as they exist objectively, are essentially the same in nature with those manifested subjectively as units of feeling, then a conceivable hypothesis remains open. Every element of that aggregate of activities constituting a consciousness, is known as belonging to consciousness only by its cohesion with the rest. Beyond the limits of this coherent aggregate of activities exist activities quite independent of it, and which cannot be brought into it. We may imagine, then, that by their exclusion from the circumscribed activities constituting consciousness, these outer activities, though of the same intrinsic nature, become antithetically opposed in aspect. Being disconnected from consciousness, or cut off by its limits, they are thereby rendered foreign to it. Not being incorporated with its activities, or linked with these as they are with one another, consciousness cannot, as it were, run through them ; and so they come to be figured as unconscious— are symbolized as having the nature called material, as opposed to that called spiritual. While, however, it thus seems an imaginable possibility that units of external force may be identical in nature with units of the force known as feeling, yet we cannot, by so representing them, get any nearer to a comprehension of external force. For, as already shown, supposing all forms of mind to be composed of homogenous units of feeling variously aggregated, the resolution of them into such units leaves us as unable as before to think of the substance of mind as it exists in such units; and thus, even could we really figure to ourselves all units of external force as being essentially like units of the force known as feeling, and as so constituting a universal sentiency, we should be as far as ever from forming a conception of that which is universally sentient.

'Hence, though of the two it seems easier to translate so-called matter into so-called spirit, than to translate so-called spirit into so-called matter (which latter is, indeed, wholly impossible), yet no translation can carry us beyond our symbols. Such vague conceptions as loom before us are illusions conjured up by the wrong connotations of our words. The expression 'substance of mind,' if we use it in any other way than as the x of our equation, inevitably betrays us into errors ; for we cannot think of substance save in terms that imply material properties. Our only course is constantly to recognize our symbols as symbols only, and to rest content with that duality of them which our constitution necessitates. The unknowable, as manifested to us within the limits of consciousness in the shape of feeling, being no less inscrutable than the unknowable as manifested beyond the limits of consciousness in other shapes, we approach no nearer to understanding the last by rendering it into the first. The conditioned form under which being is presented in the subject cannot, any more than the conditioned form under which being is presented in the object, be the unconditioned being common to the two.' [1]

V.

In the preceding paragraph we said that on the question of the relations between the physical and the moral some authors, taking the metaphysical point of view, think that the problem can be resolved, while others, basing themselves on experience, hold it to be insoluble. Further, we have seen that metaphysics fails to solve it : mechanism fails, because it reduces all to motion, which ultimately is not cognized, save on the condition of thought ; and idealism fails, because it reduces all to thought, which does not exist without an object ; so that neither of these two antithetic terms can absorb the other. The conclusion, therefore, must be that the problem is by its very nature insoluble. This, however, is not a return to a proposition long accepted, and in a manner classical. We will explain why it is not.

The commonly accepted dualism takes the metaphysical point of view ; it opposes a substance which it does not know—mind—

---

[1] *Principles of Psychology*, 2nd Edition, § 63.

to another substance it does not know—matter—without being able
to reconcile them, as is natural, for how can light be produced out
of the clash of two ignorances? On the contrary, the partisan
of experience pronounces the question unsolvable, precisely because
it transcends experience, that is to say, demonstrated or verifiable
science. The one is pent within the impotency of his metaphysics;
the other within the limits of his method. The ignorance of the
former is owing to the gaps in his philosophy; that of the latter,
to his voluntary abstention from all transcendental research.

In our times, the fine generalization known as the law of equivalence, or of the correlation of forces, has led some bold thinkers to
state in another form the problem of the relations between the
physical and the moral. Modern physics considers all the forces
of nature—heat, light, electricity, magnetism, cohesion, chemical
affinity, gravity—as capable of being reduced all to one principle,
and of being transformed into one another in accordance with
fixed rules, which are nothing else but the laws of mechanics. It
is also generally admitted that the law of equivalence governs
vital phenomena, and muscular contraction and innervation in particular. But is it also applicable to mental phenomena? Is it
possible for it to pass from nerve facts to states of consciousness?
Do mental forces enter the category of the other forces, and are
they in like manner convertible?

Some authors in our day answer affirmatively. Bain has accumulated and cited some facts from which he infers, (1) the equiva-
valence or transmutability of nervous and mental forces, and (2)
the equivalence or transformation of the mental forces into one
another. Thus, according to him, it would be possible to establish
an equivalence on the one hand between a certain nervous state
and a certain mental state, and on the other hand between the
three principal forms of mental life—sensibility, will and intelligence; so that a state of consciousness would imply the transformation and expenditure of a certain amount of nerve-force;
and an increase of sensibility would be possible only by a diminution of intelligence and will, the sum of force in the living being
remaining constant amid all these transformations. The magnificent synthesis contained in Herbert Spencer's *First Principles*
reduces all phenomena without exception to the law of equivalence.

'No thought, no feeling,' says the author, 'is ever manifested, save as the result of a physical force. This principle will before long be a scientific common place.'

They who hold this doctrine observe that nervous force, which ultimately results from nutrition, must, after it is produced, be expended in one or other of these three ways : either by acting on the viscera, the heart, or the digestive organs, as is the case in deep emotion; or by acting on the muscles and producing movements, gestures, and various expressions of the physiognomy ; or by causing the excitation to pass to some other part of the nervous system, and hence result those successive states which make up consciousness. Sensations excite ideas and emotions ; the latter in turn awaken other ideas and emotions, and so on—that is to say, the tension existing in certain nerves, or groups of nerves, when they give us sensations, ideas, or emotions, produces an equivalent tension in some other nerves, or groups of nerves, with which they are connected.

But the facts cited in support of this thesis do not appear to us to be all equally conclusive. Some of them are no doubt transformations, but then others are rather correspondences. Thus, the pain which is transformed into cries and extravagant contortions is of short duration ; pain which endures is reticent of expression. And the same is to be said of anger. But in certain cases—for example, in the cerebral excitation produced by hasheesh or opium —it is not quite certain that between the nervous state and the mental state there exists equivalence, transformation, and not simply correspondence.

This doctrine of the correlation of physical forces and thought is as yet hardly more than an outline. It is still in the qualitative period, and it is doubtful whether it will very soon enter on the quantitative period, which alone can constitute it a science. It is however a promising field, and one well adapted to exercise free and daring minds. If it could be demonstrated scientifically, it is evident that then the problem of the relations between the physical and the moral would come before us in a new aspect : it would be only a particular case of the law of the correlation of forces. We need not say that such a solution, restricted to experience, would be neither spiritualistic nor materialistic, for those at least who care for the preciseness of the terms they employ.[1]

But not to dwell upon a problem which cannot be incidentally discussed, we will endeavour to deduce a conclusion from all that has been said, which shall be based, so far as possible, on experience. It appears that all contemporary schools, when we eliminate that which appertains to the exclusive point of view of each, tend more and more to consider physical and moral phenomena as identical. This conclusion seems perfectly natural, especially to those who take the ground of experience; so that we may say—at least, so far as current language will enable us to express ideas which are opposed to current opinions—that the physical is the moral looked

---

[1] We may cite, in confirmation of what we have said, some remarkable reflections of the great English physicist, Tyndall. 'Granted,' says he, 'that a definite thought and a definite molecular action in the brain occur simultaneously; we do not possess the intellectual organ, nor apparently any rudiment of the organ, which would enable us to pass by a process of reasoning from the one to the other. They appear together, but we do not know why. Were our minds and senses so expanded, strengthened, and illuminated as to enable us to see and feel the very molecules of the brain; were we capable of following all their motions, all their groupings, all their electric discharges, if such there be; and were we intimately acquainted with the corresponding states of thought and feeling, we should be as far as ever from the solution of the problem, "How are these physical processes connected with the facts of consciousness?" The chasm between the two classes of phenomena would still remain intellectually impassable. Let the consciousness of *love*, for example, be associated with a right-handed spiral motion of the molecules of the brain, and the consciousness of *hate* with a left-handed spiral motion. We should then know when we love that the motion is in one direction, and when we hate that the motion is in the other; but the "why" would remain as unanswerable as before.

'In affirming that the growth of the body is mechanical, and that thought, as exercised by us, has its correlative in the physics of the brain, I think the position of the "materialist" is stated, as far as that position is a tenable one. I think the materialist will be able finally to maintain this position against all attacks; but I do not think, in the present condition of the human mind, that he can pass beyond this position. I do not think he is entitled to say that his molecular groupings, and his molecular motions, *explain* everything. In reality they explain nothing. The utmost he can affirm is the association of two classes of phenomena, of whose real bond of union he is in absolute ignorance. The problem of the connection of body and soul is as insoluble in its modern form as it was in the prescientific ages.' *Fragments of Science*, **vi.**

12

at from without, and that the moral is the physical looked at from within. The difference between physical and moral is subjective, not objective; it pertains not to their own nature, but to our way of viewing them. Physics has demonstrated that heat, light, and sound appear to us as different, only because each of them is addressed to a different sense, so that all the difference comes from ourselves. The psychologist ought to see that the physical and the moral appear different to us, only because the one is cognized by the external senses and under the condition of time and space, and the other by the inner sense, under the condition of time ; so that all the difference comes from ourselves. Thus the absolute, under its unconditioned form, would be entirely beyond our reach, and the conditioned forms in which it is manifested to us in experience would be opposites only by an illusion of our thought.

Perhaps we might proceed further, and draw an important deduction. If we admit the identity of physical and moral phenomena ; if we observe that all that is in the living being forms a continuous series from perfect unconsciousness, if there be such a thing, to perfect consciousness ;—if, again, there be such a thing; if it be borne in mind that the unconscious is the abyss into which everything enters and from which everything proceeds, the very root of all our mental life, and that our personality is like a wandering light on a vast and sombre lake, where it appears as though swallowed up each moment, then, perhaps, we shall be inclined to admit that the physical order and the moral order, which in our consciousness appear to be different things, are identical in the unconscious ; that conscious duality is derived from an unconscious unity, so that in the unconscious, matter and thought, object and subject, external and internal, are one. This special reconciliation of the physical and moral in man would thus lead to the reconciliation of the object in general with the subject in general, of the universe with thought.

This, it is true, is a metaphysical hypothesis, but then it is neither possible nor desirable to give up metaphysics and hypothesis. This hypothesis has been put forward by men who are as sturdy upholders of experience as are to be found, and who have treated psychology as a natural science. ' If we admit,' says Wundt, ' the identity of physical and psychical facts, then the former will come under the laws of mechanics, and the latter to those of logic, and it can be shown that these two kinds of laws are identical, and that the inner experience apprehends as a logical necessity what the outer experience perceives as a mechanical necessity.' 'This,' says he, in another place, 'is what the analysis of the process of sensation comes to, viz. that logical necessity and mechanical necessity differ not in their essence, but simply according to our way of regarding them. That which is given to us by psychological analysis as a continuity of logical operations (*Schlüsse*), is given us also by physiological analysis as a continuity of mechanical effects (*Kraftwirkungen*). . . . Logic and mechanism are identical; they are both only the form of essentially the same contents (*gleichartigen Inhalt*).[1]

CHAPTER II.

THE RELATIONS BETWEEN THE PHYSICAL AND THE MORAL. A PARTICULAR CASE.

WE have just seen how the question of the general relations of the physical and the moral presents itself in our day. We would now pass from the theory to the facts, to consider a particular case, to resolve a single question, one, however, of capital importance for the matter in hand. The question is this :—

Must it be admitted that every psychological state, of whatever kind, has always a physiological state for its antecedent?

The correlation of the physical and the moral is universally admitted, but this belief, when examined, is very vague and very inexact. The general view, and, what is more serious still, many philosophical treatises, seem to admit that this correlation holds good only in the gross, so to speak, and that frequently the body and the soul live each for itself. A few striking cases on either side are considered, all the rest being cast in the shade and forgotten. But, in fact, the thing is quite otherwise. Facts tend to

---

[1] *Menschen und Thierseele*, 12th Lecture, p. 200, and 57th Lecture. p. 437.

show more and more conclusively that this correlation is as complete as possible; that it is constant; that it is to be seen even in the most insignificant cases, and that it admits of no exception. It is of great importance for us to establish this truth here : for if we could succeed in showing it to be highly probable—as yet we cannot hope for certainty—that every psychological state supposes a physiological antecedent, a considerable advance would have been made in our inquiry into the causes. In the order of phenomena, all our science consists in demonstrating permanent coexistences and permanent successions. Suppose this permanent co-existence of a physiological and a psychological state established, we can then go further, and draw the deduction that in every individual an habitual mental state must answer to an habitual nervous state. The mental constitution of a poet and that of a mathematician imply each a physiological organization differing from the other in certain points. We can go further, and extend to the species what has just been said of the individual. The permanence of a certain turn of mind in a family during several generations supposes the permanence of certain corresponding physiological characters during the same number of generations. This leads us in the direction of the required answer, for to resolve a problem is to translate a proposition which implicitly contains a truth into another which gives a glimpse of it, and this in turn into another which exhibits it clearly.

For the present, let it suffice to establish our premisses. Evidently experience only can decide whether every psychological state is connected with a physiological state; this is a question of fact rather than of theory. Still, we cannot enumerate all possible cases; we cannot take all the states of consciousness in succession and show that they correspond, each with a particular nervous state. Such a demonstration would be endless, and it would, moreover, be in many cases impossible. We must, then, in accordance with Bacon's precept, confine ourselves to a few selected, striking, decisive facts, to *experimenta lucifera* which may serve as a basis for a sound induction. We will, then, show from examples that sentiments and ideas are referable to certain states of the organs, though at first sight they would seem to be entirely independent of them.

I.

At the lowest grade of psychological life, we meet with that infinite number of faint perceptions, scarcely conscious, of which the aggregate constitutes for every one that general feeling of existence, that *Gemeingefühl,* which is the ground on which our clear perceptions and our ideas are incessantly projected. This confused feeling, which is the resultant of a crowd of infinitesimal sensations, as the roar of the sea is the resultant of the noise of each wave, is so well described by L. Peisse, in his *Notes on Cabanis,* that we cannot do better than transcribe the passage.

'Is it quite certain that we have absolutely no consciousness of the exercise of the organic functions? If we mean a clear, distinct, and locally determinable consciousness, like that of external impressions, it is plain that we do not possess it; but we may have an obscure, dim, and, so to speak, latent consciousness of them, analogous to our consciousness of the sensations which call forth and accompany the respiratory movements, sensations which, although incessantly repeated, pass as though they were not perceived. May we not, indeed, regard as a distant, feeble, and confused echo of the universal vital labour that remarkable feeling which, without cessation or remission, certifies us of the actual existence and presence of our own bodies? This feeling is nearly always, though improperly, confounded with those accidental and local impressions which, while we are awake, stimulate and keep up the play of sensibility. These sensations, though they are incessant, make but fugitive and transient appearances on the stage of consciousness, while the feeling of which we speak endures and persists beneath those shifting scenes. Condillac well named it the fundamental sentiment of existence, and Maine de Birau the feeling of sensitive existence. In virtue of it, the body is ever present to the *ego* as *its own,* and the mental subject feels and perceives that it exists in some sort locally within the limited extent of the organism. It is a perpetual and unfailing monitor, making the state of the body ever present to the consciousness, and it manifests in an unmistakable way the indissoluble connection of psychical with physiological life. In the ordinary state of equilibrium which constitutes perfect health, this feeling is, as we have said, continuous, uniform, and ever the same, and hence it is that the *ego* does not perceive it as a distinct, special, local sensation. To be distinctly perceived, it must acquire a certain intensity, and then it is expressed by a vague impression of general well-being, or general discomfort, the former indicating simple exaltation of physiological vital action, the latter its pathological · perversion; but in thĩs case it soon is localized in the form of particular sensations pertaining to such or such a region of the body. At times it is revealed in a more indirect, though far more evident way, when it has just failed at a given point of the organism, for instance, in a limb struck with paralysis. The member in question still belongs materially to the living aggregate, but it is no longer included in the sphere of the organic *ego*, if the expression is permissible. It ceases to be felt by this *ego*, as *its own*, and the fact of this separation, though negative, is interpreted by a very special positive sensation known to all who have ever suffered a total numbness of any part of the body, produced whether by cold or by compression of the nerves. This sensation is nothing else save the expression of that sort of void or loss which occurs in this universal feeling of the bodily life; it proves that the vital state of that member was really, though obscurely, felt, and that it constituted one of the partial elements of the general feeling of life in the organic whole. Thus it is that a continual and monotonous noise, like that of a carriage in which we are shut, is soon unnoticed though it is still heard, for if it stop suddenly the cessation is at once perceived. This analogy may help us to understand the nature and working of the fundamental sentiment of organic life, which, on this hypothesis, would be but the resultant *in confuso* of the impressions made at all points of the living body by the inward movement of functions carried to the brain, whether directly by the cerebro-spinal nerves, or indirectly by the nerves of the ganglionic system.

Therefore it is not proved that, in the strict sense, the organic functions are performed absolutely without our knowledge, as Cabanis asserts.

This *Gemeingefühl*, of which the mass of men take no note, and which too many psychologists have neglected, is nevertheless the groundwork of our mental life. If in psychological analysis we could employ the microscope, it would resolve this general state into a myriad of particular states, themselves the effects of a myriad of vague excitations of the organism. Thus, then, this general feeling of existence is referable to elementary psychological states, of which each has its physiological antecedent.

II.

If from this obscure region we pass into the full light of consciousness, we have the same result. In the order of the sentiments, as in that of ideas, the phenomena that are purest, most quintessential and freest from matter, have, like others, their organic conditions. Some facts which we will cite will give us, with regard to this point, an amount of information that never could be divined by all the theories in the world unaided by experience. We will begin with the sentiments.

All must admit that many of the sentiments and passions depend upon a certain state of the organs. Most languages, indeed, employ words signifying 'heart' and 'bowels,' to denote our emotions. But it will be found that to many sentiments is attributed the privilege of being purely spiritual.

Thus, love. There is hardly any passion that is more intimately associated with the organ. Yet it has been supposed that under a certain form, called platonic, or ideal love, there arises a purely mental state, having nothing in common with the senses. The truth is, that love in man differs widely from the appetite of the brute, as in a great measure it is the work of the imagination and of the mind, because it is a complex sentiment, resulting from the fusion of many simple sentiments. An able psychologist of our own day who has analysed it, finds in it, besides a physical sentiment, a sense of the beautiful, affection, sympathy, admiration, love of approbation, self-love, love of possession and of liberty. Now we will show hereafter that all intellectual states have their physiological conditions. The physical sentiment, which is the starting-point of love, is masked by numerous states of consciousness more intense than itself; but it exists, notwithstanding, with those organic excitations peculiar to it. Facts to be found in medical works leave no doubt as regards this question, and prove that, though the spirit at first is master, the flesh at last prevails.

'A young man, devoted from an early period of his life to business, and who at the age of twenty-six had never, though occasions were not wanting, felt any desire for those pleasures which are pursued with such mad ardour by so many others, was suddenly, and without any appreciable cause, seized with a sort of amorous fury. He began to idolize all womankind, but, as he was careful to say, with the best intentions, and in all honour, not having even the slightest thought of the physical pleasure given by the possession of them. He cherished these feelings in secret, and for several months he concealed them from every one. His education and his station in life made this course obligatory on him. Soon there arose in his mind erotic fancies, of which he was inwardly ashamed, and against which he struggled with all his might. But so possessed was he with them, that his reason was not long able to resist the assault. To mental disorder there soon were added unmistakable signs of softening of the brain : a violent maniacal delirium then appeared, ending in death.' [1]

We will place side by side with this ideal form of love, mystical love, concerning which we have the same remarks to make. On reading the principal treatises on religious and philosophic mysticism, often so full of poetry, and so curious as the product of fine analyses, we cannot but recognize a variation of ordinary love, and the senses have there so active a part, that both forms often speak the same language. Spiritualistic philosophers themselves, among others Cousin, have well shown that mysticism is never nearer the senses than when it supposes itself to be very distant from them.

Moreau, in his *Physiologie Morbide*, gives a curious instance of this erratic love, which mistakes its true origin. 'I have had under my eyes for several months,' says he, 'and have been able to study thoroughly, a young woman, who in another age, and under other conditions of family and surroundings, would certainly have ranked with the Chantals and the Guyons. I will content myself with citing literally and without alteration certain passages from sundry letters written by her, which show how far she was mistaken as to the true character of the sentiments which possessed her.'

[1] Moreau of Tours, *Psychologie Morbide*, pp. 259—284.

We will quote one passage, and that not from among the strongest, referring the reader for further specimens to the book itself:—
'" I went to bed with such a swelling of all the organs that I was dull and, as it were, stupefied. .I gently kissed, like a little dog that is beaten, the hand of my Master; and then, as is my custom on every occasion of danger, I looked on that dear Master with a burning gaze of love and trustfulness, and going quite out of my own hateful personality, I reposed in him all my true life, so that I went to sleep in consequence of this practical death, and at once I was no more conscious of myself than I should have been had I died outright. I awoke, however, for a moment in the night, but as I was no better, I took refuge again in my dear Master. . . . . .
'" I meditated on the meditations of Saint François de Sales on the Song of Songs, at my morning prayer. One night, therefore, while wide awake, I felt myself in suspense in the midst of all my enjoyments, and awaiting, with a sort of terror, what the Lord would say. I saw him most vividly as he is described in the Song of Songs. . . . . . He lay down near me, put his feet on my feet, laid his hands on mine and enlarged his thorny crown, where he pressed his head to mine; then, while giving me a lively sense of the pains of his nails and his thorns, touching my lips with his own, and giving me the divinest kiss of a divine spouse, he breathed into my mouth a delicious breath, which pouring over my whole being a refreshing vigour, rejoiced it all over with an incomparable thrill, and won it for him without reserve.' [1]

We need not describe the influence of mutilation on the sentiments in general, on the direction of the mind. In the case of animals, while making them weaker, it makes them also more docile and better suited for use by man. 'It is well known,' says Cabanis, 'that eunuchs are the vilest class of the whole human race : they are cowardly and deceitful because they are weak, envious and spiteful because they are unfortunate, yet their mind is conscious of the lack of those impressions which give so much activity to the brain, and which animate it with extraordinary life.'
Then there are the hermaphrodites. All who have studied them in their moral characteristics, are aware that the individual

[1] *Ibid.* pp. 269—277.

hermaphrodite usually possesses all the psychological tastes which appertain to the predominant sex : thus the masculine hermaphrodite likes tobacco, brandy, and women. Neuter hermaphrodites have been known to engage with equal pleasure in the violent sports of boys, and in the quieter amusements of girls.[1]

We have now to consider another category of passions, which are not connected in the same way with the organs—namely, ambition, avarice, love of truth ; in a word, those sentiments which are called intellectual. These are very complex sentiments, consisting of a number of heterogeneous elements, but in which ideas play the chief part. Yet it is certain that they are accompanied by pleasure or pain, and that these two phenomena, under whatever form, are never entirely separable from the organism. Besides, ideas themselves have their physiological antecedents ; they have their condition in a cerebral state, as we shall see on looking at our problem from another point of view.

III.

Every intellectual state has for its condition and antecedent a physiological state.

First, as regards the phenomena of perception, memory, and imagination, the fact is so plain that there is no need for us to dwell upon it.

But when the question is with regard to the higher modes of thought, such as comparison, abstraction, generalization, judgment, reasoning, will, the answer is more difficult. It will be admitted that idiocy, insanity, ecstasy, general paralysis, and delirium always have their cause in a state of the brain. It will further be admitted that the development of the understanding depends on the weight, form, and chemical constitution of the brain, and on the number of its convolutions, though with regard to this point much obscurity still exists. But there is generally much repugnance in admitting that the meditation of a Newton or a Spinoza on abstract truths implies a corresponding cerebral state, and we must

---

[1] *Dictionnaire des Sciences Naturelles*, Art. ' Hermaphrodisme.' On all these questions consult Cabanis, pp. 222, 223, 253 (Peisse's edition) ; Moreau, 329 ; Coste, *Développement des Corps Organisés*, vol. i. pp. 232—239.

confess that physiology is far from being in a position to say precisely to what mode of nerve-vibration a given mode of thought answers. Yet we think that there is one fact which settles the question—that we cannot think without words. To think is to form a judgment; to judge is to abstract or generalize, and these operations cannot be performed without signs. The sign is a kind of image—the substitute for an image—and it depends on the brain, as is proved in aphasia, and all disorders of the memory which prevent our using signs. The most abstract reflections, therefore, in so far as they are connected with signs, presuppose a corresponding cerebral state.[1]

In support of these general considerations, which are based on experience, we may cite, as in the case of the sentiments, some curious facts.

Thus Dr. Dumont, a physician of the Hospital des Quinze-Vingts, has inquired into the influence of blindness on the intellectual faculties. Of two hundred and twenty blind persons with whose lives he was perfectly familiar, twenty-seven showed intellectual disorders—not including among these those affected with any appreciable cerebral lesion.

Dr. Renaudin has observed the highly instructive case of an intermittent cutaneous anæsthesia that influenced the character and the intellect of the patient. 'A youth, Arthur ——, had always given perfect satisfaction to his parents. Gifted with ordinary understanding, he had begun his elementary studies with some success. Suddenly his faculties lost their energy, and he became so unruly that he was expelled the school. He might have been considered an ordinary bad boy,' says M. Renaudin, 'but as I continued my investigation I found in him a complete insensibility of the skin, and I concluded that this was the pathological explanation of the fact. Nor was I mistaken, Arthur has since been sent to Maréville, and from direct observation I have become still more confirmed in this opinion, because the cutaneous anæsthesia being somewhat intermittent, it has been

---

[1] We can think without language, but not without some mode or other of physical expression. The famous Laura Bridgman was always moving her fingers in her dreams and during her waking reflections.—(Maudsley, p. 417.)

easier to appreciate its influence on the mind of the patient ; when
it ceases, he is docile and affectionate.   When it reappears, his
evil instincts return, and we have had reason to know that they
might have led him even to murder.'

It has been observed that when there is perfect physical similarity
between twins, which is not rare, it is always accompanied with
moral similarity.   Moreau saw at Bicêtre two young men who were
so much alike that one would be taken for the other.   They both
possess the same monomania, the same dominant ideas, the same
hallucinations of hearing ; they never speak to any one, nor do
they communicate with one another. 'An exceedingly curious fact,
often observed by the attendants and by myself, is this : from time
to time, at irregular intervals of two, three, or more months,
without appreciable cause, and by the entirely spontaneous action
of their malady, a very marked change occurs in both brothers at
the same period ; often on the same day they quit their habitual
state of stupor and prostration and earnestly entreat the physician
to give them their freedom.   I have seen this repeated even when
the two brothers were separated from one another by a distance
of several miles.' [1]

The phenomenon of suggestion also, as produced in magnetized
subjects, and in the state of catalepsy or hypnotism, supplies
decisive facts in support of our proposition.   Ordinarily, the ideas,
sentiments, and volitions suggest the sign, and are interpreted by
it ; here, on the contrary, the sign suggests the idea, the sentiment,
the volition.   The phenomenon is reversed.   Thus, by placing
the magnetized person on his knees, the thoughts of humility and
reverence are suggested ; by lifting up his lips and his eyelids in a
certain way, he is rendered proud and haughty ; by raising his arms
into the air, or clasping his hands on some object, he is made to
think that he is climbing.   Carpenter has collected a number of
facts of this kind.

It may therefore be said that experience supplies decisive facts
to confirm our proposition, that every psychological phenomenon
has a physiological antecedent.   It cannot be asserted on sound
logical grounds that this is certain.   To make it so, the proposition

---

[1] *Op. cit.*, p. 172.   See an analogous fact in Trousseau, *Clinique Médicale,*
i. 253.

should either be strictly deduced from some unquestionable biological law, or else it would have to be possible to give experimental proof of it in all possible cases. We can do neither of these things. But we hold that this thesis possesses all the probability that accompanies the inductive process; we hold that were our science sufficiently advanced, we could, the state of the brain being given, thence deduce the corresponding thought or sentiment; and, conversely, the sentiment or thought being given, we could deduce the state of the brain. Leibnitz, whose genius was all-penetrating, had a glimpse of this truth at a period when science scarce allowed a suspicion of its existence. 'All that ambition led Cæsar's mind to do is represented also in his body; there is a certain state of the body which answers even to the most abstract reasonings.'

We might have deduced our proposition from what was before said; for if it be admitted that the physical and the moral differ not objectively but subjectively—not in their nature, but as to the mode in which they are known to us; if vital phenomena are on the one hand specially mental, and on the other specially physical, but yet such that each of them, taken in its totality, is ever both physical and mental; then it is plain that every psychological phenomenon supposes a corresponding physiological state. But we have thought it best to establish this truth directly, and by experience, independently of all hypotheses. We need only add that here, as everywhere, our solution is restricted to phenomena, and has nothing to do with the ultimate reasons of things.

CHAPTER III.

PHYSIOLOGICAL AND PSYCHOLOGICAL HEREDITY.

I.

IF we sum up what has been said in the two foregoing chapters, we shall see that in consequence of these researches the problem, What is the cause of psychological heredity? is very much simplified.

In the first place, we endeavoured to show that the general

relations of the physical and the moral may be conceived as a relation of equivalence, so that in the last analysis there exists only one species of phenomena, neither material nor spiritual, but which, from a purely human point of view, we call physiological when we grasp them from without and through the senses, and psychological when we grasp them from within and through the consciousness. As we have remarked, however, this is but an hypothesis, the value of which will be better and better determined in the progress of the sciences; but the fate of which is of no importance for the experimental portion of our thesis.

In the next place, passing from speculation to facts, from metaphysics to biology, we showed, on the ground of experience, that it is extremely probable, if not certain, that every mental state implies a corresponding nervous state, and *vice versâ;* so that, were our science more perfect, we might from the mental state of a being infer the nervous state, and from the nervous state infer the mental state.

If these premisses be accepted, the problem of the cause may be more clearly stated. In fact, all our science consists in apprehending relations between simple phenomena or groups of phenomena. We have here two groups of phenomena, the one physiological and, above all, nervous, the other psychological; from the standpoint of heredity there can only subsist between these one or other of these three relations :—

1. A simple relation of simultaneity, physiological and psychological heredity being parallel, though entirely independent of one another.

2. A relation of causality, psychological heredity being considered as the cause, and physiological heredity as the effect.

3. Another relation of causality, but with physiological heredity as the cause, and psychological heredity as the effect.

We will not stop to examine the first hypothesis, which appears to us to be an artificial question. It rests on the strange notion of two substances, the body and the soul, perfectly distinct, entirely different, and so alien to one another, that it is matter for surprise to find them travelling together and in constant relations with one another. The question might have been put in this form in the seventeenth century, but in the present state of science it is no longer acceptable; and it would not be rash to assert that the great minds who in that age professed this dualism would now be the first to reject it. We have seen that in our time there is a growing tendency to admit an intimate correlation, a mutual interchange between the two orders of phenomena, so that the difficulty is not to unite but to separate them; and we could not explain why this radical dualism is still so accredited, did we not know that it is yet more difficult to extirpate an old error than to bring a new truth into acceptance.

Without insisting on this hypothesis, which in itself alone includes all the difficulties of both the others, let us proceed to examine them.

1. It might be held that psychological heredity is the cause of physiological heredity. This proposition is evidently the one that is maintained by the idealists and the animists. We are not aware that they have laid it down in precise and explicit form, and this no doubt because they have been very little concerned with the problem of heredity, which is chiefly physiological. And, indeed, it is worthy of remark that while spiritualistic philosophy has been much occupied with the future destiny of the soul, it has bestowed very little thought on its origin. It has always inquired whither we are going, and but seldom whence we come. And yet these two problems are intimately connected, and are both equally mysterious.

Theologians have taken more pains to work out this question. It is one that is closely connected with the foundation whereon Christianity rests, the transmission of original sin. Their opinions are not very harmonious, but are of no importance here. They may be reduced under two heads.

Some have taught that God, the only and the immediate origin of souls, creates, at the instant of conception, a special soul for the body which comes into being.

Others hold that all souls are sprung, like all bodies, from the first man, and that they are propagated in the same way—that is, by generation. This would seem to be the opinion of the majority. Tertullian, St. Jerome, and Luther held it, as also two philosophers, Malebranche and Leibnitz. The latter held it to be 'the only doctrine wherein philosophy can harmonize with religion.'

If we might be allowed to have an opinion on this subject, we should say that the second opinion would appear the more orthodox. But we will take the philosophical point of view, and since the idealists say nothing about the relation between the two forms of heredity, we shall have to indicate that relation ourselves. In their system, their logic would lead us to view this relation as follows :—

We will start with the fertilized ovum, that source of everything that lives. This ovum is not merely an aggregation of molecules, which the physiologist studies under the microscope ; it is also, and above all, a force, that is to say, a manifestation of the soul. Admit if you will (for we idealists have no great liking for this hypothesis) that this soul inherits from its parents certain determinate forms of sensitive, intellectual, and voluntary activity, and that it contains these virtually. The soul thus constituted now sets about fashioning its body. Follow its labours from that moment which caused Harvey so much astonishment, when he saw slender threads like those of a spider's web, stretch out from one corner to another of the matrix, and then saw this network forming a sac which held a white liquid in which appeared the *punctum saliens.* Follow this evolution, whose aspect changes sometimes from hour to hour, and whose instability affects the most essential no less than the most accessory portions, so that it might be said that the unseen workman is feeling his way, and that he completes his work only after many a mistake. Pursue your observations to the moment when embryonic life is at an end and extra-uterine life begins, and then see how evolution still goes on, until the being is fully constituted ; and you must confess, perhaps unwillingly, that all this is wonderful work, which, in spite of errors, anomalies, and deviations, is not the effect of chance, and that it is not without intelligence, though without consciousness. And observe: here the soul is the cause, the organism the effect; consequently, the conclusion is quite natural that the nature of the soul implies that of the body, and that the ground of physiological heredity is to be sought in psychological heredity.

Thus, as we believe, and without weakening it at all, this proposition might be maintained. As for transcendental idealism, which regards as simply physiological all that does not appertain to pure intellect 'beyond time and space,' we have already spoken of it when treating of the heredity of the intellectual faculties.

If we examine this doctrine, we shall find that it is with it as with all metaphysical hypotheses ; we might refute it, but we cannot extirpate it. The great objection appears reducible to this: that the idea of generation, which is its basis, is utterly unintelligible from the idealistic point of view. The idea of generation, in the psychological sense, might be understood in the hypothesis of the equivalence or mutual transformation of two groups of phenomena which are regarded as essentially identical. But that is not the thesis of the idealist. In his view there exists but one only substance, thought, and of this all others are the manifestations. The idea of generation and hereditary transmission results from experience, and can be given only in experience ; if these phenomena are full of mystery they are none the less real, since we may track their course, their evolution. But when you apply them to the ideal, the supersensual order, they represent nothing ; they are but metaphors, empty words, hollow abstractions, since there are no concrete things to which they may be referred.

About a century ago, Wollaston, a spiritualistic, even a Christian philosopher, justly said in his essay, *The Religion of Nature Delineated*, that in the purely ideal order, the fact of generation is unintelligible. 'We should have to explain clearly,' says he, 'what we mean, when we say that a man can transmit the soul, as it is not easy to conceive how thought, or how a thinking substance, could be produced like the branch of a tree. Indeed, we do not see how the expression can be employed, even in a metaphysical sense. We should have to define whether this generation proceeds from one, or from both of the parents. If from both, then it follows that one branch may be the product of two different trunks, a thing unexampled in all nature ; and yet such a supposition would be more naturally made with reference to vines and plants, than to intellectual beings, which are simple and incomposite substances. . . . From these considerations we are led to the conclusion that there is no other substance save matter ; that the soul, resulting only from the disposition of the body, must be born with it, of father or mother, or both ; and that the generation of the soul is a consequence of the generation of the body.' Wollaston regards this conclusion as materialistic, and, as always occurs in such a case, he sacrifices facts to hypotheses, and argues against heredity. But, as we need have no fears of that bugbear, let us examine the last remaining hypothesis.

2. This hypothesis regards physiological heredity as the cause of psychological heredity. Of course, we speak here only of the immediate and secondary cause, of cause in the order of phenomena—that is to say, the invariable antecedent. So understood, this solution appears to us the only one that can be accepted.

No one questions the influence of the physical on the moral, only it is commonly regarded as transitory, momentary, or at least constantly variable. Thus an excessive absorption of alcohol will produce confusion of thought ; a certain nervous state will cause delirium ; the introduction of hasheesh into the organism will give a feeling of beatitude. These and similar phenomena are very striking, though, in fact, of no great importance. But it *is* of importance to remark that to that habitual, customary state of the organism which we call temperament, or constitution, there must correspond an habitual, customary state of the mind. This admits of no doubt, but it is forgotten. But if we bear in mind the truth that the influence of the physical on the moral is permanent ; that it is exerted by means of infinitesimal, but incessantly renewed acts; that there exists a necessary correlation between those two orders of existence which we call body and soul, and this no less as regards secondary and transient, than as regards fundamental and permanent states, which are, as it were, the ground on which phenomena are projected : we shall see that, a permanent physiological state implying a correspondent psychological state, physiological heredity must imply psychological heredity. It were puerile to object here that oftentimes a person resembles one of his parents in feature, form, and temperament, though differing in mind ; for plainly the important point here is the heredity of the organic conditions of the mind, *i.e.* the brain. As we have seen, the organism is not always transmitted entire, and its transmission presents many puzzling anomalies.

Physiological heredity will be admitted without hesitation. It seems perfectly natural that the organism which is begotten should be like that which begat it. This all understand, or think they understand. But why not view psychological heredity in the same way? Apart from prejudice, routine, and preconceived ideas, which will not give way, the reason is that, rightly enough, people find the idea of generation, as applied to the soul, unintelligible. But all becomes plain if we connect psychological heredity, as effect, with physiological heredity, as cause.

We see, then, that this relation of causality between the two heredities is only a particular case of the relations of physical and moral. Its only peculiarity is, that here psychical heredity corresponds with permanent tendencies, not only in the individual, but also in the race, the family. Further, whereas physiological heredity is immediate, psychological heredity is indirect, mediate. The organism is transmitted directly; and if, together with the organism, the nervous diathesis of the parents is transmitted, their mental aptitudes are likewise transmitted by this intermediary.

It will, perhaps, be asked, seeing that we assert a perfect correspondence between nervous and psychical phenomena, why we consider mental heredity as an effect of physiological heredity. Might we not reverse the proposition?

We have already combated that thesis. But, independently of the negative reasons given, there is one which seems to us positive. It is, that experience shows mental development to be always and everywhere subject to organic conditions, while it does not show the converse to be true in a general way.

If there is any order of phenomena that is unequivocally worthy of being called *psychological*, it is the facts of consciousness. But consciousness presupposes for its production definite organic conditions. If they do not exist, there is no consciousness; and when they disappear, consciousness is at an end. And it may be remarked, that as regards the brain, consciousness does not stand in any vague, general relations. Though physiologists still debate as to whether the important point in the brain, considered as a psychological organ, is its weight, or its chemical constitution, or the number of its convolutions, or its form, or its type, it is likely that each of these conditions possesses a special importance of its own. Thus, it may be affirmed that an adult human brain weighing less than two pounds induces that mental state which we call idiocy.

When, therefore, we say that mental evolution depends on cerebral evolution, and, consequently, that psychological heredity depends on physiological, we state a plain truth of experience, a generalization drawn from an immense number of facts. Logically, then, the *onus probandi* lies with idealism; it is for the idealists to upset our proposition, not for us to disprove theirs. This is a point in logic too often overlooked, to which we would for a moment call attention. It sometimes happens that a good cause is compromised, because we bring all our strength to bear against the opposite opinion, instead of simply defending our own. A metaphysician, reviving an opinion of Descartes, might hold, as I have heard men hold, the hypothesis of animals being mere machines, and might defy us to prove its falsity. It is possible; but it is enough for us to reply that the metaphysician has to prove it. Every doctrine that is based on experience and analogy, and that is in accord with the general laws of the universe, must be regarded as true until the contrary is proved. Of course it may be false, but, at least, it has in its favour presumptions that it is true, and its upholders are under no obligation to refute the opposite doctrines, so long as they are only likely or probable. Such, we take it, is our position in regard to the idealistic thesis. That is, our doctrine rests on experience, against which an *a priori* theory is of no weight.

Still, we should not be surprised if to some it savours strongly of materialism. To this difficulty, we might in the first place reply, that if it is true it must nevertheless be accepted, whatever its character; that it is impossible to protest too strongly against an unphilosophical tendency which would judge doctrines, not according to their worth, but according to the brand they bear; and that philosophy cannot approve such a tendency without postponing truth to something else—that is to say, without committing suicide. We might also remark that, for us, materialism is only a phantom that disappears so soon as you face it resolutely; it is like ghosts, which alarm only those who believe in them. But it is better to meet the difficulty face to face, and to show that the objection is without force.

In the first place, it is clear so long as we confine ourselves to the investigation of second and immediate causes—and we shall again repeat that our investigation goes no further—the given solution cannot be either materialistic or spiritualistic. To connect psychological with physiological heredity is simply to state a fact, and it is for experience alone to say whether the affirmation is true or false.

But if it be desired at all hazards to raise the insoluble question of the ultimate cause, this is our answer : A materialistic doctrine is no doubt one that desires to explain all things, and in particular the phenomena of mind, by the properties of matter, matter being regarded as the sole reality. But we have shown that such a doctrine is an utter illusion, inasmuch as the concept of matter is finally resolved into notions of force, resistance, colour, motion, and so forth, all of which are data of consciousness; so that it might, without paradox, be asserted that the substructure of matter is mind.

We may remark that our solution is perfectly reconcilable with this metaphysical hypothesis—that is to say, with the extremest idealism. In fact, the only difference between us is one only of position; we reason from the standpoint of experience, the idealist from the standpoint of the absolute. We debate the question only within the strict bounds of experience ; the idealist goes in search of perfect integration, because, to his eyes, nothing is known so long as we know only the relative.

Further, it is said that materialism is that doctrine which from the inferior deduces the superior, from the worse the better. Is not this what we have just been doing, when subordinating mental heredity to organic ?

If the nature of the matter be considered, it will be seen that this question has no place here. Our subject is only one case in the vast science of the relations between the physical and the moral. That science does not inquire what is body, or what spirit, nor is it required to subordinate either of these to the other. It is naturally divided into two parts: the influence of the organism on mental manifestations, and the influence of mental manifestations on the organism. To the first part belongs the question of heredity. It is thus only a small portion of a very extensive science, which itself lies outside of metaphysics.

Heredity, thus understood, appears to us to be merely one of the many physiological influences to which mental development is subject; but it is a mistake to suppose that this implies a metaphysical solution. It is true that by the law of heredity, the higher is subordinated to the lower; but it would be to go beyond experience, and to risk a wholly gratuitous assertion, to assert that heredity absolutely proves the dependence of the higher on the lower, of the better on the worse.

II.

Thus to the question originally stated, 'What is the cause of psychological heredity?' we may reply, not transcending the domain of experience, 'Physiological heredity.' Because the organism, and in particular the nervous system, is transmissible, therefore the various modes of sensation, instinct, imagination, intellect, sentiment, are also transmissible. Psychological heredity being thus referred to physiological, as to its immediate cause, we have to inquire the cause of this latter, and to ask how physiological heredity is produced.

In the present state of biology we cannot hope for any positive explanation of heredity. We are reduced to hypothesis. The most recent of these, and the best wrought out, is that of Darwin, in his *Variation of Animals and Plants under Domestication*, the broad outlines of which are found in Spencer's *Principles of Biology.* It bears the name of pangenesis.

To understand it aright, we must first remember that contemporary physiology looks on every living body, regardless of its unity, as an aggregate of cells in prodigious numbers, each of which has a life of its own, and possesses the fundamental properties of life—nutrition, by which it is ever assimilating and disassimilating; evolution, by which it grows in volume and becomes complicated into more perfect and more numerous parts; reproduction, in virtue of which each cell can produce another, that cell a third, and so on. Virchow has shown that a single cell may be diseased; so that it may be said that this automatic element plays in the organism the same part as the individual in the State, having a certain degree of independence, though constituting an integral part of the body social.

A curious instance of the power of reproduction in the cell is found in the *begonia phyllomaniaca.* If a piece of the leaf of this plant be taken, and planted in suitable soil, maintained at a proper temperature, a young begonia will spring from it ; and so small is the fragment that is capable of producing an entire plant, that a single leaf may produce about one hundred plants.[1] Nor is this all, for each plant so produced in turn develops on its shoots and on its leaves myriads of similar cells, inheriting the same property of becoming, in their turn, like plants. Thus the original cell, on leaving the mother plant, inherits not only the power of self-reproduction, but multiplies it, and distributes it without any diminution of its energy to all the cells of the plant it produces, and this for countless generations.

To explain this power of reproduction and hereditary transmission in living beings in general, Darwin offers the provisional hypothesis of pangenesis, 'which implies that each of the atoms or units constituting an organism reproduces itself.'

It is almost universally admitted, he tells us, that the cells, propagated by spontaneous division, preserve the same nature and are ultimately converted into different substances and bodily tissues. Alongside of this mode of multiplication, I suppose that the cells, prior to their conversion into formed and perfectly passive material, emit minute grains or atoms which freely circulate through the entire system, and when they find sufficient nutrition afterwards develop into cells like those from which they came. These atoms we will call gemmules. We assume that they are transmitted by parents to their descendants, and that usually they develop in the generation immediately following, though for several generations they may be transmitted in the dormant state and develop at a later period. It is supposed that gemmules are emitted by each cell or unit, not only during its adult state, but during all its states of development. Finally, we assume that the gemmules have a mutual attraction for one another, and hence their aggregation into germs and sexual elements. Thus, strictly speaking, it is not either the reproductive elements or the germs

---

[1] Herbert Spencer, *Principles of Biology*, vol. i. § 65.

that produce new organisms, but rather the cells themselves, or units constituting the whole body.[1]

It may be observed that no valid objection can be drawn from the extreme minuteness of these gemmules, our notions of size being purely relative. When we bear in mind that the ascaris may produce about 64,000,000 ova, and a single orchid nearly as many million seeds; and that the organic particles emitted by scent-secreting animals, and the contagious molecules of certain diseases, must be of excessive tenuity, the objection will not appear very weighty.

Hence, ' we must consider each living being as a microcosm, made up of a multitude of organisms capable of self-reproduction, of inconceivable minuteness, and as numerous as the stars of heaven.' This hypothesis enables Darwin to explain a great number of phenomena, very different in appearance, which, however, physiology regards as essentially identical. Among these we may name gemmiparity, or reproduction from buds, fissiparity, where reproduction is effected by spontaneous or artificial division, sexual generation, parthenogenesis, alternate generation, the development of the embryo, repair of the tissues, growth of new members in place of those which are lost (as occurs in the case of the lobster, the salamander and the snail)—in short, all modes of reproduction whatsoever, and all the modes and all the varieties of heredity.

We have seen that a distinction may be drawn between characters which are developed and those which are simply transmitted. Transmission may take place without development, as is proved by the very numerous facts of atavism and reversional heredity, whether under the direct or the collateral form. This phenomenon, which we have compared with alternate generations, is very well explained by Darwin's hypothesis. The common fact of a grandfather transmitting to his grandson, by his daughter, characters which she does not or cannot possess, can only be understood on the supposition that in the daughter they exist in the latent state; or, to give a physiological basis to this idea, gemmules

---

[1] Darwin, *Variation, etc.*, vol. ii. chap. xvii.

are transmitted to the second generation, and preserved there, which are developed only in the third.

Darwin also explains how modifications of bodily or mental habits may be hereditary. 'According to our view, we need only suppose that certain cells come to be modified, as well in their structure as in their functions, and then they give out gemmules similarly modified . . . When a psychic attribute, a mental habit, or insanity is hereditary, we must hold that there has really taken place a transmission of some effective modification, and this, on our hypothesis, would imply that gemmules springing from modified nerve-cells are transmitted to the descendants.' Of course these modified habits become fixed only in time, since the organism must subsist amid novel conditions for a considerable period, so that these may act upon it, modify its cells, and make possible the transmission of a larger and larger number of modified cells.

In the preceding remarks we have reasoned only from physiological data. But we know that in the question of heredity the antithesis of psychological and physiological is a simple difference of standpoint. These cells and gemmules are not brute, inanimate matter ; they are possessed of force, of life, of tendencies, and we have seen that it is as difficult to conceive of the material without the spiritual as of the spiritual without the material. Therefore the hypothesis is applicable as well to mental as to organic heredity, and if it holds good for the one, it holds good also for the other. It may, in fact, be seen how well the two orders appear to correspond.

In the physiological order, at its lowest stage, we have as an irreducible element the cell, or physiological unit, possessed of a life of its own. From the consensus of countless lives of this kind results the general life of the being whose unity appears to us as a resultant, a harmony. This harmony, in proportion as we ascend the scale of organisms, tends more and more to perfect unity, without ever reaching that ideal.

In the psychological order, at its lowest stage, we have as the irreducible element or psychological unit, force as it exists in every cell, or, at least, nerve-power as it exists in every nerve-cell. From the consensus of all these infinitesimal psychical acts, centralized in the ganglia, and afterwards in the brain, results psychological

13

life, which, in proportion as we ascend the scale of being, passes from the simultaneous to the successive form—which is the necessary condition of consciousness—and tends more and more toward perfect unity, personality, the *ego*, without ever attaining it absolutely.

Thus the parallelism is complete between these two orders of facts, which at bottom are only one ; and so we can understand, or at least suspect, how the two orders of heredity may flow from the same cause.[1] Enough, however, has been said hypothetically, and we must conclude.

To sum up : we think we have proved that psychological heredity has its cause in physiological heredity, and that this cannot be reasonably disputed. The two heredities, being thus reduced to one, we again sought for the cause of heredity, and found only a hypothesis, probable indeed, but which, lying beyond the limits of experience, cannot be verified. The definite result of these researches—and the point is so important that it must be again and again repeated—is that heredity is identity as far as is possible ; it is one being in many. 'The cause of heredity,' says Häckel, ' is the partial identity of the materials which constitute the organism of the parent and child, and the division of this substance at the time of reproduction.' Heredity, in fact, is to be considered only as a kind of growth, like the spontaneous division of a unicellular plant of the simplest organization.

Having studied the Facts, the Laws, and the Causes, we have now to look at the practical side of heredity, the Consequences.

---

[1] Compare the very bold and ingenious hypothesis of Herbert Spencer (*Psychology*, 2nd Edition, § 139), of which the following is the substance. Our sciences, our arts, our civilization, all social phenomena, however multitudinous and complicated, are reduced on final analysis to a certain number of feelings and thoughts. These in turn are referred to the primitive sensations, to the data of the five senses. The senses are reducible to touch. Physiology goes far to confirm the saying of Democritus, that all the senses are modifications of touch. Touch itself has its basis in those primordial properties which distinguish organic from inorganic matter. And many facts point to the conclusion that sensibility of all kinds takes its rise out of those fundamental processes of integration and disintegration, in which life in its primitive form consists.

PART FOURTH.

THE CONSEQUENCES.

Thus out of savages come at length our Newtons and Shakespeares.

Herbert Spencer.

CHAPTER I.

I.

THE idea of progress is quite modern. Its originators in the seventeenth century were Bacon, Descartes, Pascal, and, above all, Leibnitz. In the eighteenth century it was the object of a lively faith for all the philosophers of that period. In the nineteenth century it has become almost a commonplace. Still, in its current form, it is vague and incomplete.

First, it is vague. The word progress has no very definite meaning. For some it represents merely the act of advancing, for others it means improvement, which is a very different thing. Moreover, the common view accepts progress as a fact, without inquiring after its law, its cause. Is it a chance product, or has it a law, and if so, what is the law? What is the hidden form in the nature of things? What the productive power that determines its being? These questions are not even asked.

It is incomplete, and this is a still graver defect. By an unscientific illusion, but one that is perfectly natural to man, we look at progress only from the human point of view. In the view of nearly every one progress means the transition from bad to middling, from middling to good, from good to better—in short, improvement. As history shows that humanity generally advances from the less to the more perfect, as we see that as time goes on manners tend to become milder, life easier, habits more moral, social institutions more just, political institutions more liberal, knowledge more diffused, and beliefs more reasonable, we conclude that in spite of all retrogressive movements, in spite of exceptions, illusions, and disappointments, the victory after all is with progress— that is to say, the improvement of man and his moral surroundings ;

and we say with Herder, that humanity is like a drunken man, who, after many a step forward and many a step backward, yet at last reaches his destination. Progress, so understood, is a human fact, restricted to the sphere of the moral and political sciences, and limited to history, as having the same bounds as liberty.

A more exact, and at the same time a broader, view would lead us to see in human progress only a part of the total progress, and to substitute for this equivocal expression the more appropriate terms, evolution or development. This substitute is highly important, for in the place of a human, subjective, hypothetical opinion, it sets a cosmic, objective, scientific system. Progress no longer appears as the law of humanity only, but as the law of universal nature.

The idea of evolution in this wide and true sense will doubtless ever be considered one of the grandest philosophic conceptions of the nineteenth century. Born of the study of the natural sciences, of religions, languages, history, of all that changes and lives, it has in turn given to these studies a new meaning, has quickened and renovated them. Hegel was the first to attempt the grand synthesis which must one day reduce all things under the law of a perpetual coming into being. His metaphysical hypothesis may have perished, as so many more have perished, but the radical idea of his system remains. Better still, new aspects of the law of evolution have since appeared in the whole field of science. To cite only one instance, the bold hypothesis which takes its name from Darwin has given a new shape to the question of the origin of species, and has brought it to bear on the highest problems of philosophy.

The latest essay in philosophical synthesis based on the idea of evolution is the work of Herbert Spencer. This synthesis, the outlines of which are given in his essays, while its definite form is given in his first principles, is intended to cover and explain in detail the phenomena of biology, psychology, sociology, and morals. It not only possesses the merit, as being recent, of including a larger number of facts and of partial doctrines; its true merit consists in substituting for Hegel's subjective, metaphysical method an objective, scientific one—the method of the natural sciences. Thus the law of evolution—stripped of all teleological ideas, and

having as its result not man's welfare but the necessary development of the cosmos ; not progress in the purely human sense, and
our advance toward perfection, but the advance of the universe
toward an ever-increasing complexity—may be referred to the
laws of mechanics, to the ultimate laws of motion ; and thus the
problem of the universe, considered from the standpoint of
evolution, becomes a problem of dynamics.

It would carry us beyond our subject to sketch this antithesis
here. It will suffice for us to note its chief features, and to indicate
the *cause* and the *law* of evolution.

Considered in general, every evolution may be defined as an
integration ; and this explains, in a certain sense, how it is always
a transition from less to greater. Its law is the transition from
the homogeneous to the heterogeneous, from the uniform to the
multiform, from the less to the more coherent, from the indefinite
to the definite—these various expressions indicating the various
aspects of one and the same change, which is essentially identical.
Thus it is that in astronomy evolution explains the transition from
the almost homogeneous primitive nebulæ to our solar system, with
its planets and satellites varying so widely in density, velocity and
distance from the centre ; in geology, the transition from the relatively homogeneous primitive igneous mass to the earth as it is,
the surface of which alone appears to us so heterogeneous ; in
biology, the transition from the inferior organisms of the primitive
ages to the multiform fauna and flora of the present ; in psychology, the transition from undeveloped and embryonic forms of
mind to states more and more complex ; in sociology, the transition
from the simple societies of primitive times to the most complicated
and most heterogeneous societies of our epoch ; in history, the
development of languages, mechanic arts and fine arts, and their
ever multiplying subdivisions.

Thus evolution consists in an integration, a transition from
simple to complex. But this uniform process presupposes some
fundamental necessity from which it results. This universal law
implies a universal cause. The reason of this universal transformation of homogeneous into heterogeneous is this, that every
active form produces more than one change, and every cause more
than one effect. Thus a shock will produce motion, sound, heat,

and light. A little small-pox virus in the organism will produce very numerous morbid phenomena. An economic reform will .lead to many industrial and social consequences. Everywhere, in short, even when the cause is simple, the effects are manifold.

Evolution thus understood, and both as to its law and as to its cause reduced to ' a purely physical interpretation ' of phenomena, offers a scientific character which is not possessed by the current doctrine of progress. Then, too, the latter, being concerned only with human welfare, and considering that as the final cause of all change, finds itself much embarrassed in view of sundry incontestable facts which show that humanity at certain periods stays and retraces its steps. Evolution explains these facts. The development theory, as Lyell well observes, implies no necessary progression. It is possible for a new race to be of simpler structure, and of less developed understanding, than those which it displaces ; a slight advantage is sufficient to insure it the victory over its rivals. The law of evolution accounts equally well for progress and for what is called degradation—that is, a retrograde movement towards an inferior structure, or a lower form of dynamism. It is sufficient if a being so degraded, whether physically or morally, is better adapted to its new conditions of existence than a being more highly endowed.

Now that we have fixed a precise meaning on the words evolution, development, and progress, we can see how this law governs the whole question of the consequences of heredity. In this portion of our work we propose to show how heredity has contributed to the formation of certain intellectual or sensitive faculties, and of certain moral habits. We can now have a glimpse of this truth. Heredity and evolution are the two necessary factors of every stable modification in the domain of life.

Suppose evolution without heredity, and every change becomes transitory : every modification whatever, whether of good or bad, useful or hurtful, disappears with the individual. Evolution confined within these narrow limits, loses all significance and all force ; it is nothing but an accident, without any value.

Suppose heredity without evolution, and there is nothing but the monotonous conservation of the same types, fixed once for all. Physiological characters, instincts, intellectual and moral faculties, are preserved and transmitted without modification. Nothing increases, nothing diminishes, nothing changes.

On the other hand, suppose both evolution and heredity, and then life and variation become possible. Evolution produces physiological and psychological modifications; habit fixes these in the individual, heredity fixes them in the race. These modifications as they accumulate, and in course of time, become organic, make new modifications possible in the succession of generations; thus heredity becomes in a manner a creative power. This fact of the heredity of acquired modifications has made its appearance often in the course of the present work; though we shall have to examine it in detail further on, it will be useful to dwell upon it here for a little while, as it will give us a better understanding of the relations between heredity and the law of evolution.

In the physiological introduction we showed that acquired modifications can certainly be transmitted. We have seen, for instance, that animals artificially made epileptic transmit that morbid disposition to their descendants. We have also seen that this point is possessed of some difficulty, for facts seem to show that these deviations from the type tend to return to the normal state, and that the law is, that accidental states are not perpetuated, but that, after subsisting for a few generations at longest, they first grow fainter, and then disappear. Thus we should return to the difficulty we met at the outset, that we should have evolution without heredity, or at best with only a restricted heredity, yielding no results of any importance. The difficulty, however, is only an apparent one. Even were we to accept the hypothesis of a return to the primitive type, which is the one most at variance with our theory, it will be observed that this return has no place except when a race is left to itself. The experience of breeders shows that certain physiological characters can be thoroughly fixed and perpetuated by continual selection, notwithstanding some exceptions and cases of reversion; but education acts upon the mental faculties precisely as the breeder's art acts on the organism and its functions. We shall see that the capacity for seizing abstract ideas, and for complying with the conditions of civilized life, becomes fixed only after a considerable length of time in certain races; these, left to themselves, return also to the primitive type. Thus there is established in the individual, between the heredity of the natural characters and that of the acquired characters, a conflict, in which nature must win if art does not counteract it. Bacon's saying is true of heredity, as of all natural laws : *Natura non nisi parendo vincitur.* But with the aid of art, under the constant influence of education, or of the same moral environment, acquired characters become fixed; and then there is established in our psychical constitution a second nature, so intimately blended with the former, that usually they cannot be distinguished.

To sum up : without the law of evolution, nothing is simpler than to determine the consequences of heredity. It would not be worth while to study them separately, for they would consist only in the indefinite conservation of the same specific characters. But with evolution all is different. The living being tends incessantly to be modified by causes both internal and external. The internal causes determine those spontaneous modifications of the organism and of the dynamism which, as we have seen, some authors explain by a law of spontaneity, such as a new physical character, or a new mental aptitude. By external causes we mean the action of circumstances, which have as strong an influence on the moral as on the physical being, and which in time tend to fashion it in a certain manner. In the battle of life, the struggle for existence, that great biological fact which Darwin has so well established that his adversaries themselves have accepted it, these modifications constitute for the individual a probability of its survival, if by them it is better adapted to new conditions. They render it possible for the living being in the first place to subsist, and then to perpetuate itself. Heredity, which is essentially a conservative force, tends to transmit to the descendants the whole nature of their parents ; as well every deterioration, physical, mental, and moral, as every physical, mental, and moral amelioration. The blind fatality of its laws regulates not alone progress, but also decay.

Man, therefore, as he comes into the world, is not the impressionless statue dreamt of by Bonnet and Condillac. Not only is he possessed of a certain constitution, a certain nervous organization, which predisposes him to feel, to think, and to act after a manner which is peculiar and personal to himself, but we may even affirm that the experience of countless generations slumbers in him. So far is he from being homogeneous, that all the past has contributed to his constituents. The present state of his mechanism and his dynamism is the result of innumerable modifications slowly accumulated ; and it may be affirmed that were heredity to act alone, and were there no crossings, no spontaneous variations, no psychical combinations or transformations, the secret of which we cannot penetrate, the descendants would be necessarily inclined to feel and to think as their ancestors.

II.

This hasty statement shows that heredity is one of the chief factors of the law of evolution ; that by accumulating slight differences, heredity produces effects apparently out of all proportion with the original causes. The living being is subject to the action of its environment and modified by it ; nor does man, considered as a thinking, sentient being, escape this law. Hence we see at one time an amelioration, at another a deterioration of his faculties. Chance, but especially education, may develop his intellect, his character, his imagination, his sentiments; and—since these acquired modifications are sometimes transmitted by heredity, and, in fact, taking everything into account, are mostly transmitted— we may say that the evolution of the psychical faculties is a law of the intellectual world, and that the gain made by each generation is to the advantage of those which follow. But where man has discovered a law—that is, an invariable rule—which governs a group of phenomena, if these phenomena are within his reach, or come under his control, he can modify them, because he holds in his hands the mainspring that moves and governs them. Thus he is acquainted with the laws of heredity : he knows that they exist and act, notwithstanding many exceptions which mask their action. Can he turn them to account ? Can he employ them for the perfecting of his species ? Let us put the question in clearer and more explicit terms. The starting-point is a race of medium intelligence, morality, and artistic and industrial capacity. The goal is a race, quick of comprehension and expert in action, well-disciplined, of gentle manners, and easily adapting itself to the complicated forms of civilization. The problem is, how we are to raise the masses to the level of those who, at the outset, were greatly above them. Can this be done?

We would observe, first of all, that so far is this aspiration from being chimerical, that every effort of civilization has it and it alone in view. But the end is attained by means of education, an external agency, different from heredity, which acts from within. As we view it, education is unequal to this task. There remains, in some natures, a substratum of unintelligent savagery which may be overlaid by civilization, but never done away. Hereditary transmission alone could modify them. We will return to this point hereafter.[1]

From the psychological standpoint, therefore, the only one that concerns us here, the question takes this form : Can we, by means of selection and heredity, increase in a race the sum of its intelligence and morality?

Heredity is an effect—it depends on generation, and generation depends on the nature of the agents; it is, therefore, at the root of the matter. How assort the parents with a view to the amelioration of the race? This question, simple as it appears, has given rise to inextricable disputes, which we thus summarize :—

Suppose a large family, gifted physically and morally, its members healthy, strong, intelligent, active; assign to them all some one talent, that for the stage, for instance, as in the Kemble family. Ought the members to intermarry with one another in order to fix this talent definitively, and to make it organic, so to speak? Some will call such a union desirable, others detestable. There is an eager contest in our day over this question of consanguineous marriages. Ancient legislation, evidently giving expression to the prevailing opinions, and which must have been based as well on experience as on prejudice, is not at all unanimous on this point. Consanguineous marriages are condemned by the laws of Manu, the Mosaic code, the laws of Rome, the decrees of the Christian councils, and the texts of the Koran. Thus opinion has been adverse to them among nearly all civilized peoples; yet the ancient laws of the Persians and of the Egyptians permitted the marriage

---

[1] See chap. iii. § 2.

of the nearest relatives. In Syria consanguineous marriages were common, at least in the reigning families, from the earliest times down to the end of the Seleucidæ. As for savage races, such as the Samoiedes, Tartars, Caribs, American Indians, etc., their customs in one place allow such marriages, in another proscribe them. Passing from the practical domain of customs to the theoretic domain of science, we meet with the same state of indecision.[1]

According to Darwin, the consequences of close interbreeding in animals, carried on for too long a time, are generally believed to be loss of size, of vigour, and of fertility. He cites the opinions of several breeders in confirmation of this. Yet 'with cattle there can be no doubt that close interbreeding may be long carried on advantageously with respect to external characters, and with no manifestly apparent evil as far as constitution is concerned.' Bates, a well-known breeder, says that 'interbreeding with bad stock is ruinous and disastrous, but with first class cattle it may be practised safely within certain limits.' A flock of sheep has been kept up, in France, during sixty years without the introduction of a single strange ram. With pigs on the other hand long continued interbreeding is attended with the most disastrous results. 'Mr. J. Wright, well known as a breeder, crossed a boar with his daughter, granddaughter, and great-granddaughter, and so on for seven generations; the result was, that in many instances the offspring were sterile, others died, and among those which survived a certain number were idiotic, incapable of sucking, or walking straight.' As regards birds, Darwin finds a considerable number of proofs which condemn unions between the same blood. He refuses to consider the question as it concerns man, 'since it is there surrounded by prejudice,' still he seems not to be in favour of consanguineous marriages.

Other authors condemn them without reserve, among these Prosper Lucas and Dr. Boudin. The latter, taking his stand on a great number of facts and figures, considers them as the undoubted cause of very many morbid phenomena, several of which concern

---

[1] Lucas, vol. ii. p. 903 ; *Bulletins de la Société d'Anthropologie,* vols. i. iii. iv. and vi. ; Darwin, *Variation, etc.,* vol. ii. ch. xvii.

the mental life, as, for instance, deaf-muteness, idiocy, and epilepsy. In his view, consanguinity is of itself essentially baneful, and determines, without the concurrence of any other morbific cause, the appearance of many grave diseases and infirmities.[1]

' History,' says Lucas, 'witnesses to the disastrous consequences which it brings on man.' 'Aristocracies obliged to recruit their numbers from among themselves become extinct,' says Niebuhr; 'in the same way often passing through degeneracy, insanity, dementia and imbecility.' Esquirol and Spurzheim, at least, give this reason for the frequency of mental alienation and of its heredity among the great families of France and England. Deaf-muteness in humbler families appears also to have the same origin.

It would not perhaps be rash to see an effect of consanguinity in the premature decline of the Lagidæ, and of the Seleucidæ. The Lagidæ from Ptolemy Soter down to Cleopatra and Cæsarion (—323 till 30) reckon sixteen sovereigns, and the Seleucidæ, from Seleucus Nicator to Antiochus Asiaticus (—311 till 64) reckon twenty. They often married their sisters, their nieces, or their aunts. Moreover, when the marriages were not consanguineous, alliances were formed between these two effete families, the Lagidæ nearly always marrying Seleucidæ, and the Seleucidæ marrying Lagidæ. Now, it is certain that these races were in a state of perpetual decay, in proportion as they became more remote from their two or three first founders.

To these many reasons against consanguineous marriages nothing but exceptional cases seem to be opposed. Burdach attributes good results to consanguinity, but only among animals. Dr. Bourgeois wrote the history of his own family, which was the

---

[1] *Memoir de la Société d'Anthropologie.* According to Dr. Boudin, the danger of consanguineous marriages is shown by the following facts. In Berlin there were

        in 10,000 Catholics   3 deaf-mutes
        in 10,000 Protestants 6   ,,
        in 10,000 Jews   27   ,,

In the United States, in 1840, the negro population, who were given to promiscuity, showed in Iowa 91 times as many deaf-mutes as the whites. These figures, and the inferences drawn from them, have been questioned See *Bulletins de la Société d'Anthropologie*, vols. iii. and iv.

issue of a union in the third degree of consanguinity. In the course of one hundred and sixty years there were ninety-one marriages in that family, sixteen of them consanguineous, and yet there resulted neither infirmity nor sterility. Similar facts are cited by MM. Voisin and Dalby. There are two small French islands, Batz and Bréhat, in which consanguineous marriages are very frequent, yet the population is healthy and vigorous.

The two opinions may, perhaps, as M. de Quatrefages observes, be reconciled. The tendency of heredity is to reproduce the whole being; the child is only a resultant, a compromise between the tendencies of both the parents. If these tendencies are the same, they are all the more evident in the product. If the parents enjoy perfect health, consanguinity will tend to preserve it in their descendants, and then, so far from being prejudicial, it will have good results. But that perfect equilibrium which constitutes physical and moral health may easily be disturbed in the parents, and then the consequences will become more and more evident in the children. Now, in consanguineous marriages the chances are many that this disturbance of equilibrium will be of a like nature in both of the parents. Hence it follows that in many cases such unions will be injurious, and all the more dangerous in proportion as the morbid predispositions common to both parties are more marked. 'The consequence we are to draw from all these facts would appear to be, that near relationship between father and mother is not in itself hurtful, but that, in virtue of the laws governing heredity, it oftentimes becomes so; and hence, in view of the eventualities to which consanguinity leads, it is at least prudent to avoid consanguineous marriage.'[1]

It would therefore appear that the 'in and in' method adopted for the improvement of the lower races would have little likelihood of success if applied to man, and that we must renounce this plan of fixing and of making organic certain intellectual aptitudes. The process of crossing families would probably be better. This would consist in selecting a pair out of two different families, both possessed in a high degree of the particular quality, talent or tendency, which it is desired to transmit to the progeny in increased propor-

[1] Quatrefages, *Rapport sur les Progrès de l'Anthropologie*, p. 461.

tion. This proposed selection has but rarely been attempted, and never uninterruptedly. Instances of it might be found in mediæval times, in the golden age of the aristocracy. Often then, when an alliance was about to be formed, there was required on both sides not only well-authenticated noble descent, but also vigour, valour, courage, loyalty, piety—in short, all the chivalric virtues which it was desired to transmit to the children. It can hardly be doubted that if this selection were carried out methodically it would lead to good results for the improvement of the human race. Of course there would be many exceptions, many failures, many unforeseen anomalies, produced by chance, or by reversional heredity ; the phenomena of heredity are too complex and too delicate to be produced with the mathematical regularity of a machine ; but it. is probable that the general result would nevertheless be excellent.

Still, it may be objected that any such method as this would be only half successful. Grant that in this way we could perpetuate for the common good a nearly constant sum of eminent, illustrious, or merely notable men, or grant, even, that the number of such could be increased, there would still remain a far larger number of inferior minds of which heredity would perpetuate the deficiencies, just as, *ex hypothesi*, it perpetuates the superior qualities of the others. Must we dream that the case admits of no remedy ? Must we admit that here the law of competition is in force, and that it will in course of time stamp out whatever does not rise to a certain level ? May we hold that crosses judiciously contrived between one class and another might raise up that which is beneath, without lowering that which is above ? Would civilization be the gainer ? Or would such crosses only produce a uniform level of mediocrity ? These questions may be debated, but not resolved.

Some writers hold that a physically and morally superior race, when united with an inferior one, lowers itself without raising the other, so that all such alliances would constitute a loss to civilization. This opinion is enforced with a hardy logic by the author of a voluminous work on the *Inequality of Human Races.*[1] In his

---

[1] De Gobineau, *Essai sur l'Inégalité des Races Humaines*, 4 vols. 8vo.

view, there are three races of men, perfectly distinct and different, not by any mere external difference, but by a radical and essential one; the blood of one race is as different from that of another 'as water is different from alcohol.' These three races are the black, the yellow, and the white. The black race, which is unintellectual, sensual, passionate, abandoning itself to its instincts, represents, according to M. de Gobineau, the female element. The yellow is the male element; it possesses a positive mind, a narrow intellect, a love of comfort, utilitarian tendencies, and totally lacks artistic aptitude. The white is the noble race, gifted with superior faculties, and possessing aptitudes for poetry, sciences, and politics. Of this noble race the noblest branch is the Aryan, and of this branch the noblest family is the Germanic.

The first two races, left to themselves, are totally incapable of attaining to civilization. This power is possessed only by the white race. But in lifting the other two out of barbarism the white race itself is degraded by contact with them. What the other two races gain the white loses, just as when an exquisite wine is mixed with wines of inferior quality. Nor is this all; not only is the mongrel race inferior to the white, but also, inasmuch as every cross is in itself a cause of degradation, it follows that the white blood, though it does not change in quantity, yet loses its virtues on occasion of every new cross. From all this the reader will conjecture what our author thinks of modern civilization. An epoch which, by travel and by the multiplied needs of commerce and civilization, brings all peoples into mutual contact, and brings about alliances of every description, is, in his eyes, a 'horrible confusion.' The white race, which was uncontaminated in the time of the gods, still pure enough in the heroic age, already tainted in the days of the aristocracy, has now entered 'the era of unity.' When the confusion becomes complete, and when the white blood in every human creature shall bear to that of the other races the ratio of one to two, then 'the nations, or rather the human herds, oppressed by a gloomy somnolence, will live swallowed up in their nullity, like buffaloes ruminating in the stagnant puddles of the Pontine Marshes. Our shameful descendants will surrender to vigorous nature the universal dominion of the earth, and the human creature will be no longer her master, but only a guest,

like the inhabitants of the woods and waters.' Humanity will
have existed from twelve to fourteen thousand years.[1]

If we accept M. de Gobineau's doctrine, and apply to families
what he says of races and peoples, the conclusion to be drawn
from it is evident enough. We should say to them : Beware of
all admixture, and preserve your blood pure at any cost. Do not
try to bring up to your own level inferior members of the human
race, men, peoples, or races, for you would lose far more than
they could gain. But this conclusion appears to us very rash ;
and though on this point there are many hypotheses and conjectures, and but few truly scientific assertions, though the facts are
so contradictory as to warrant every possible interpretation, still
it seems to us that there are some very good arguments against
this theory of pure races, this horror for all admixture.

In the first place, I do not think that, with perhaps the exception of China, history presents a single instance of any great
civilization, without a preliminary mingling of peoples and races.
Take the Arabs, originally Asiatic. So long as the race remained
pure, it made little or no progress. Mahomet appeared, and then
they overran, as conquerors, Asia, Africa, and Spain, giving rise to
the great civilization of Persia, Damascus, Bagdad, and Cordova.
The Jewish people, rigidly exclusive as they were, had to admit
some Syrian, Persian, Phœnician, and Greek elements, in order to
work out their own civilization. Nor were the indigenous civilizations of the New World exempt from this law. The Incas of
Peru were a superior race that came to that country at a late
period in its history, probably in the thirteenth century. The
Aztecs in Mexico, who were conquered by Cortes, had been preceded by the Chichimecs and the Toltecs. But not to multiply
instances, it is evident that civilization, being by its nature a complex state, a harmony, many dissimilar and even unequal elements
were needed to form it. The more we advance in the knowledge

---

[1] M. Gobineau's view has been held in a very mitigated form by M. Périer,
who, in his *Essai sur les Croisements Ethniques*, takes chiefly the physiological
standpoint. He also inclines to the opinion that any race that is endowed
with any natural gift loses much by crossing. The author, notwithstanding,
admits that 'the people of purest blood is not therefore the least civilized, and
vice versâ.'

of nature, the more convinced do we become of this truth : that the highest phenomena of thought and life are also the most complex, and that, as a general rule, the inferior is always the simpler. Civilization has everywhere grown by contact, mixture, union. 'The more elements a people gains,' says M. Serres, 'the more it advances; the life of a people augments in proportion as its characteristics are multiplied.' Nor is there anything to prove that when two families or two races combine the mixture is rudely made, as in the mingling of wines. It may be that talent, characters, and new aptitudes may be revealed by the mere fact of cross-breeding, just as in chemistry two bodies which combine form a third possessing new properties. But ethnic chemistry is not sufficiently advanced to warrant this opinion, and therefore we must be content with simple conjecture.

We now return to our original question : When two elements cross, one inferior and the other superior, does the latter finally get the mastery, so that in the end there is a clear profit for the human race ? This problem is far from being solved, especially in its psychic aspects, as psychologists have studied it only cursorily and in a general way.

Half-breeds have furnished the chief materials for this study, for in them it is more easily pursued. The mixed elements being widely different—usually blacks and whites—are naturally magnified, so that we can study them, as it were, through a microscope.

Some naturalists regard these mixed races as doomed to disappear, either because the race has but little fecundity, or because the individual possesses but little vital resistance. Yet, according to M. Omalius d'Halloy, if we take the whole population of the globe as 750,000,000, the half-breeds would count at least 10,000,000. In Mexico and in South America they have in three centuries risen to be about one-fifth of the total population. D'Orbigny, who has closely studied man in America, is a strong partizan of cross-breeding between nations. 'Among the nations in America,' says he, 'the product is always superior to the two types that are mixed.' Finally, in Polynesia, and in the Marquesas Isles in particular, while the indigenous population is falling away with fearful rapidity, the half-breeds are increasing in numbers, so that this region seems destined to be re-peopled by a race half

European and half Polynesian. If we admit, with scme authors, that it needs several generations, or even several centuries, for a crossed race to adapt itself to its surroundings, and for the reversional heredity, which goes back to the primitive types, to be firmly established, we can foresee the time when the number of half-breeds will be far larger than it is at present.

But what is their mental value? Do they stand much above the inferior race or much below the superior race?

Darwin notes in some half-breeds a return towards the habits of savage life; but this, as it seems to us, may be only a mere phenomena of atavism. 'Travellers speak of the degraded state and savage disposition of crossed races of man. That many excellent and kind-hearted mulattoes have existed no one will dispute; and a more mild and gentle set of men could hardly be found than the inhabitants of the island of Chiloe, who consist of Indians commingled with the Spaniards in various proportions. On the other hand, many years ago, long before I had thought of the present subject, I was struck with the fact that in South America men of complicated descent between Negroes, Indians, and Spaniards, seldom had, whatever the cause might be, a good expression. Livingstone, after speaking of a half-caste man, on the Zambesi, described by the Portuguese as a rare monster of inhumanity, remarks, "It is unaccountable why half-castes, such as he, are so much more cruel than the Portuguese; but such is undoubtedly the case." An inhabitant remarked to Livingstone, "God made white men, and God made black men, but the devil made the half-castes." When two races, *both low in the scale,* are crossed, the progeny seems to be eminently bad. Thus the noble-hearted Humboldt, who felt none of that prejudice against the inferior races now so current in England, speaks in strong terms of the Zambos, or half-castes between Indians and Negroes; and this conclusion has been arrived at by various observers. From these facts we may perhaps infer that the degraded state of so many half-castes is in part due to reversion to a primitive and savage condition, induced by the act of crossing, as well as to the unfavourable moral conditions under which they generally exist.' [1]

Variation, etc., ii. p. 46.

There are other half-breeds, however, who are at least equal in point of intellect to their parents of the superior race. In 1789, nine English sailors mutinied, deserted their captain, and settled on Pitcairn Island with six Tahitans and fifteen Polynesian women. A quarrel soon arose among them. Five of the white men were killed, and the women murdered the Tahitans. The four white men and the ten surviving women lived in a complete state of polygamy. Strife broke out afresh between the four Europeans. Two were killed, and the remaining two resolved to live in peace, and to regenerate this little community, born amid an outburst of every wild passion. Captain Beechy visited the island in 1825; he found there a population of sixty-six individuals, remarkable for their fine proportions, their strength, their agility, their quick and ready intelligence, their great desire for instruction and for moral qualities, of which he gives a touching example. This community, consisting entirely of half-breeds, was superior at least to the vast majority of the elements which had given birth to it.

In Brazil, where, as the prejudices of colour are less strong than elsewhere, half-breeds may aspire to position in society, they have shown a decided artistic superiority over the two original races. 'Nearly every painter and musician in Brazil is a half-breed. They possess, also, a turn for science, and many of them have become medical practitioners of high distinction.'

In Venezuela, says M. de Quatrefages, mulattoes have been distinguished as orators, publicists, and poets. One of them, formerly Vice-President of New Grenada, was a prominent writer and a good administrative officer.

Authors who are by no means favourable to half-breeds admit that, particularly in America, they possess considerable intelligence, wit, and imagination.

We can draw no decisive conclusion from these facts, to which we might easily add many others ; not so much because the opinions are mutually contradictory, as because they are vague. Anthropologists, who usually are so minute and exact in their physiological distinctions, so soon as they come to consider mental characters, the complexity of which is so great, confine themselves to general phrases, which are almost always the same. Some naturalists, however, have supposed that from all these facts of cross-breeding we might deduce a law which would give the answer to the question proposed in the present chapter. It may be thus stated :—

The mixture of two unequal races tends to efface the less perfect of the two. When a white man marries a negress, their child is a mulatto. When two mulattoes of equal blood intermarry, their child is whiter than themselves. This fact is an application of a general law of nature, in accordance with which mixed forms have a tendency to return to the types from which they are sprung, and in the struggle for life the more perfect type prevails.[1]

Cases of unilateral crossing give some curious results. When the white is united to the black, and then with the half-bred progeny, the white type is seen to predominate more and more in every generation. The pure type reappears in the fifth generation. When this unilateral crossing takes place with the pure negro on the one side, and successive generations of mulattoes on the other, less time is required to bring back the perfect negro type. It reappears in the third generation.

In a large part of South America (Brazil, the Argentine Republic, Paraguay, etc.) a fact of great importance is found occurring with considerable uniformity. From numerous and trustworthy testimonies it appears that 'in that vast region, where these two races are crossed in so large a scale, the European type always prevails in the long run. In Brazil, men of "mixed blood," of all degrees of hybridization, are numerous, forming a new population, which is ever growing more indigenous and coming nearer to the white type, and, judging from what is taking place all over South America, they will finally absorb all the other elements of the population.' M. de Quatrefages is not clear whether this fact is to be taken as a proof of the ascendancy of race. He is rather inclined to suppose that it is due to conscious selection in cross-breeding, the process being as a general rule unilateral, and in favour of the white race. However this may be, 'it is a result of great importance, for in this struggle between races, the victory

[1] Except where it is impeded by the action of its surroundings, as appears to be the case in Peru, where the half-breed population has a strong tendency to return to the indigenous type.

will at last be with that race which possesses the superior elements.'

Should the future verify these prognostics, should the white race, after eliminating the two others, restore the cross races to its own type, it will have performed, in its own way, a work of regeneration; then the question with which we began will be definitely settled, and the mean level of humanity will have been greatly raised, still more perhaps by hereditary transmission than by the external action of education and custom.

III.

As we have seen, evolution in living beings, though it generally implies amelioration, progress, transition from worse to better, still, in its scientific sense, implies only the transition from simple to complex, from homogeneous to heterogeneous; and hence, instead of progress, it sometimes leads only to diminution of force and to decay. We have now to consider heredity under this latter aspect, as related to the law of evolution.

Everything that has life also declines and becomes extinct. It it doubtless because of this too evident truth that the belief in the law of progress appeared so late in man's history. First the individual disappears, then the family, then the nation; and just as the individual makes use of many bodies before he finally becomes extinct, so, too, the family makes use of many individuals, the nation many families, the human race many nations. Perhaps humanity itself must disappear at last, made use of by some mightier force. It may be that in the evolution of the universe humanity is but one term in an endless series, one link in an endless chain.

If we glance at any family that has acted a part in history, we see the following facts. Its origin is so obscure that usually we have to imagine or invent it; it comes into prominence, grows, and attains its climax in one, two, or three generations at most; it then declines and becomes extinct. Take the second race of Frank kings. It starts with Saint Arnoul, Bishop of Metz, follows an ascending series, Pepin d'Heristal, Charles Martel, Pepin the

---

[1] Quatrefages, *loc. cit.* p. 457.

Short, Charlemagne ; in the latter it attains its most perfect development, and then it declines.   The third race starts with Robert the
Strong, Count of France, reaches its climax in Philip Augustus,
St. Louis, and Philip the Fair, and then it becomes extinct in
three obscure kings.   It is much the same with the Valois branch,
sprung from Charles de Valois, son of Philippe le Hardi, and
with the Angoulême branch, sprang from Louis d'Orléans, son of
Charles V., which ended with the feeble sons of Catherine de
Médicis.   Then come the Bourbons, whose climax is indicated
by Henri IV. and Louis XIV., and who ever since have been on
the decline.   So, too, with the Guises, Condé's, etc.   Nor are those
families exempt from this law who have acted a great part, only on
a small stage, in their own province or their own city.   Indeed, it
would not perhaps be inexact to say, with Dr. Lucas, that ' the
ascending movement of the exalted faculties of most founders of
families is nearly always arrested at the third generation, seldom
goes on to the fourth, and hardly ever transcends the fifth.'   So it
is, too, with nations.   Their origin is obscure , they grow, attain the
full measure of their power, and then their fate brings them to
that period where they belong only to history ; and their decadence
is due, not so much to those vague causes to which it is commonly
attributed by historians, as to a definite cause: the decay of the
faculties, physical, intellectual, and moral (and of the organic
functions which are their condition), if not in all the citizens, at
least in the majority of them.

Heredity plays its part in this decline.   Though by itself, as we
have seen, it can do nothing, being merely a conservative tendency,
still it is heredity alone that makes progress possible during the
ascendant epoch of evolution.   But then, on the other hand, after
evolution has entered on its downward period, heredity confirms
and regulates the decline.   One by one it laid—fatefully, blindly
—the courses of the edifice, and one after another it removes them
with the same blind fatality.

The influence of heredity is either direct or indirect.

Its direct influence is exerted through the state of marriage.   It
is not a rare occurrence for a man of note to marry a woman of
indifferent capacity, out of family or social considerations, or from
chance or caprice.   It has been observed that great men often

leave descendants unworthy of them; in fact, advantage has been
taken of this fact in order to call in question hereditary transmission, whereas we should rather perhaps find in it a striking confirmation of the law. Galton, in his work on English judges,[1]
observes that of thirty-one judges raised to the peerage previous to
the close of the reign of George IV., nineteen are still represented
in the peerage by their descendants, and twelve peerages are
extinct. Having minutely investigated the cause of this extinction,
he discovered them in social reasons, in motives of convenience
which led to ill-assorted unions : those peers whose families soon
disappeared 'married heiresses.' Even when unequal matches do
not produce such grave results as these, it is not to be doubted
that, in virtue of the laws of heredity, they must cause a degeneration, which, being again and again repeated, must of necessity
bring about the extinction of a gifted family, or, what is worse, its
mediocrity. It is evident that a son may take after his indifferently
gifted mother as readily as after his illustrious father, and that, as
in any case he must be the resultant of the two, the chance of his
being inferior to his father is as two to one.

Considered as an indirect cause of decline, heredity acts by way
of accumulation. Every family, every people, every race brings
into the world at their birth a certain amount of vitality, and of
physical and moral aptitudes, which in course of time will become
manifest. This evolution has for its causes the continual action
and reaction between the being and its surroundings. It goes on
until the family, people, or race has fulfilled its destiny, brilliant
for some, distinguished for others, obscure for the majority. When
this sum of vitality and of aptitudes begins to fail, decay commences.
This process of decay may at first be of no moment, but heredity
transmits it to the next generation, from that to the following one,
and so on till the period of utter extinction, if no external cause
interferes to stay the decay. Here, then, heredity is only an
indirect cause of degeneration, the direct cause being the action
of the environment, by which term we understand all action from
without—not only climate and mode of life, but also manners,

---

[1] Pages 130-132. See the concluding chapter of the work, with regard to
the question whether great men leave no posterity.

14

customs, religious ideas, institutions, and laws, which often are very influential in determining the degeneration of a race. In the east, the harem, with its life of absolute ignorance and complete indolence, has, through physical and moral heredity, led to the rapid decay of various nations. 'We have no harem in France,' says a naturalist, 'but there are other causes, quite different in their origin, which tend ultimately to lower the race. In our day, paternal affection, with the assistance of medical science, more certain, and possessed of more resources, makes more and more certain the future of children, by saving the lives of countless weak, deformed, or otherwise ill-constituted creatures that would surely have died in a savage race, or in our own a century or two ago. These children become men, they marry, and by heredity transmit to their descendants at least a predisposition to imperfections like their own. Sometimes both husband and wife bring each a share to this heritage. The descendants go on degenerating, and the result for the community is debasement, and, finally, the disappearance of certain groups.'[1]

The only way of getting a clear idea of a case of psychological and moral decay, hereditarily transmitted, is by finding for it some organic cause. The physiology and anatomy of the brain are not yet sufficiently advanced to explain it; we cannot say to what change in the brain such and such a decay of intellect, or such and such a perversion of the will, is to be attributed. But cerebral phenomena and psychical phenomena are so closely connected that a variation of the one implies a variation of the other.

This being assumed, let us take a man of average organization, physically and morally. Let us suppose that, in consequence of disease, outward circumstances, influences coming from his surroundings or from his own will, his mind is impaired, to only a trifling extent it may be, but yet permanently. Clearly heredity has nothing to do with this decay; but then, if it is transmitted to the next generation, and if, further, the same causes go on acting in the same direction, it is equally clear that heredity in turn becomes a cause of decay. And if this slow action goes on with each new generation it may end in total extinction of intellect.

---

[1] *Revue des Cours Scientifiques*, vol. vi. p. 690.

These remarks also apply in every respect to nations and races: all that is required is that the destructive influences should bear, not on an isolated individual, but upon a mass of individuals. The mechanism of decay is identical in the two cases; and we are justified in the conclusion that the causes which, in the narrow world of the individual and the family, produce a considerable diminution of the intellectual forces, must produce the like effect in that agglomeration of individuals which constitutes a society. .

Historians usually explain the decline of nations by their manners, institutions, and character, and in a certain sense the explanation is correct. These reasons, however, are rather vague, and, as we see, there exists a more profound, an ultimate cause—an organic cause, which can act only through heredity, but which is altogether overlooked. These organic causes will probably be ignored for some time to come, but our ignoring them will not do away with them. As for ourselves, who have, for purposes of our own, attempted to study the decay of the Lower Empire—the most amazing instance of decay presented by history—tracing step by step this degeneration through a thousand years: seeing, in their works of art, the plastic talent of the Greeks fade away by degrees, and result in the stiff drawing, and in the feeble, motionless figures of the Paleologi; seeing the imagination of the Greeks wither up and become reduced to a few platitudes of description; seeing their lively wit change to empty babbling and senile dotage; seeing all the characters of mind so disappear that the great men of their latter period would elsewhere pass only for mediocrities—it appears to us that beneath these visible, palpable facts—the only facts on which historians dwell—we discern the slow, blind, unconscious working of nature in the millions of human beings who were decayed, though they knew it not, and who transmitted to their descendants a germ of death, each generation adding to it somewhat of its own.

Thus, in every people, whether it be rising or falling, there exists always, as the groundwork of every change, a secret working of the mind, and consequently of a part of the organism, and this of necessity comes under the law of heredity.

Here we bring to a close our general study on the consequences of heredity. We must next look at the details. In order to proceed with the inquiry methodically, we will proceed from causes to effects, that is to say, from sentiments and ideas to acts, and from acts to social institutions. We will therefore study the influence of heredity, first on the constitution of the human soul, on its intellectual states, its sentiments and passions, then on the acts which give outward expression to these inner states; lastly, on the institutions which result from these acts, and which not only regulate, but also consolidate them. Thus we shall have to consider, successively, the psychological, the moral, and the social consequences of heredity.

CHAPTER II.

THE PSYCHOLOGICAL CONSEQUENCES OF HEREDITY.

I.

The study of the psychological consequences of heredity must begin with the instincts. We will not here discuss a question already treated,[1] since it will be enough to state briefly the certain or probable results already obtained.

If heredity acted merely the part of a conservator, its consequences, psychological or otherwise, would present no difficulty whatever. On the hypothesis of individual types created once for all with their physical and moral attributes, the only consequence of heredity would be the indefinite repetition of these types, with some accidental deviations—unimportant facts of spontaneity. But the case is very different. Notwithstanding the character of immutability usually assigned to instincts, they may vary as we have seen, and their variations are transmissible. Hence the first consequence of heredity, that it renders possible the acquisition of new instincts. This consequence rests on facts, and is certain and indisputable.

Another consequence, one that is merely possible, and which we have stated only as an hypothesis, is the genesis of all instinct whatever by way of heredity. Instincts, regarded as hereditary

---

[1] See Part I. ch. i.

habits, would be the result of the accumulation of psychical acts
which, originally very simple, have, in virtue of the law of evolution, passed from the simple to the complex, from the homogeneous to the heterogeneous, thus giving rise to those highly
complex acts which seem to us so wonderful.

Hitherto we have restricted ourselves to looking simply at the
bearings of this doctrine; we are now to meet with it under
another form, and we shall study its bearings here also.

II.

The same question, in fact, arises with regard to the intellect.
Here some assign to heredity only a secondary influence, asserting
that it allows the transmission and accumulation of certain characters, and makes the development of the intellect possible, in the
individual and in the species.

Others go much farther, and attribute to heredity an actual
creative power. According to them, the genesis of the constituent
forms of intellect and of the laws and conditions of thought is the
work of heredity.

We will first examine this latter doctrine, the most radical, the
most recent, the least known out of England. There it has been
held by a few contemporary philosophers, and has given an
entirely new shape to the famous problem of the origin of ideas.
If this doctrine be true, it gives so important a part to heredity
that we must here discuss it fully.

It is one of the great merits of the school of sensationalists that it
early perceived the importance of questions of genesis. Through
all its researches into the origin of our cognitions it was really
concerned with the embryology of mind. It does not, however,
appear to have been at first clearly conscious of this, or it would be
impossible to explain the conception of a statue by Condillac
and Bonnet—an actual adult individual, whose genesis could
not but be illusory and artificial. This is as though the physiologist were to take man at his birth, without concerning himself
about the embryonic period which preceded it. It is singular
to see how superficial, external, and imperfect are the processes
of Condillac, and with what simplicity he thinks the most involved and complex phenomena may be explained and produced.

Condillac's system, however, has been excellently criticized already, and that by his own school.[1] But whatever its defects, we have reason to be thankful that it took the wrong course, as it led to finding the correct one, by suggesting the necessity of an embryology of mind.

In Condillac's day, the various hypotheses of naturalists with regard to the fact of generation might be reduced to two chief hypotheses, one holding the pre-existence of germs, and the other epigenesis.

The doctrine of the pre-existence of germs was the older, and, in some sense, the orthodox hypothesis. Vallisnieri, Bonnet, and Spallanzani maintained it in the seventeenth century; Haller also held it. It asserted that the ovum contains the animal or the man already formed, though of infinite minuteness, that all beings, each with its proper structure, have been contained in ova from mother to mother ever since the moment of creation; that the act of generation merely gives them life and makes them capable of growth and development. 'They are,' says Maupertuis, in his *Vénus Physique,* 'only little statues, enclosed one within another, like those works of the lathe in which the carver shows his skill with the chisel by making a hundred boxes shut up one within another.'

The doctrine of epigenesis, on the other hand, then represented by Buffon and Wolff, held that the being is formed in all its parts in the act of generation. The embryologists of the nineteenth century have shown that originally the germs of all organisms are

[1] Cabanis, p. 521, *Peisse's Edition.* It is interesting to compare Condillac's rude embryology with that of the great psychologists of the present time. It is given in its completest form by Mr. Herbert Spencer in his *Principles of Psychology.* The analysis begins with the most complex cognitions, and by successive decompositions arrives at the simplest act of thinking—viz. the perception of a difference. The synthesis, a very different affair from Condillac's artificial process, starts from reflex action, passing through instinct and memory, and arrives at the operations of reason, sentiment, and will. The author thus ascends from the conditions of a psychic state to the state itself, from the lower to the higher, from vague and general modes of mental activity to those that are precise and more and more determinate, from the simple to the complex. The comparison between the two methods is instructive; it just marks the difference between a truly scientific method and a purely verbal process.

structureless and alike, and that the development of each germ consists in acquiring the structure peculiar to its species. Some of them, even, such as Menckel and Serres, discovered in the temporary and transient forms of the embryogeny of man and the other vertebrates the arrested and permanent forms of invertebrate organisms. At least this much is certain, that at a certain point of their development the embryos of all vertebrates, whether birds or fishes, reptile or man, present only the most general and the simplest features of the vertebrate type. Nothing could differ more widely than this from the hypothesis of 'little statues' fully formed.

In our opinion, if we look at the theories on the origin of our cognitions, that is, the embryogeny of mind, in the light of these two hypotheses as to the embryogeny of the body, the philosophic question assumes a new aspect.

The spiritualistic or rationalistic school holds, after its own fashion, the pre-existence of germs. Whether, with Descartes, we accept innate ideas, or, with Leibnitz, hold that arithmetic and geometry exist in us virtually, and that there are graven on the soul truths which it has never known, is to hold that the soul, so long as it has existed, has possessed all its constituent elements. Experience perfects and completes it, but gives to it very little indeed, compared with what it receives. Just as, in the hypothesis of the pre-existence of germs, the minute being is developed, but does not undergo any change in its essential parts, or in the relations between them, merely attaining greater size, filling up gaps and acquiring a few accessory organs; so in the spiritualistic hypothesis, experience merely causes us to adapt ourselves to the fundamental forms and laws of the human soul, to those ideas and judgments which constitute it, so to speak, and which are to the mind what the cerebro-spinal axis is to the body. This analogy will appear still more evident when we remember that Leibnitz compares the human soul, previous to experience, to a statue outlined by the veinings in a rough block of marble.

As for epigenesis, its counterpart in philosophy is not, we take it, ordinary sensationalism, but a new system which we are about to describe in the words of Spencer, Lewes, and Murphy, and which lays much stress on heredity.

These philosophers have, in the first place, made an excellent, radical, and decisive criticism of the old empiricism. ' To accept,' says Spencer, ' the untenable assertion that prior to experience the mind is a blank is to overlook the very root of the question, viz. Whence comes the faculty of organizing sensations? . . . If at birth there exists nothing but a purely passive receptivity of impressions, why could not a horse receive the same education as a man? . . . Why should not the cat and the dog, subjected as they are to the same experiences obtained in domestic life, attain to the same degree and the same kind of intelligence? Under its current form, the experience hypothesis implies that the presence of a nervous system organized in a certain way is an unimportant circumstance, a fact that need not be taken into account, yet it is the most important fact of all.'[1]

Cognition is necessarily the product of two factors : first, we have what is presented to the mind, the internal or external phenomena, form, colour, agreeable or disagreeable sensations, etc. ; and then we have what the mind itself offers—the laws of thought, which connect the phenomena, and reduce to order this indisciplined and confused mass. This was clearly seen and well shown by Kant. But the philosophers of whom we speak, while they admire him, reproach him with having regarded the laws of thought as ultimate, irreducible, and inexplicable facts, instead of investigating their genesis. ' Kant and his disciples,' says Mr. Lewes, ' taking up the adult human mind, considered its *constituent forms* as *initial conditions.*' ' These forms,' say they, ' are implied in each individual experience.' Certainly, for if they were not so implied they never could be got out of them. This explanation is logically perfect, but it is of no service for psychology, which has to resolve a question of origin. Reasoning *à priori*, we might say that the vertebrate type is the necessary form which makes the vertebrate possible. This will do in anatomy, but it is false in morphology, which shows that the typical form results from the successive phases of the animal's development. Kant anatomized cognition well enough, but he disregarded its morphology.

What, then, are these mysterious forms of thought? Like the

---

[1] *Psychology*, 2nd ed., § 208.

forms of life, they are evolutions, not preformations. While they are the laws of experience, they are at the same time its results—results of the experience of the race, and not of the individual; they are the product of heredity. Let us get a clear idea of this doctrine.

I hear a bell ring. This fact, apparently so simple, is nevertheless highly complex; it consists of a group of sensations, inductions, and sense-images, each one of which is in itself a group. Not to speak of the primitive elements, which is not here necessary, and noting only the simple, rough, well-known facts, the sum of which makes up for us the phenomenon, we can tell the quality of the sound of a bell which is rung; whether the bell is large, small, or medium sized; whether it is near or distant, whether it is sounded by a hammer or by a clapper, whether it is in this church or in that, etc.; finally, whether the sound continues for a long time or not. This last fact, the *continuance* of the sensation, I take to be one of the elements of the group,—in fact, an essential and fundamental element, and, so to speak, the ground on which all the others are projected. Again, suppose I have a tooth drawn. This fact also consists of a group of sensations, sentiments, and ideas, far more complex than the preceding; and here, too, we find that duration is an essential element. Take any fact, any experience whatever, and you will always find groups of sensations, and among the elements of each group you will find duration, or time —that is to say, duration in its abstract and universal form, considered objectively.

I open my eyes, and see before me a fresh sown field. This fact, too, is a group of sensations and ideas (colour, form, distance, etc.), and in this group there is one attribute which, in like manner, is regarded as essential—viz. that continuity which, uniting together all the countless points of the field, makes of them one extended whole. This quality of extension I find coupled with other variable qualities, in an immense number of objects which I call material. Hence I regard extension or space, *i.e.* abstract, simple, possible extension, as a permanent attribute of all bodies.

I approach the fire, and it warms me; I smell an alkali, and it catches my breath; I see a cannon ball fired, and it knocks down the wall it strikes. In these, and countless other cases like them, the first fact is always followed by the second. The phenomenon, taken in its totality, is presented to us as something made up of two groups, so arranged that the first always necessitates the second; in other words, in the sum of qualities and relations which make up this inseparable pair we find, as an essential element, the relation of constant succession between the first and the second—the property that the first is always followed by the second. This fundamental property, which is also found in many other pairs, is denominated *causality*.

The foregoing analyses are not borrowed from the English philosophers, but we think they exactly represent their views. Now, if with them we hold that the mind is formed as well by the action of external objects upon it as by its reaction on external objects; if we hold that accidental, variable, changeable attributes must produce in the organism, and hence on the mind, accidental, variable, changeable modifications, but that fixed and essential attributes must have permanent modifications answering to them; if we observe that the attribute of duration being found in all the groups, that of extension in nearly all, and the relation of causality in a very large number of couples, they must recur millions of times during the life of each, and so, by repetition, tend to become organic; if, finally, we observe that these modifications are hereditarily transmitted to a new individual, who in turn experiences the same fixed and permanent impressions, and by him to another and another without limit, we shall then be able to understand the part played by heredity in the genesis of the forms of thought, and to see how heredity may produce, in the second or third generation, a mental habitude so deeply rooted as to be rightly called innate, provided it be borne in mind how it has come to be so.

'We have seen,' says Herbert Spencer,[1] 'that the establishment of those compound relief actions, called instincts, is comprehensible on the principle that inner relations are, by perpetual repetition, organized into correspondence with outer relations. We have now to observe that the establishment of those consolidated, those indissoluble, those instinctive mental relations constituting our ideas of space and time, is comprehensible on the same

---

[1] *Psychology*, 2nd ed., § 208.

principle. For if even to external relations that are often experienced during the life of a single organism, answering internal
relations are established that become next to automatic—if such
a combination of psychical changes as that which guides a savage
in hitting a bird with an arrow becomes, by constant repetition, so
organized as to be performed almost without thought of the process of adjustment gone through ; and if skill of this kind is so
far transmissible that particular races of men become characterized
by particular aptitudes, which are nothing else than partially organized psychical connections—then, if there exist certain external
relations which are experienced by all organisms, at all instants of
their waking lives—relations which are absolutely constant—there
will be established answering internal relations that are absolutely
constant, absolutely universal.   Such relations we have in those of
space and time. . . . As the substrata of all other relations in
the non-*Ego*, they must be responded to by conceptions that are
the substrata of all other relations in the *Ego*.   Being the constant
and infinitely repeated elements of thought, they must become the
automatic elements of thought—the elements of thought which it
is impossible to get rid of—the ' forms of intuition.'

From this brief statement of the question it is easy to see that
it is one of the highest in all philosophy, as being concerned with
the genesis of thought itself.   Here we arrive at a first cause : we
leave facts and enter on metaphysics.

Thought is, in fact, one of the forms of the unknowable—indeed,
the most mysterious of them all.   A little reflection suffices to
show this.   It is certain that the exterior world, the object, is
knowable only in so far as it is reducible to thought; that it has
no existence for us, save on that same condition ; that in it we
see only a sum of phenomena governed by laws ; and as the
phenomena are resolved into perceptions, and the laws into ratiocinations, therefore the whole universe may be resolved into
psychological states.   To say, with the idealists, that thought is
the measure of all things, so that the limits of our thought are
also the limits of reality, is certainly a gratuitous hypothesis ; for
we cannot be certain that beyond all actual or possible cognition
of ours there are not actual existences for ever unknowable, and
we have no warrant for making human thought the absolute

thought. But when we say, in a purely relative sense, that our thought is for us the measure of being, we enunciate an unquestionable truth, almost a truism; and from this purely human point of view we may affirm that the world has no existence for us, except in so far as it is thinkable. The world is a system of unknown qualities which we explain with the assistance of another unknown quality, thought; the latter, however, still remains the x of an unsolvable equation.

If, then, we see that thought is both an ultimate cause in metaphysics and an ultimate principle in logic, we must not be surprised at finding it impossible to answer that apparently simple question, What is thought? We are utterly unable to go beyond external and superficial explanations, and to get at the essence of thought.

Under its phenomenal form, thought is a simplification. To think is to simplify, to reduce plurality to unity. All the objects of our states of consciousness must be either concrete or abstract, and we cannot get at either of these but by a process of simplification. In the first place, those objects which we call concrete— a house, a man, a star—are extended, and yet can enter into our thought only under the form of a simple series, only under the condition of time. We know not how an act which has no extension can represent an extended object—how time can for us take the place of space. But it is certain that concrete objects are knowable for us only on this condition, and that to refer space to time is to refer the complex to the simple—to simplify.

To obtain our abstract cognitions we must abstract, generalize, induce and deduce, and all these operations in the last analysis amount to classification according to resemblances and differences, or to simplification. Thought, therefore, is the unifying principle which reduces to order the chaos of the universe. To think is to unify.

But this unification is but the process, the mechanism of thought. When we speak of our cognition of thought, we mean only the forms of thought. We cannot go beyond this, nor can we know how, by means of our consciousness, there is formed in our minds a world answering to, though not resembling, all that is without us. All discussion, therefore, with regard to the nature of thought, is concerned only with its forms; and when we assert that these forms are the result of heredity, we assert that thought itself, as a phenomenon, is a result of heredity.

As we have seen, the associationist school, while agreeing with Kant as to the necessity of certain fórms (time, space, causality) in order to connect experience and to constitute thought, differs from that philosopher by holding these forms to be the result of an evolution. The difference is more radical than would at first sight appear, for in Kant's hypothesis it is the forms of the subject that give shape to the object, while in the other hypothesis the object gives shape to the subject: in the view of the one the universe is dependent on thought, in that of the other thought is dependent on the universe. We would observe, by the way, that the criticism made in France on the association psychology is not well founded. The law of the association of ideas, it is said, having been discovered first, the only originality of this system of psychology is that it has generalized that law, and endeavoured to bring under it all the operations of thought. But this is a misconception in regard to the true originality of this school, which is very different. To assert, as this school does, that the cause of our internal *nexus* exists in *nexus* which is external; that when two phenomena are rarely associated in the object they are also rarely associated in the subject, and that when they are always associated in the object they are always associated in the subject, is to assert, in opposition to Kant, that the laws of cognition depend absolutely on the laws of nature, to import mechanism into the intellect, and to subject the intellect itself to mechanism as the ultimate law governing its phenomenal development.

Moreover, the hypothesis of a genesis of the 'forms of thought' by continuous evolution is not characteristic of the whole associationist school, but only of those adherents of it who accept universal evolution. We regard it as a simple hypothesis, and only desire to show that it is not so inadmissible as it may at first appear.

Starting from the hypothesis of a primordial nebula, we see that the universe must have endured thousands and thousands of years, during which nothing existed but physical and chemical phenomena. We cannot tell when or how, or by what series of blind attempts and essays life could be produced. Neither do we know how the transition was brought about from the physiological to the psychological epoch—from the period of no thought to the period of thought. The development school, however, is bound to maintain this ascending evolution. This was perceived even by Lamarck, and he boldly supposes the existence of a primitive race of non-sentient animals. 'In producing life,' says he, 'nature did not abruptly set up so high a faculty as that of sense. Nature did not possess the means of creating this faculty in the imperfect animals belonging to the earliest classes of the animal kingdom.'[1]

When we consider from the biological point of view the phenomena of mental activity, and compare them with purely vital facts, we find that both possess in common this essential point, that they are a correspondence. Herbert Spencer has shown how physiological life consists of a correspondence between a being and its environment,[2] and how in the sum of actions and reactions which constitute life there is a continual adjustment of internal to external relations, so that the degree of life varies as the degree of correspondence, perfect life being perfect correspondence. But mental life is, like bodily life, a correspondence. To think, or to have a cognition, is to have in our mind a certain state corresponding to a certain state without; and this correspondence also is found in all possible degrees, from the zoophyte to man, so that the degree of cognition is measured by the degree of correspondence. Between life and thought, therefore, there are other differences than that between a partial and a total correspondence, between a correspondence imperfectly unified (life) and a correspondence perfectly unified (consciousness); finally, and here is the mystery, between an unconscious and a conscious correspondence. If we could know how the simultaneous becomes successive, and how plurality becomes unity, then we could tell how thought results from life.[3] They suppose that they have explained this

---

[1] *Philosophie Zoologique*, Discours Préliminaire, 7.

[2] *Principles of Biology*. For instance, there must be in a plant certain changes answering to the changes of its environment (humidity, dryness, etc.).

[3] An author who holds the genesis of the forms of thought through evolution has developed the singular hypothesis that it is possible to 'think in space.' (Murphy, *Habit and Intelligence*, ch. xxxvii.) For this, says he, it would suffice that a mind, in place of thinking as our mind does, with words succeeding one

metamorphosis by heredity. Though we do not mean to give any advantage to this theory, still we must observe that thought is impossible except with the aid of certain forms to serve as schemata; that if these forms are annexed to a certain state of the brain, as is probably the case, and if this state of the brain is itself the result of a gradual evolution, then the conclusion is all but inevitable that the forms of thought are the result of an evolution in the species. Gratiolet, whose immaterialism (*spiritualisme*) has never been called in question, used to say that to him ' it was evident that the ontological analysis of philosophers, and especially that prime distinction between the ideas of time and space, were inscribed in advance among the preordinations of the animal organism.' Admit evolution also, and development has nearly gained its cause.

On this hypothesis, thousands and thousands of years rolled away before thought could appear on earth. Neither animals unprovided with a nervous system (bryozoa), nor those whose ganglia are nearly independent of one another (asterias), nor those in which there is just a beginning of unity, could have arrived at conscious-ness : their physical life must be a confused state in which the subject is not distinguished from its object. It is only in the higher animals, and perhaps in man alone, that the brain, resulting from a gradual evolution, and shaped by countless actions and reactions which have been preserved and transmitted by heredity, could become the instrument of thought.

Thus the doctrine of development rigorously applies to the world of thought the same hypothesis as to the world of life. On the one hand, it deduces all species from three or four primitive types, or it may be from only one. On the other hand, from a few very simple psychical acts, it may be from only one, it deduces the endless variety of instincts and intelligences of sentiments and passions. We have endeavoured to show how this hypothesis

---

another in time, should think by means of figures traced in space. But even in that case we should have thinking in both time and space, and not in space alone. It is useless to dwell upon an hypothesis of which the verification is impossible, and which, farther, is in contradiction with the essential condition of thought, viz. unity.

is to be understood, and on what grounds it rests; for our own part, we neither accept nor reject it.

If we are to accept it, it must be verifiable by experience, or demonstrable by logic. Experimental verification would consist in showing that it agrees with all the facts, and that it can be brought entirely under their control; but it is impossible to show any such thing. Logical demonstration would consist in showing that this one hypothesis, exclusive of all others, explains the facts; but this demonstration *per absurdum* is impossible.

If we are to reject it, the hypothesis must involve some logical contradiction; but this is not the case. It is true that it is difficult to understand how no-thought can become thought, but without attempting to explain this, we may bear in mind that this transition is progressive, and that life and thought share in common this *essential* character, that they are a correspondence produced by a series of actions and reactions. Moreover, this evolutional genesis of the forms of thought, which the doctrine of development applies to the species, is admitted by all as applying to the individual. The individual cannot think (in the proper sense of the word) until his brain is developed; and if thought, in its true sense, possessed of all its constituent forms, comes into being in an instant—which is doubtful—we do not see why this bright flash in the night of the unconscious should not have lighted up the species also, at some definite instant. To say that the objects of the constituent forms of thought—space, time, causality—could not have modified the brain, because they have no concrete existence in nature, as have a stone or a dog, is not to present a difficulty; for if, with Leibnitz, we regard them as relations it is quite natural that the brain should be modified, not only by things, but by the relations between things.

These two opposite theories—the one regarding thought as the essential causality to which nature is a secondary causality, and the other regarding nature as the essential causality and thought as secondary—might perhaps be reconciled by admitting the identity of mechanism and logic, of intelligence in nature and intelligence in thought. We have already alluded to this doctrine, but this is not the place to set it forth.

III.

We have now seen how, on certain hypotheses, heredity contributes towards the creation of intelligence. We now propose to turn aside from this radical solution, and to inquire how it contributes towards its development. We here use the word intelligence in a sense at once common and philosophic, as that faculty of judgment, ratiocination, and abstraction which in conduct is denominated prudence, good sense, tact, dexterity, penetration; in art, inventiveness, taste ; in science, the faculty for discovery, for generalization, and for detecting relations. Having already proved by sundry facts from normal and morbid psychology and from history the existence of intellectual heredity, we will take it for granted here as an empiric law, and we will investigate its consequences.

If we consider heredity under purely ideal conditions, nothing can be simpler than to determine its consequences : it fixes and preserves the modes of intelligence as they appear. Thus some variety of the intelligence—humour, for instance—appears in an individual either by spontaneous variation, or by that chance concurrence of causes which has been called spontaneity : now if heredity alone were at work it would transmit this mental modification uninterruptedly to all the succeeding generations. But, as we have seen, it meets with hindrances of every description, which tend to weaken or even to destroy it. Yet if, instead of considering isolated cases where heredity appears to be at fault, we consider a large number of cases ; if we invoke what has been called the law of numbers, the exception disappears, the accidental vanishes, and the law, or, in other words, the essential character, takes the chief place. Thus it is that heredity contributes to the formation of national character. A certain turn of mind may easily fail to be perpetuated in a family; but if it is common to a tribe, a people, a race, it is safe to say that it must be perpetuated. We have seen how closely at bottom the French mind resembles the Gallic mind, as described by Strabo, Diodorus Siculus, and other ancient historians. Thus, in the formation and conservation of the special character of a family or of a nation, heredity is a very important factor. But not to dwell here on this

point, which is not so much a consequence of heredity as the law
itself, under its most perfect form, we pass on to the consideration
of another still more curious point, not so well known, and more
difficult to prove, but which, from its bearing on intelligence, constitutes an important consequence of heredity. It may thus be
stated under an ideal form, that is, without taking into account the
exceptions : heredity, acting by way of accumulation, augments
intelligence in successive generations, and thus makes it capable
of fresh developments.

This we will now endeavour to prove.

We will first point out the physiological grounds of the fact
under consideration.   It is well known that every organ is
developed by exercise : in the blacksmith the muscles of the
arms ; in the pedestrian, those of the legs.   The organ produces
the function, but the function in turn reacts on the organ and
develops it.   We can scarcely doubt that this holds good with
regard to the brain, that it grows by exercise, and that this augmentation is transmissible by heredity.   Dr. Brocas, on the
strength of various researches, says that the capacity of the skull,
and consequently the volume of the brain, corresponds with the
degree of intelligence of the different races : the largest are found
in the white race, then in the Caucasian, next in the negroes of
Africa—the Australian negro holds the last rank.   Albert, of
Bonn, says that having dissected the brains of several persons
who had for years been accustomed to mental work, he found in
all the cerebral substance very firm, and the grey matter and the
convolutions highly developed.   'The augmentation of the mass
of the brain,' he says, 'is proved partly by the difference existing
between cultured and uncultured people, and partly by the increased volume of brain which results from the progress of
civilization in Europe ; an increase which accumulates, by reason
of heredity, in a degree which admits of demonstration.' *(Mit
Hülfe der Vererbung sich so weit summirt, dass es constatirt werden
kann.)*   In fact, we find that among the educated classes the
size of the head is usually large, and that the contrary is the
case among the uneducated.   Finally, there is a fact which directly
concerns the question in hand : excavations made in cemeteries
show that the size of skulls has increased since the Middle Ages.

Dr. Broca compared together one hundred and twenty-five skulls from the crypt of the old church of Saint-Barthélemi, in Paris (twelfth century), one hundred and twenty-five skulls from the Cimetière des Innocents, used from the thirteenth to the eighteenth century, and one hundred and twenty-five skulls from the old Cimetière de l'Ouest, open from 1788 till 1824.

Here are the results of this comparison, so far as regards the mean capacity of the crania.

		Mean Capacity.		
Skulls of the twelfth century	84·777	cubic inches
„	Cim. des Innocents	83·783	„	„
„	Nineteenth century	86·901	„	„

It will be seen that the mean capacity of the skulls belonging to the present century possesses a decided superiority. As regards the inferiority of the skulls from the Cimetière des Innocents to those of the twelfth century, Dr. Broca explains it by observing that the crypts of the church of the 'Cité' were used by the upper classes ; while as for the crania from Les Innocents, it is beyond doubt that they belong to the lower classes, Philip Augustus having presented that plot of ground to the city of Paris as a burying place for the poor.

Resting on these physiological data, Gall and his disciples, as also Auguste Comte, Pritchard, and others in more recent times, have held that the mental faculties are capable of augmentation, inasmuch as they are transmissible. The conclusion appears logical. Intelligence has for its condition, for its chief organ, the brain ; the brain grows by exercise, and this growth is transmissible by heredity. Hence it is perfectly fair to conclude that every modification, every improvement of an organ, imports a modification, an improvement in function, and that consequently the development of the brain implies development of the intelligence.

But this important fact, that progress of the intelligence is possible, not only in the individual, but also in the race; that heredity transmits and accumulates trifling modifications, we should wish to establish directly by psychological arguments, and not by resorting to physiology, as we have just done. It is a difficult task, and we can only attempt it.

We will first try to understand upon what condition the progress of intelligence takes place in the individual. It proceeds by a gradual evolution. The mind can at first grasp simple facts, then more complex ones, next simple relations, and then relations more and more complicated. Each stage of this progress has its condition in an anterior progress, which must have been realized previously, and which alone makes the following one possible. The intelligence may be compared to a building, in which each course of masonry must be laid securely in order to receive another. Or, if with certain contemporary philosophers we compare the act of cognition to a correspondence between the internal states of the subject and the external states of the object, we may say that the mind must first correspond with very simple relations in order to rise to those which are highly complex.

This difference, about which there is no question in theory, is forgotten in practice. Doubtless where there are problems strictly dependent on one another, as in mathematics, the mind cannot but follow the natural course; but in the domain of the social and political sciences, nothing is more common than for people to begin at the end. Hence so many vain theories and erroneous doctrines, the mind being unable to understand what is complex, since it has not first grasped what is simple. For it is a mistake to suppose that it is sufficient to bring a gifted, intelligent mind face to face with such and such facts, and that it will understand them at once. A thousand instances prove the contrary. Let a person, intelligent, but of imperfect culture, read Grecian or Roman history, and we are surprised, amazed, at the misinterpretations he will make of it. The Middle Ages abounded in blunders of this sort whenever an attempt was made to describe a world different from that which then existed. See how the Trojan war, Cæsar and Alexander are travestied in the poems of chivalry, or in the quaint pictures of the fifteenth century.[1] This is shown still better by an example from savage life. A native of New Zealand, intelligent and curious, connected with the chief families of his country, accompanied an English traveller to London for educa-

---

[1] For example, see at the Campana Museum the adventures of Theseus and Ariadne, with cavaliers, pages, churches, gothic houses, narrow streets, battlements, etc.

tion, but owing to the imperfect development of his mind he could understand nothing of our European civilization, and interpreted everything according to the notions of a savage. Thus, when a rich man passed, he would say, 'That man has a good deal to eat,' unable to understand wealth in any other way.

The mind must certainly be first moulded by previous culture in order to enter on complex questions, and this is true of the species no less than of the individual. In the individual all progress of the intellect becomes, when fixed by memory, the basis and the condition of further progress; in the species all progress of the intelligence becomes, when fixed by heredity, the basis and the condition of further progress. Heredity plays, in regard to the species, nearly the same part that memory plays in regard to the individual.

If in our literary history we make some unexpected comparison —as, for example, between men of letters of the fifth century and those of the eighteenth; between Gregory of Tours and Tredegarius, etc., and Voltaire, Diderot and the whole Encyclopedistes; or between the court of Charlemagne and our romantic movement of the nineteenth century—the discord is so complete, the contrast so great, that the comparison seems to be simply whimsical. There is, between the intellectual forms of the two epochs compared, an immense difference, which it is usually said proceeds from progress and civilization.

We are told, and it is proved to us, how the French mind reached its apogee after much groping and many efforts and failures. But this progress is explained altogether by external causes— the influence of Christian beliefs, the crusades, great discoveries, Greek and Latin culture, the Renaissance, etc. But there is also, it seems to us, an internal cause of which we hear nothing; the gradual transformation of the intelligence by heredity. The average French mind in the sixth and ninth centuries was capable only of a certain degree of culture; beyond that it understood nothing, and distorted everything, after the manner of the New Zealand savage. But this average mental constitution, improved by culture, was bequeathed, principal and interest, to the next generation, and so on for ten or twelve centuries.

This is no mere hypothesis, although it would be difficult to establish it to demonstration. Yet, if we open the *Collection des Historiens de Gaule et de France*, and if, glancing at the chronicles and memoirs of the Middle Ages, we disregard the subjects which have specially engaged the minds of historians—accounts of battles, sieges, captures of hamlets, alliances and treaties of peace—and direct our attention to what they often regard as of no importance for history—that is to say, anecdotes, miracles, and dreams which give every minute and individual detail—we cannot fail to arrive at the conclusion that the state of the intellect was not then the same as to-day, and that the difference between the two epochs is constitutional, organic. It is, however, difficult to define in what the difference consists. It would require an acute mind, well acquainted with medical science, and possessed of good psychological insight, to define it exactly. In general terms, it may be said that it consists in this, that the Middle Ages felt what the eighteenth century has thought; that in the one the affections predominated, in the other reason; that a brain in the Middle Ages was full of sensations and images, in the eighteenth century it was full of abstractions and ideas.

Certainly in no period have men dwelt more in the region of imagination, sentiment, and dreams. This is abundantly shown in Gothic art, in chivalry, in the writings of Dante and of the various schools of mystics.[1] With the exception of a few extraordinary minds and a few dry school-men, that whole period lived altogether in sentiment. The circumstances of the times were favourable to this state of things—constant wars, battles, sieges pillage, violent emotions of every kind. The sentiment, continually excited and quickened, became exaggerated like an hypertrophied organ. Hence this curious result, that the excessive development of sensitiveness checked the development of the intelligence. In this feverish storm of emotions and impressions, cool, calm judgment appeared at a disadvantage. Then were the minds of children in the bodies of men. Whereas we find ourselves, from the period of infancy, in an atmosphere of science,

---

[1] *E.g.* the schools of St. Victor, St. Bernard, Gerson, etc., and the great German mystics of the 14th century, Eckardt, Tauler, and Henry Suso. We might mention also Raymond Lulle, whose life was so romantic and eccentric.

reason, method and rational explanations, whose special effect is to develop the mind; they, on the contrary, were the prey of wild passions, tossed from pole to pole of thought, from orgies to ecstasies, by some conversion sudden as a thunderclap. As they felt much and thought little, they knew nothing even in old age, whereas we even in childhood know much. They died young, we are born old.

Hence it is that their chroniclers give those accounts of miracles, prodigies, apparitions and dreams which succeed each other without end or truce, sometimes touching and poetic, oftener extravagant and puerile. They are at home in this world of imagination; to them a prodigy appears perfectly simple, an apparition quite natural; miracle is, for them, matter of course. These things they recount simply, and without the shadow of a doubt, as they do a siege or battle. The universe, which for us is an infinitely complex mechanism, ruled by fixed laws down to its minutest details, was for them a wondrous stage, whereon mysterious personages moved the scenes. If, now, we bring all these facts together, and endeavour to trace them to their cause—that is, to the habitual state of the human soul which produced them—we shall, without much difficulty, find that the chief characteristic of the Middle Ages was lively imagination, internal vision. But experimental psychology proves, beyond the possibility of a doubt, that the difference between lively imagination and hallucination is only a difference of degree; so that, indeed, every great artist, every *seer*, is more or less subject to hallucination. Hence we are led to conclude that the Middle Ages were ever on the border of hallucination, if they did not overstep it. In several of these chroniclers' stories we also meet with the oppression of nightmare, and with the painful visions accompanying it; for generally the visions are painful, though usually so distinct, so full and minute in detail, that we feel that this has been *seen*.[1]

---

[1] Marvellous stories abound in nearly all these chronicles, and we might mention in particular, Gregory of Tours, Frodoardus, Mathew of Westminster, Raoul Glaber, and Guibert de Nogent in his *Life*. The two latter authors are specially interesting from our present point of view. It would be impossible to find hallucination better characterized than in the two following narratives :—

We are now, after a long circuit, able to resolve our problem and to reach a conclusion. It may be remembered that we have already endeavoured to show that for every habitual mental state there is an habitual state of brain, and thence deduced the fact that for the mediæval state of semi-hallucination there must have been a corresponding cerebral state, and another for the precise, accurate mind of the eighteenth century. This transition was effected by a slow progress—that is to say, that education and culture produced in the mind and brain trifling though stable modifications, which were handed down, preserved, and accumulated by heredity. Thus was formed an average intellectual constitution, more and more able to conceive abstract ideas, and consequently less and less able to perform mental operations by means of visions and impressions.

It has often been observed that among the inferior races children who are sent to school, or whom an effort is made to instruct, at first show a surprising facility, but this suddenly ceases. Thus, the Sandwich Islanders have an excellent memory, learn by

---

'One night, before matins, I saw before me, at the foot of my bed, an ugly little monster in human form. He appeared to me to be of middle stature, with skinny neck, slender figure, deep-black eyes, narrow, wrinkled forehead, flat nose, wide mouth, swollen lips, short, weak chin, goat's beard, narrow pointed ears, unkempt, lank hair, teeth like those of a dog, sharp pole, prominent chest, a hump on his back, pendant buttocks, and dirty garments. He seized the side of the bed whereon I lay, shook it with fearful violence, and kept saying: You have not long to remain here. Suddenly I awoke in alarm. . . . I leaped out of my bed, ran to the monastery, threw myself at the foot of the altar, and there remained prostrate for a long time, frozen stiff, as it were, with fright.' R. Glaber, Book v. ch. i.

He saw the same devil on two other occasions. We find all the horror of nightmare in the following narrative from Guibert de Nogent :—

'On a certain night, having been awakened by my sufferings—it was in winter, I believe—as I lay in my bed, thinking I should be in greater safety owing to the proximity of a lamp which gave a bright light, lo, all of a sudden, amid the profound silence of the night I thought I heard several voices from above. At the same moment my head received a shock as though I were dreaming; I lost the use of my senses, and thought I saw a certain dead person appear, the while some one shouted out that he had died in the bath. Alarmed at this apparition, I leaped from my place and uttered a cry; I saw that my lamp was out, and amid the fearful gloom discerned the demon, in his proper shape, standing erect, and beside the dead man.' Guibert de Nogent, i. xv.

heart with wonderful rapidity; but cannot use their thinking faculties. 'In childhood,' says Sir Samuel Baker, 'the young negro is more advanced than the white of the same age, but his mind does not bear the fruit of which it gave promise.' 'In New Zealand,' says Thompson, 'children of ten years are more intelligent than English children; still, very few New Zealanders are capable of receiving, in their higher faculties, a culture equal to that of the English.' One of the reasons given in the United States for not educating negro children with the whites is, that after a certain age their progress does not correspond; the intelligence of the negro appearing to be incapable of going beyond a certain point. Now if these facts are not to be attributed to an incurable defect of the nature, we have here an argument in favour of heredity. These savage minds are, as it were, uncultivated lands, which can only be broken up by the continuous toil of generations. Hence it is that in India the children of Brahmins, sprung from a class that has long been cultivated, display intelligence, insight, docility; while, according to the experience of missionaries, children of the other castes are considerably their inferiors in these respects. Again, a nation cannot with impunity be robbed of the most intelligent and the bravest of its population, for that is a selection in the wrong way, and its consequences are deplorable. 'By martyrdom and imprisonment,' says Galton, 'the Spanish nation was drained of free-thinkers at the rate of 1,000 persons annually, for the three centuries between 1481 and 1781; an average of 100 persons having been executed and 900 imprisoned every year during that period. The actual data during those 300 years were 32,000 burnt, 17,000 persons burnt in effigy (I presume they mostly died in prison or escaped from Spain), and 291,000 condemned to various terms of imprisonment and other penalties. It is impossible that any nation could stand a policy like this without paying a heavy penalty in the deterioration of its breed, as has notably been the result in the superstitious, unintelligent Spanish race of the present day.'

Not to accumulate further examples, we may now conclude with the remarkable words of Herbert Spencer, which sum up the intellectual consequences of heredity no less than its organic conditions: 'The human brain is an organized register of infinitely

15

numerous experiences received during the evolution of life, or, rather, during the evolution of that series of organisms through which the human organism has been reached. The effects of the most uniform and frequent of these experiences have been successively bequeathed, principal and interest; and have slowly amounted to that high intelligence which lies latent in the brain of the infant—which the infant in after life exercises, and perhaps strengthens or further complicates—and which, with minute additions, it bequeaths to future generations. And thus it happens that the European inherits from twenty to thirty cubic inches more brain than the Papuan. Thus it happens that faculties, as of music, which scarcely exist in some inferior human races, become congenital in superior ones. Thus it happens that out of savages unable to count up to the number of their fingers, and speaking a language containing only nouns and verbs, arise at length our Newtons and Shakespeares.'

IV.

All that has been said of the intelligence may be applied to the sentiments. We have, even, in some measure anticipated that subject, for it was impossible to borrow facts from history which should not be concrete, synthetic—that is to say, mixed with sentiments and ideas; it is only the analytic method of psychology which separates these two elements, almost always intimately united.

If I think of any triangle, a sphere, a parabola, an algebraic operation, or any other mathematic truth, the result for me is a cognition, and nothing more. But most of the objects of which we think, or which we perceive, produce in us an agreeable or a disagreeable state—*i.e.* a sentiment—simultaneously with their cognition. Though we class them under the general heads of pleasure and pain, the sentiments are infinite in number, in shades, in intensity, etc. It may be said that every sentiment— not including those altogether inferior modes of sensitive action which are little more than instincts—implies at least an indistinct cognition. In that low region of the unconscious, sentiment and thought seem blended in indiscriminate unity, where they cannot be reached directly by any of our means of cognition. But so soon as consciousness awakens, sentiment has always an object; it is always referable to a known or to a supposed cause; it accompanies cognition; it wraps it round; it is, as it were, its radiation. Thus the evolution of intelligence and that of senti- ment are parallel. Just as intelligence begins with slight per- ceptions, both very simple and very gross, and by a process that goes on for ages becomes able to embrace the system of the uni- verse, and to state some complex problem in social philosophy; so sentiment starts with a very simple and very general manifesta- tion, as the instinctive love of an animal for its young, and thence rises to the most refined, exquisite, and cultured forms—the religious sentiment of Schleiermacher, and the æsthetic sentiment of Goethe or Heinrich Heine. And this transition from simple to complex is brought about, in the case of sentiment as in that of intelligence, by an integration, a fusion into one harmonious whole of many simple sentiments. It would require a power of analysis such as not even contemporary psychology yet appears to possess, to trace back, by successive decompositions, the sen- timent of nature, as found in the great poets of the nineteenth century, to the very simple sentiments and perceptions which are its basis.

Certain forms of sentiment are totally wanting among primi- tive peoples. In the Australian language there are no words to translate justice, sin, crime. These people understand neither generosity, pity, nor clemency. They regard revenge as a duty. The reason is that their understanding cannot grasp the highly complicated moral relations from which these notions are derived. It has also been observed that certain sentiments of a refined nature, such as melancholy, charity, and the profound sentiment of nature, have their rise at a later period in history. The reason of this is easy to find: they presuppose the acquisition of many notions, each one of which is highly complex. The human soul must first have the idea of the infinite, of a vague and mys- terious beyond, to feel the painful depression and the refined emotion which that idea excites. It must have got beyond the narrow, local ideas of antiquity with regard to the tribe, the city, or the country, in order to experience a broader sentiment em- bracing all humanity. The sentiment of charity also—which is, however, very ancient among Buddhists in the east—had its rise among a few chosen souls, philosophers or poets, then broadened out and developed, and during the first three centuries of the Christian era it spread out into the world under the influence of the broader ideas and the gentler characters which then prevailed. Humboldt, in his *Cosmos,* shows that the 'sentiment of nature' is a thing known only to the moderns in the west.

We might endeavour to show, were this the proper place, that under each of these complex sentiments there are many real or imaginary ideas, each one of which produces in the human soul a simple sentiment; that out of the fusion of these simple sentiments there is formed a total sentiment; but for our present purpose it is enough to have shown that the evolution of sentiment is closely connected with that of the intelligence. The conclusion is, that if heredity is the condition of the specific development of intelligence, and if the evolution of sentiment is in strict accord with that of intelligence, then the sentiments too depend on heredity. And here again progress is secured, not only by the external influence of manners and customs, but also by the internal influence of heredity.

Among acquired sentiments which have been hereditarily augmented, we may mention that of fear in many wild animals. Thus, 'when the Falkland Islands were first visited by man, the large wolf-like dogs (*Canis antarcticus*) fearlessly came to meet Byron's sailors, who, mistaking this ignorant curiosity for ferocity, ran into the water to avoid them; even recently a man, by holding a piece of meat in one hand and a knife in the other, could sometimes stick them at night. On an island in the Sea of Aral, when first discovered by Butakoff, the saigak antelopes, generally very timid and watchful, instead of flying from the men, looked at them with a sort of curiosity. So again, on the shores of the Mauritius, the manatee was not at first in the least afraid of man; and thus it has been in several quarters of the world with seals and the morse. The birds of several islands have very slowly acquired and inherited a dread of man. At the Galapagos Archipelago I pushed with the muzzle of my gun hawks from a branch, and held out a pitcher of water for other birds to alight on and drink.'[1]

---

[1] *Variation, etc.,* vol. i. ch. i.

The sentiment of music is reckoned by Herbert Spencer among those which are formed by hereditary accumulation. 'The habitual association of certain cadences of human speech with certain emotions, has slowly established in the race an organized and inherited connection between such cadences and such emotions. The combination of such cadences, more or less idealized, which constitutes melody, has all along had a meaning in the average mind, only because of the meaning which cadences had acquired in the average mind. By the continual hearing and practice of melody, there has been gained and transmitted an increasing musical sensibility.' When we call to mind that Mozart, Beethoven, Hummel, Haydn, and Weber, were the sons of distinguished composers and musicians, and if we note the surprising instance of the Bachs, we can hardly consider these facts to be spontaneous variations. They 'can be ascribed to nothing but inherited developments of structure, caused by augmentations of function.'[1]

And Galton, assuming the standpoint of the heredity of the sentiments, with its consequences, passes this severe judgment on the Middle Ages. 'The long period of the dark ages under which Europe has lain is due, I believe, in a very considerable degree, to the celibacy enjoined by religious orders on their votaries. Whenever a man or woman was possessed of a gentle nature that fitted him or her to deeds of charity, to meditation, to literature, or to art, the social condition of the time was such that no refuge was possible elsewhere than in the bosom of the Church. But the Church chose to preach and exact celibacy; the consequence was that these gentle natures had no continuance; and thus, by a policy so singularly unwise and suicidal that I am hardly able to speak of it without impatience, the Church brutalized the breed of our forefathers. She acted precisely as if she had aimed at selecting the rudest portion of the community to be alone the parents of future generations. She practised the arts which breeders would use who aimed at creating ferocious, currish and stupid natures. No wonder that club law prevailed for centuries over Europe; the wonder rather is, that enough good remained in

---

[1] Spencer, *Biology,* i. § 82.

the veins of Europeans to enable their race to rise to its present very moderate level of natural morality.' [1]

Without dwelling any longer on the part played by heredity in the evolution of the sentiments, we will now consider certain curious phenomena of reversion, or atavism.

We are sometimes astonished to see how obstinately the warlike and nomadic instincts which characterize savage life persist in certain civilized persons, and how difficult it is for certain natures to adapt themselves to that complex environment, the result of a host of opinions and habits, which we call civilization. Here we cannot but recognize a root of primitive savagery, preserved and vivified by heredity.

Thus, the taste for war is a sentiment very general among savages : for them life is warfare. This instinct, common to all primitive people, has been of service in the progress of humanity, if, as we may well believe, it has insured the victory of the stronger and more intelligent races over those less gifted. But these warlike instincts, preserved and accumulated by heredity, have become a true cause of destruction, of carnage, and of ruin. After having served to create social life, they are no longer of any use but to destroy it; after having assured the triumph of civilization, they now only contribute toward its overthrow. Even when these instincts do not bring two nations into conflict, they manifest themselves in ordinary life in certain individuals, by a quarrelsome, contentious disposition, which leads often to revenge, to duels, and to murder.

So, too, with regard to the love of adventure: savage races possess this to such a degree that they launch out into the unknown with all the thoughtlessness of children. No doubt this love of adventure has still a rightful place even in the most advanced civilizations, and it would be a great misfortune for humanity were it to disappear. Yet it cannot be denied that this enterprising, reckless spirit, serviceable as it is at first in opening new worlds to commerce, travel, science, and art, has for some men been only a source of vain or ruinous excitement, the only one which circumstances permit them—like gaming, speculation, and intrigue, or the selfish, turbulent ambition of conquerors, who sacrifice whole nations to their caprice.

---

[1] *Hereditary Genius*, p. 357.

'We sometimes see the reappearance, in remote descendants, of ancient race-instincts that for many generations have lain dormant or hidden, but which now come to light as an unaccountable return to the moral type of the ancestors. The higher classes of society furnish us with the most striking instances of this; as if the leisure and independence which their wealth assures to them, exempting them from the influence of the local environment and the present conditions of the life of their race, set at liberty psychical forces which are held in check among their contemporaries. Thus an irresistible instinct for theft not only is sometimes manifested among the children of cultivated races, in whom it is usually soon corrected by education, but even at times persists in adults, and with irresistible force betrays women belonging to our ancient noble castes into offences hardly excusable by their inability to conquer fate or evidently fatalistic character—unhappy heiresses of the old instincts of our barbarous conquerors.

'So, too, with that passionate love of hunting, which is no longer of use under our present social conditions; which exists more or less as an instinct in every child; which even persists and develops so readily in every adult possessed of the means of indulging it, and inspires all our fashionable youth, and the remnants of our territorial nobility ; it can only be explained by the blind and predestined heredity of race-instincts that have long survived their utility, in the descendants of peoples for whom these same instincts were long essential conditions of life. Here, then, we have merely phenomena of atavism, which preserves, or bring to light at intervals, the psychical characteristics of remote ancestors.'[1]

It would be hard to find a more striking example of the tenacity of savage instincts, and of their tendency to reappear, than is found in the following narrative from a voyage to the Philippine Islands :—

'These savages have ever been distinguished from the other Polynesian races by their unconquerable love of freedom. The repugnance of the Negritos (as the Philippine Islanders are called) to everything that could subjugate them or make them live by rule, will make them always objects of interest to the traveller. Here is an instance of their love of independence :—

---

[1] *Origine de l'Homme et de Sociétés, par Mme. Royer*, ch. iv.

'In a raid made on the Isle of Luçon by native soldiers, under the orders of a Spanish officer, a young black about three years old was taken prisoner. He was carried to Manilla. An American having offered the authorities to adopt him, the boy was baptized and named Pedrito.

'When he was of proper age to receive some instruction, an effort was made to give him as good an education as is to be got in those remote regions. Old residents in the island, who knew the Negrito character, laughed in their sleeves at the attempts made to civilize Pedrito. They predicted that sooner or later the young savage would go back to his mountains. His adopted father, aware of the jests made on his care for Pedrito, was nettled by them, and announced his intention of taking the boy to Europe. He took him to New York, Paris, and London, and only brought him back to the Philippines at the end of two years' travelling.

'Gifted with all the readiness of the black race, Pedrito spoke with equal fluency Spanish, French, and English; he would wear on his feet nothing but fine, polished boots, and every one at Manilla to this day remembers the grave air, worthy of a "gentleman," with which he met the first advances of persons who had not been introduced to him. Scarcely two years after his return from Europe he disappeared from the house of his protector. The mockers triumphed. We should probably never have learned what became of the philanthropic Yankee's adopted son were it not for the singular meeting a European had with him. A Prussian naturalist, a kinsman of the celebrated Humboldt, resolved to make the ascent of Mount Marivalis, not far from Manilla. He had almost reached the summit of the peak when he all at once found himself in presence of a swarm of little blacks. . . . The Prussian was preparing to sketch a few portraits when one of the savages drew near to him smiling, and asked him, in English, if he was acquainted at Manilla with an American of the name of Graham. It was our friend Pedrito. He told his entire history; when it was ended, the naturalist tried, but in vain, to induce him to return with him to Manilla.'[1]

In missionary narratives we find abundance of similar facts.

---

[1] *Revue des Deux Mondes*, 15 Juin, 1869.

Thus the missionary societies sometimes adopt Chinese infants and have them educated in European institutions at great expense : they go back to their own country with the resolve to propagate the Christian religion, but scarcely have they disembarked when the spirit of their race seizes upon them, they forget their promises, and lose all their Christian beliefs. It might be supposed that they had never left China. [1]

To sum up, the consequences of heredity have been found to be twofold. Now it builds for the future, making possible, by the accumulation of simple sentiments, the production of sentiments more complex. Again it goes back towards the past, setting up again forms of sensitive activity once natural, now in disaccord with their environment. For there exist in the bottom of the soul, buried in the depths of our being, savage instincts, nomadic tastes, unconquered and sanguinary appetites which slumber but die not. They resemble those rudimentary organs which have outlived their functions, but which still remain as witnesses to the slow, progressive evolution of the forms of life. And these savage instincts, developed in man during the past, whilst he lived free amid the forests and streams, are from time to time recalled by heredity, by some trick which we do not understand, as though to let us measure with the eye the length of road over which we have travelled.

CHAPTER III.

MORAL CONSEQUENCES OF HEREDITY.

I.

AT the first step in every study of morals we meet the inextricable problem of free-will. We are the less able to avoid it here, since it touches our subject at more than one point. We have already often directed attention to the fatalistic character of hereditary transmission, and the reader must see that what we give to heredity we take from free-will, and that heredity offers an abundant

---

[1] A. Réville, *Revue des Deux Mondes*, 4ᵉ Septᵇʳᵉ 1869.

source, though hitherto but little explored, of arguments in favour
of fatalism.   This much is certain, that heredity and free-will are
two opposite and irreconcilable terms.   The one creates in us
the personality, the character; it is the peculiar mark which distinguishes us from what is not ourselves; it is that in us which is
most essential, most intimate.   The other tends to substitute the
species for the person, to blot out what is individual, and to subject all to the impersonal fatalism of its laws, so that we are
necessarily destined to feel, think, and act as our fathers, whose
thoughts, apparently extinct, re-live in us.   In a word, by free-
will we are ourselves, by heredity we are others.

We have, therefore, to consider the question of free-will.   This
we will endeavour to do very briefly, dismissing all solutions that
have been disproved, and simply exhibiting the question as it
stands in the present state of science.

The partisans and the opponents of free-will may contend for
ever without agreeing, provided each side stands on its own ground
and will not quit it.   Those who hold the affirmative proceed
subjectively, saying : I have an inner sense of my freedom of will,
therefore I am free.   Those who hold those negative proceed objectively, saying :   All things are regulated according to laws ; moral
as well as physical science proves this, therefore free-will is an
illusion.   Each occupies a point of view totally different from that
of the other.

The argument of the former seems at first view decisive, but on
reflection it is found less conclusive.   If, with the greater part of
the philosophers in the last two centuries, we consider psychological life as limited to the domain of consciousness, and if we identify
the soul with the *ego*, then we may hold that the various motives
of which we are conscious are counsel, advice, reasons, subjects of
deliberation, but they are not that which deliberates, compares,
selects ; and that, consequently, a voluntary act supposes, besides
motives, something more.   But if we may hold, as we may with
truth, that besides the conscious life there is also an unconscious
life whose influence is very great on our sentiments, our passions,
our ideas, our activity in general, who can tell what part this unconscious agent may play in our determinations?   Hence the assertion, I have a consciousness that I am free, therefore I am free,

loses much of its value, because consciousness supplies only a portion of the elements of the problem, and by no means supplies them all. Furthermore, this unconscious agency, which is over-looked, may be, as we shall see, the very groundwork, the essence, and, as it were, the root of the will.

As for those who, regarding the testimony of consciousness as secondary, adopt an objective method, they derive their arguments chiefly from two sources, physical and physiological phenomena, and historical and social facts.

The physical world, say they, is subject to the laws of a determinism which allows no exception. Experience proves, and science demands this. Science is explanation; to explain is to determine, and to determine a phenomenon is to refer it to its immediate conditions, or to its laws. We have no intelligible idea of a phenomenon that is produced spontaneously, with nothing to determine it to be, or to be in one way rather than in another. That would be a creation *ex nihilo*, a miracle. Leibnitz, and after him Laplace, have very forcibly expressed this truth. Physics and chemistry having demonstrated that nothing comes into being and that nothing perishes—neither matter nor force—that there occur only transformations, which themselves are determinable, the idea of universal determinism has become a scientific common-place. The principle of the correlation or equivalence of forces is the highest expression of this belief in determinism. Thus Mr. Herbert Spencer, taking his stand on this principle of equivalence, reduces all phenomena, without exception, to transformations of motion ; according to him, social facts arise out of certain psychological states, and these out of certain physiological conditions, life itself resulting from the play of physical forces : ' And if it be asked, whence these physical forces which through the intermedium of the vital forces produce the social forces ? we reply, as we have all along, from solar radiation.'

In a world where all things are so firmly linked together, what place is there for free-will ? What right have you, say the determinists, to break up the series of effects and causes, for the purpose of bringing in an unintelligible spontaneity ? You say, when I wish to move my arm I move it; but this movement is not, as you suppose, a creation—it must have already existed in your organism under a different form ; and the very act whereby you form your resolution is conditioned, is subject to determinism. There is ground for believing that every mental state is determined by organic conditions, and that consequently it comes indirectly under the laws of universal determinism. Even though you dispute this, you are in no better case, for at least you must concede that this mental state depends on those which precede it, and that it is subject to the laws of association, called into existence by association; but these laws of association are only one form of determinism.

It has been thought that this difficulty may be obviated by taking the ground that, supposing the voluntary act to be an effect, it is not therefore a necessary effect, and that causality does not always imply constraint, nor, consequently, necessity. To us this explanation seems not to go to the root of the question. The problem is not whether motives have or have not the character of coercion, but whether there is, besides motives and determining causes, a spontaneity which belongs to the individual himself. We might, indeed, regard our ideas, sentiments, and passions as forming a system of forces, each of which tends to pass over into action. There would occur between them action and reaction, attractions and repulsions, some of them combining to act in unison, others warring with one another, while others again are mutually neutralized wholly or in part. On this hypothesis the voluntary act —the final result of a conflict of forces—would not appear to be a constrained effect, and yet it would not have even the shadow of free-will. It would be so far from being free that, given the elementary forces, we might calculate the act as a problem in mechanics. If free-will exists, it can only consist in that property of the subject whereby it reacts against the determining causes, and in consequence of this reaction determines certain acts.

Before we examine more closely this obscure question, which will bring us unexpectedly back again to heredity, let us briefly consider the difficulties raised against freedom of will by the moral sciences.

Considerations drawn from the general course of history and from the sequence of historical facts are always somewhat vague. The study of social phenomena, classified and computed in statistics, gives a firmer ground for objections. As Quetelet, Buckle, Wundt,

and Littré,[1] have observed, all acts commonly regarded as resulting from free-will—such as murders, thefts, crimes and offences of
all kinds, marriages, divorces, suicides—reach about the same
figure year after year in a given country.   Thus, in Belgium, in the
five years 1841—5 the average number of marriages in cities was
2,642 per annum, the utmost deviations being + 46 and —136.
In France, during the long period between 1826 and 1844, the
number of criminals per annum varied from 8,237 to 6,299, and
so on.

It is certain that we cannot glance at the statistics of the various
human acts without being struck with the regularity of their occurrence.   This proves that man's causality is governed by laws
which admit very little variation, but it in no wise proves that such
causality does not exist.   We entirely believe in the existence of
social and historical laws, but statistics cannot teach us whether
these laws stand alone, or whether there is not besides an indeterminate number of causes.   As Wundt very well remarks, when we
extend our observations from one man over a whole population,
we eliminate all those causes which appertain only to the individual,
or to a small portion of the population.   We adopt the same procedure as the physicist, who, in order to eliminate all accidental
influences, always brings together a great number of observations
and thence deduces a law.   But when the statistician, having thus
put aside the individual influences, concludes that they have no
existence, it is as though the physicist were to conclude that the
accidental influences he eliminated in the general did not exist in
the individual.   The physicist may disregard these, since for him
they have no significance ; but as for the psychologist—who raises
the question whether besides the social influences there exist
causes of volition of an individual nature—he, of course, may not
overlook those deviations proper to each particular case, for they
indicate the existence of individual causes.[2]

From what has been said we get little more than negative
notions about free-will, and, indeed, it is perhaps impossible to go

---

[1] The reader will find some curious statistics in the *Révue de Philosophie
Positive*, for Sept. 1868.
[2] Wundt, vol. ii. ch. 56.

any further. For our part, we are inclined to regard free-will as a *noumenon*, and therefore an insoluble enigma. Still, taking their stand on the ground of experience, and without any pretensions of penetrating to ultimate principles, the most recent psychologists (of the school which treats psychology as a natural science) have given this question of free-will a new aspect, which enables us better to apprehend its relations with heredity. They all recognize the necessity of admitting in man a proper spontaneity, and this some of them hold to be chiefly physiological, others chiefly psychological. In England the chief exponent of these views is Bain, in Germany Wundt.

According to Bain,[1] the germ of the will is to be found in that spontaneous activity which has its seat in the nerve-centres, and which needs no impressions from without, nor any interior feeling whatever to bring it into play. No psychologist before him had ever spoken of this spontaneous activity, or of its essential connection with voluntary acts. The first mention of it is in Müller. That physiologist observes that the fœtus performs movements that evidently cannot depend on the complex causes which determine the movements of the adult. The cause of these movements can exist only in the nerve-centres; and as the nervous force is not equally distributed all over the body, but is accumulated in certain centres, these differences determine the fœtus to move in one way rather than in another. Hence the germ of will-power is a spontaneous excitation; it is a primordial fact of our nature; and the stimulus proceeding from our sensations and sentiments does not supply the internal power, but merely determines the mode and the measure of action.

While we admit the psychological importance of this discovery, and the merit of having clearly put it forward, we do not think that it helps us much. Mr. Bain tells us nothing about the origin of this nervous force, or of the causes which determine its accumulation in one place rather than in another. But he elsewhere has asserted, and as strongly as any one, that 'the true source, the true antecedent of all muscular power, is a liberal expenditure of nervous and muscular energy, which in the last resort derives from

---

[1] Bain, *Emotions and Will.*

a good respiration and a good digestion . . . . that what carbon in a state of combustion is to a steam-engine, food and air are to the living organism, and that consciousness, which is produced by the expenditure of power, is no more the cause of this power than the light from the furnace is the source of the movement of the engine.' Nor is it easy to believe that this spontaneity does not itself come under mechanical laws. Nerve-force can be only the transformation of some prior physical force. The inequality of its distribution over the body must also depend on physical or mechanical causes. Hence we do not see what becomes of this 'spontaneity,' acted on as it is on all sides by mechanical laws.

Wundt, in a very remarkable and important work, full of facts and ideas, which unites to the experimental and positive method of English psychology a certain German boldness without rashness, puts the question of free-will under a different form. We have already seen that he protests against conclusions drawn from statistics, showing that in human acts there is a variable element which statistical science may rightly enough overlook, but which the psychologist must endeavour to reassert; that, moreover, if statistics disclose to us the external causes of voluntary activity, they leave us in absolute ignorance of its internal causes. These internal causes constitute what Wundt very well denominates the personal factor (*der persönliche Factor*).

External factors, he says, we denominate motives, but not causes of will. 'Between motive and cause there exists an essential difference. A cause necessarily produces its effect, not so a motive. It is true that a cause may be neutralized by another cause, or transformed into its effect, but in this transformation we can always track the effect of the prior cause and even measure it. A motive, on the other hand, can only either determine or not determine the will; in the latter case, we have no means of knowing its effect. The uncertainty of this connection between the motive and the will is based solely on the existence of the personal factor.'[1]

---

[1] *Vorlesungen über die Menschen und Thierseele*, vol. ii. pp. 414, *seq.* See also, *Annalise Fisiologica del Libero Arbitrio Umano*, by Dr. Herzen, Florence. 1870.

What, then, is this personal factor which thus mysteriously breaks in on the series of causes and effects? It is 'the internal essence of the personality, the character.' There we must look for the root of will. 'Character is the sole immediate cause of voluntary activity. Motives are always only indirect causes. Betwixt motives and the causality of character there is this great difference, that motives either are or may readily become conscious, whereas this causality is ever absolutely unconscious.' Hence character—personality—must for ever remain an enigma, so far as its inmost nature is concerned; it is the indeterminable *Ding an sich* of Kant. 'The motives which determine the will are a part of the universal concatenation of causes; but the personal factor, wherewith will commences, does not enter into this concatenation. Whether this inmost essence of personality, upon which, in the last resort, rests all the difference between individuals, is itself subject to causality, we can never decide on the ground of direct experience.'

'When it is asserted that the character of man is a product of air and light, of education and of destiny, of food and climate, and that it is necessarily predetermined by these influences, like every natural phenomenon, the conclusion is absolutely undemonstrable. Education and destiny presuppose a character which determines them: that is here taken to be an effect which is partly a cause. But the facts of psychical heredity make it very highly probable that, could we reach the initial point of the individual life, we should there find an independent germ of personality (*Selbständiger*) which cannot be determined from without, inasmuch as it precedes all external determination.' [1]

We readily accept this doctrine of Wundt. It possesses the advantage of showing, on the one hand, that free-will, considered in its essence, is a noumenon; and on the other hand, that on the ground of experience the fatalistic and the ordinary view are not irreconcilable; but, inasmuch as the ultimate roots of the will repose in the unconscious, we may suspect such a reconciliation, but we cannot establish it. We will abide by this conclusion. We have elsewhere endeavoured to show—and we will not repeat

---

[1] Wundt, vol. ii. p. 416.

our argument—that psychology, even experimental psychology, must admit a certain element which comes before us as a fact; this we call the *ego*, the person, the character : no other word will designate it properly, but of it we can only say that it is that which in us is inmost, and which distinguishes and differentiates us from what is not ourselves; this it is by which our ideas, our sentiments, our sensations, our volitions are given to us as ours, and not as the phenomena of something outside ourselves. And we put the question, whether the instinct of self-preservation, which is so strong in animals, may not be this individual principle, cleaving stubbornly to existence, and struggling to maintain its hold on life?

If now we study the part played by personality, not now in psychology, but in history, the problem occurs in the same terms, and seems resolvable in the same way. The individual is subject to the laws of nature, both physical and moral, and is governed by them. But beyond the almost boundless field of determinism we have had a glimpse of the possibility, and even the necessity, of an autonomy, a spontaneity. So, too, in history, where the action of natural laws is great, where, indeed, it is nearly everything, we must also assign its due part to personality, as represented especially by great men. 'The expedition of Alexander and the poetry of Homer are both due to individuals. But had Alexander never lived it is probable that the course of history would have been other than it has been; and if Homer had not lived perhaps the religion and the manners of the Greeks would have taken another form. . . . Individual will, therefore, exerts a great influence . . . yet this influence is but a momentary cause. Homer changed the manners of the Greeks only because the Greeks made his poetic creations their own; and Alexander could never have made his mark so deeply in history, were it not that his will had the same ground as the general will.'[1]

Both history and psychology, then, appear to lead us to the conclusion that determinism does not suffice to explain everything. But if we push our inquiries still further, we are met by a fresh difficulty. With regard to this personality—whose true

---

[1] Wundt, *ibid.* p. 408.

nature we despair of knowing, because it rests in the unfathomable depths of the unconscious—do we at least know whence it is, what is its origin ?

Clearly, there can be but two hypotheses : either we must say that at every birth there is an act of special creation, which places in each being the germ of its character, of its personality; or we must admit that this germ is the product of preceding generations, and that it necessarily comes from the nature of the parents and from the circumstances of the generative act.

The first hypothesis is so unscientific that it is hardly worth discussing. Hence we have to consider only the second.

Here, then, we find ourselves at the very heart of the matter. We imagined we were escaping from heredity, and now we meet with it in that very germ which is the one thing in us which is inmost, most essential and most personal. After having shown, by a long enumeration of facts, that the sensitive and intellectual faculties are transmitted—that we may inherit an instinct, a passion, a variety of imagination, as well as consumption, or rickets, or long life—we expected that at least one portion of psychological life would be found to lie beyond the reach of determinism, and that character, personality, the *ego*, would be found exempt from the law of heredity. But heredity, or in other words determinism, meets us on every side, from within and from without. Nay, even if with the evolutionists we recognize in heredity a force which not only preserves, but which also creates by accumulation, then not only is the character transmitted, but it is the work of fate, made up bit by bit, by the slow and unconscious but ever accumulating toil of generations. The question becomes perfectly inextricable—an enigma within an enigma.

We are not so simple as to attempt its solution. We touch here upon that region of the unknowable to which every inquiry into first causes inevitably leads. Here science ends, and it is as little scientific to hold with the fatalists that there exists in the universe only an absolute determinism, without exception, as to say with their opponents that determinism is only a lower mode of existence, lying outside of and beneath free-will. Though the former school may show very well that free-will is governed by fixed laws, they can bring forward no fact to decide whether the final cause of all things is mechanism or free-will. To this end the physiological and psychological phenomenon of generation would have to be without mystery, whereas such is not the case. On the other hand, when Schopenhauer and his followers assert that free-will lies without the categories of causality, time and space, by the aid of which we think, and that these forms of thought are inapplicable to it because that in its essence it is not a phenomenon, and therefore cannot fall into the universal concatenation—they advance a metaphysical hypothesis, perhaps true, certainly ingenious and specious, but for which verification is impossible; they offer a possibility as a reality.

But taking, as we do, the humble standpoint of experience, we can only say that if character—what Kant calls empiric character—is inherited, it is so only with many exceptions; that this heredity is even harder to prove than that of a simple mode of psychical activity; and that in proportion as we descend towards the unconscious, which is the groundwork of the character, this affirmation becomes more and more hypothetical, without, however, being stripped of probability.

We can now reach a practical conclusion. The basis of morals is responsibility; can it be said that heredity suppresses this? There is no universal reply to this question, but we may reduce all the particular cases under two principal heads.

One of these comprises all those cases where inherited tendencies do not possess an irresistible character. Man inherits from his ancestors certain modes of sensation and of thought, and is therefore disposed to will, and consequently to act as they did. This heredity of impulses and tendencies constitutes an order of internal influences, in the midst of which the individual lives, but which he has the power of judging and of overcoming. They do not, any more than any other internal or external circumstances, imply the suppression of free-will, the abolition of the personal factor, or the irresistible necessity of acts. 'In a word, it is for heredity, as for spontaneity, to give a more or less sensible inclination to good or evil, and consequently more or less disposition to commit faults. But vice or virtue does not depend on either; vice or virtue is not self-existent—they do not consist in the fatal nature of the internal or external impulses acting on us, but in the mental and executive agreement of the will. For all these reasons they are personal—they depend on free-will, and are not hereditary.'

The second case is that in which inherited tendencies possess an irresistible character. Not to speak of those states of well-defined insanity in which the individual is *alienus a se,* where personality disappears, assailed and finally overcome by fatal impulses or fixed ideas, we have seen indisputable cases where the tendency to vice and to crime is a heritage which descends with the certainty of fate. The personal factor has then no strength to react against these interior impulses. Let the reader recall the many instances of this kind cited under the head of Heredity of Sentiments and Passions. In such cases there is no responsibility.

In this unceasing conflict which goes on within us between individual and specific characteristics, between personality and heredity, and, in more general terms, between free-will and fate, free-will is more frequently overcome than is commonly supposed. But this is often not admitted, and as Burdach well observes, with the excellent intention of proving to man that he is free, we too often forget 'that heredity has actually more power over our mental constitution and our character than all external influences, physical or moral.' This we shall now see under another form, when we inquire into the relations between education and heredity.

II.

Great stress has recently been laid on the influence of the physical environment. It has been shown how the climate, the air, the character of the soil, the diet, the nature of the food and drink—all that in physiology is comprised under the technical terms *circumfusa, ingesta,* etc.—shape the human organism by their incessant action ; how those latent, silent sensations which do not come into consciousness, but still are ever thronging the nerves of sense, eventually form that habitual mode of the constitution which we call temperament.

The influence of education is analogous. It is a moral environment, and its result is the creation of a habit. We might even affirm that this moral environment is as complex, as heterogeneous and changeable, as any physical environment. For education, in the full and exact meaning of the term, does not consist simply of the lessons of our parents and teachers : manners, religious beliefs, what we read, what we hear, all these are so many silent influences which act on the mind, just as latent sensations act on the body, and which contribute to our education; that is to say, they cause us to contract habits.

But we must not exaggerate. Some—such as Lamarck and his daring predecessors—have attributed so much to the influence of the physical environment as to make it simply a creator ; and so great power has often been attributed to education, that the individual character would be its work, to the exclusion of all native energy. Thus the expression of Leibnitz was bold: Entrust me with education, and in less than a century I will change the face of Europe. Descartes too, attributing to his method what was the fruit of his genius, goes so far as to say that ' sound understanding (*bon sens*) is the most widely diffused thing in all the world, and all differences between mind and mind spring from the fact that we conduct our thoughts over different routes.' The sensist school, in its abhorrence for everything innate, has exaggerated even this view. According to Locke, ' out of one hundred men more than ninety are good or bad, useful or harmful to society, owing to the education they have received.' Helvetius, carrying this view to its extreme, holds that ' all men are born equal and with equal faculties, and that education alone produces a difference between them.' With astonishing obstinacy he propounds the incredible paradox that men do not differ from one another in acuteness of sense, reach of memory, or capacity for attention, and that all possess in themselves the power of rising to the highest ideas ; differences of mind depend entirely on circumstances.[1]

It is highly important that we ascribe to education only what belongs to it, and that we vindicate against it the rights of spontaneity, for the cause of spontaneity is our own. To us spontaneity and heredity are one. Whether certain psychic qualities result from spontaneous variation, or from hereditary transmission, is a question of no importance. We have only to show that they exist before education, which may at times transform them, but never creates them ; and that the opponents of heredity err when they explain by the external cause of education what results from the internal cause of character. Their argument often consists in stating this dilemma, which to them appears decisive : Either children do not resemble their parents, and then there is no law of heredity, or they do resemble them morally, and then there is no need to look for any other cause than education. It is perfectly natural that a painter or a musician should teach his art to his son, that a thief should train his children to theft, that a child born amid 'debauchery should bear the impress of his surroundings.

We must do Gall the justice to admit that he clearly saw and proved, in the teeth of the prevailing prejudices, that the faculties which occur in all the individuals of a species exist in the various individuals in very different degrees, and that this variety of aptitudes, propensities and characteristics is a universal fact common to all classes of beings, independently of education. Thus, among domesticated animals, all spaniels and pointers by no means exhibit the same acuteness of scent, the same skill in tracking, etc.; shepherd dogs are by no means all gifted with the same instinct ; racehorses of the same stock differ from one another in speed, and draught horses of the same race differ from one another in strength. The same is true of wild animals. Singing birds have by nature the note peculiar to their species, but they differ from one another in the style, the depth, the range, and the charm of their voice. Pierquin has even discovered among horses and dogs imbeciles, maniacs, and lunatics.

In the case of man, a few well chosen instances will suffice to show the part played by spontaneity, often only another name for heredity, and to cut short the incomplete explanations drawn from the influence of education. The reader will remember how D'Alembert, a foundling, brought up by a poor glazier's wife, without means or advice, derided by his adoptive mother, his comrades, and his master, who did not understand him, still went his way without losing courage, and became at twenty-four a member of the Académie des Sciences ; and this was only the beginning of his fame. Suppose him brought up by his own mother, Mademoiselle de Tencin, admitted at an early age to that famous salon where so many men of note were wont to assemble, initiated by them into the problems of science and philosophy, refined by their conversation : in such case the opponents of heredity could not fail to see in his genius the product of his education. The lives of most great men show that the influence of education on them was in some instances of no moment at all, in others injurious, generally trifling. If we take great captains, that is to say, the men whose entrance into life is most easily fixed because it is the most brilliant, we find Alexander entering on his career as a conqueror at the age of twenty; Scipio Africanus (the elder) at twenty-four, Charlemagne at thirty, Charles XII. at eighteen, Prince Eugène commanding the Austrian army at twenty-five, Buonaparte the army of Italy at twenty-six, etc. And the same precocity in many thinkers, artists, inventors, and men of science, shows how small a thing education is, compared with spontaneity.

We restrict education, as we think, within its just limits, when we say that its power is never absolute and that it exerts no efficacious action except upon mediocre natures. Suppose the various human intelligences to be so graduated as to form a great linear series, rising from idiocy, the bottom of the scale, to genius, which is at the top. The influence of education is at its minimum at the two ends of the series. On the idiot it has hardly any effect: unheard of exertions and prodigies of patience and ingenuity often produce only insignificant and transient results. But as we rise towards the middle degrees this influence grows greater. It attains its maximum in average minds, which, being neither good nor bad, are much what chance makes them ; but as we ascend to the higher forms of intelligence we see it again decrease, and as we come nearer to the highest order of genius it tends towards its minimum.

So variable is the influence of education that we may doubt whether it is ever absolute. It is needless to cite facts from history, which tells only of men of eminence or distinction—we need only appeal to every-day experience. It is not rare to find children sceptical in religious families, or religious in sceptical families ; debauched men amid good examples, or ambitious men in a family of retiring, peaceable disposition. Yet we are speaking only of ordinary people, whose life passes away on a restricted stage, who die and are forgotten.

Education is a sum of habits : among civilized nations it builds up an edifice so skilfully contrived, so complicated, so laboriously raised, that we are astonished if we examine it in detail. Compare the savage with the accomplished gentleman, and how great is the difference. The fact is that six thousand years and more stand between the two. Many of the habits which we contract through education have cost the race centuries of effort. Education has to fix in us the results achieved by many hundreds of generations. Millions of men have been needed to invent and bring to perfection those methods which develop the body, cultivate the mind, and fashion the manners. Consider what is implied in the words 'a complete education.' To know how to walk, to run, to wrestle, to fence, to ride, and all other bodily exercises; to know several languages, to make verses, and study music, drawing, painting ; to reflect and reason; to be conformed to the customs, usages, and conventionalities of society. Each of these acts, and many others, must needs have become a habit, an almost mechanical mode of life in us, and a perfect education results from the fusion of these habits. There must needs have been formed in us, by many artificial processes, a second nature, which so envelops our original nature as to seem to have absorbed it. Most commonly, however, such is not the case. It is not rare in our own times to find in families of high, and even princely station, individuals overlaid with such an education as this, but it is only a very thin covering indeed—a glossy varnish that on the slightest friction scales off, and then the true, that is the brute, nature appears with all its savage instincts and unbridled appetites; in an instant it bursts all the bonds which civilization has imposed upon it, and finds itself, as it were, at home in barbarism. We are sometimes amazed at seeing nations highly civilized, gentle, humane, charitable in time of peace, giving themselves up to every excess so soon as war has broken out. The reason of this is that war, being a return to the savage state, awakens the primitive nature of man, as it subsisted prior to culture, and brings it back with all its heroic daring, its worship of force, and its boundless lusts.

As Carlyle has said, civilization is only a covering underneath which the savage nature of man continually burns with an infernal fire.

We must ever bear in mind these facts, and be careful not to believe that education explains everything. We would not, however, in the least detract from its importance. Education, after centuries of effort, has made us what we are. Moreover, to bear sway over average minds is in itself a grand part to play; for though it is the higher minds that act, it is mediocre minds that react, and history teaches that the progress of humanity is as much the result of the reactions which communicate motion, as of the actions which first determine it.

III.

We are now in a position to inquire into the part which heredity plays in the formation of moral habits. Our task were easy enough if the genesis of moral ideas and the history of their development had been discovered. Had some one, taking for his standpoint the doctrine of evolution, shown through what successive phases human morality must needs have passed in order to rise from the lower forms of savage life to the higher forms of our present civilization; had the various stages of this progress been so marked that we might see their logical dependence, and understand why one precedes and another follows, and wherein the former is the condition of the latter—we could then readily discover the place of heredity as a factor in this development. Unfortunately, the genesis of moral ideas has never been traced with anything like perfection, and it is a work to be attempted only by some master hand. While we wait for this to be done by Mr. Spencer in his *Principles of Sociology*, we are compelled to attempt here a coarse and imperfect sketch.

In doing this there are two possible methods. We might proceed analytically, starting from current moral ideas, as now manifested in the usages, laws, and opinions of civilized nations; then, tracing back the course of history, we would eliminate all sentiments of new formation, thus by successive simplifications reaching the basis, the essential condition of all morality. Or we might proceed synthetically, starting from the rudest state of society, and

16

then, with the aid of anthropology, psychology, philology and history, determining the evolution of moral ideas and their steady progress from the simple to the complex. There is of course a point where history fails us. History, being the consciousness of civilized nations, necessarily implies continuity of tradition, whether oral or written; and such continuity could not be found among people without arts, without monuments, and whose records are only from day to day. But where history falls short, anthropology may yet serve as a guide.

Yet we will not inquire whether the human race has ever had a 'purely physiological period.' It suffices for us to begin our investigation with that primitive epoch which we call the savage state. The savage is like the child : all travellers are unanimous on this point. He is chiefly characterized, psychically, by the exclusive predominance of sensibility and imagination (under their lower forms), and consequently, from the moral point of view, by the most absolute individualism. Their impressions and their ideas possess an extraordinary mobility, which finds expression in an exuberance of gesture, exclamations, contortions, and monkey-tricks. They act less with design than by caprice. The portrait drawn by Dumont d'Urville of the natives of Australia, answers in every respect to children, even in the minor details, especially the childish pronunciation of certain letters, such as *s* and *r*. It is impossible that they should possess anything more than the merest outlines of morality. As each individual is at every moment carried away by violent and sudden outbursts of passion, as his life is only a whirlwind of caprices, and as, in the absence of reflection, there is never a moment's interval between desire and act, the result is a turbulent and sanguinary existence, without anything like order or reason.

The first progress is made under the pressure of authority. The wisest, speaking as kings or priests in the name of a God, or of a supernatural power—which alone has any control over those wild natures—impose restrictions on this absolute liberty of the individual. These ordinances, though frequently violated, are nevertheless the first germ of social justice ; and so soon as some regard for property is established we discern the first lineaments of a civilization. Such were, half a century ago, the inhabitants of New Zealand and the Tonga Islands. The former, who were superior to the average Australian, more thoughtful and more intelligent, already had clear notions about the rights of property, and even about the rights of nations—they put trust in the word of their enemies. Theft was rare among them. Marsden says that a chief was angry with a man who had stolen some old iron, and he gives other instances of their honesty.[1]

Any tribe that is incapable of rising to this idea of justice and of reciprocal duties, or of incorporating it in their manners, is fated to perish by the inevitable logic of events. This leads us to estimate at its true value a doctrine still largely diffused, which regards morality as simply conventional. The philosophers of the eighteenth century were disinclined to see in it anything more than an artificial production, based on a primitive contract. Before their time, Pascal had advanced this theory in a famous passage, where he himself did but express a thought previously uttered by Montaigne: 'They do but trifle when, in order to give certitude to laws, they say that some of them are stable, perpetual, and immovable, which they call natural laws.'

This scepticism has been opposed only by denunciation and denial, based on vague proofs. Perhaps if its opponents had accepted the evolution of moral ideas they would have found a better answer, because that analysis, penetrating to the very basis of morality, shows its nature and its stability. We might say that morality is natural, as is proved by the fact that it is an absolute condition of man's existence, and might establish our position thus :—man, considered as an intelligent being, can only live in a society ; this is proved by the most positive facts ; in a state of isolation man is without a mind. On the other hand, society, even in its simplest form, can only exist on certain definite conditions. Suppose a society whose members hold it to be right, or else simply indifferent, to murder and pillage one another; where parents abandon their children, and children maltreat their parents—it is quite clear that such a society cannot subsist ; it will perish by a vice inherent in its very constitution. As well

---

[1] For the particulars see Dumont d'Urville, tomes iii. and iv., *Pièces Justificatives.*

might we say that an acephalous or hydrocephalous monster can live and breed—which would be a physiological absurdity. It is inevitable that every monster and every organism outside of the normal conditions of existence shall perish; and this is true also of the body social. But morality reduced to its essentials—that is, to those natural laws which excite Montaigne's merriment—consists in those essential conditions without which man disappears. Thus, to sum up, without morality no society, and without society no human race. Therefore we have here no convention, and we may truly say morality is natural, since it is a necessary consequence of the very nature of things. Further, we may say that it is immutable, necessary, imperative; not employing these terms in the vague, transcendental and incomprehensible sense usually given to them, but in a precise, positive, and unambiguous sense; for they signify that morality is as stable as nature, and its necessity is that of logic.

Thus the idea of evolution, though it looks like empiricism, leads to unexpected results. If we could dwell upon the point, it would also, doubtless, give us a little better understanding of what is meant by progress in morals. Usually, in treating this subject, it is deemed sufficient to state that morality is immutable in substance, but variable in accidents; which is true, but vague. To hold, on the one hand, that it is wholly subject to change is to deprive it of all stability, of all authority, and to deny what is unquestionable—that morality is inherent in the nature of things. On the other hand, to assert that it is subject to no change is to give the lie to history, to mutilate facts, to give a partial explanation for a complete one, to juggle with difficulties instead of resolving them. It is very evident that the moral ideas of the France of to-day do not resemble those of the Franks in the time of the long-haired kings; and that no bishop of our day would judge the crimes of Clovis as did Gregory of Tours, though he sprang from a saintly family and was himself almost canonized.

Unfortunately for us, this investigation has never been made. If the invariable in morals had been clearly discriminated from the variable, the primitive from the acquired, it would be easier to ascertain the influence of heredity, for it can act only on the variable element, which is subject to the law of evolution. Much has been said about this invariable basis, but very little has been fixed. Without actually attempting to do so here, it is enough to state how the question presents itself to us. In the first place it is evident that if this common basis exists—if there be a certain number of moral truths serving as a foundation for all the rest, however diverse and complicated, and as a criterion to qualify our own acts and those of others—then this ultimate law must be very general in its character, and consequently very vague. Since, *ex hypothesi*, it must be found at the root of every moral act, present, past and future, actual or possible, and as consequently it applies to an incalculable number of facts, it can only be abstracted by a very elaborate process; and the operation whereby we thus pose it *in abstracto* is, though it has a certain scientific utility, really artificial. The law is not thus presented to us simply and nakedly; we always find it as an integral part of a whole. But those ultimate elements which seem to lie at the root of every moral act, and which abstraction isolates, are these: seek your own good—seek the good of others. These formulas may be thus translated : respect yourself—respect others ; but this latter expression is more concrete and consequently less general than the other. These formulas alone appear to us to be ultimate, because they alone are natural ; and they appear natural to us because they are those absolute conditions of existence of which we have already spoken.

If this be admitted, we are, perhaps, in a way to draw a sufficient line of demarcation between the invariable and the variable in morals. These ultimate precepts represent only a very small part of the acts which we call moral ; they are only one element among many. Every moral act, such as is every moment performed among civilized people, may be likened to some very complex compound, to some highly complicated motion, or to some organic product. The moral element proper enters into it as a component part, but it must combine with a great number of other elements to produce the total act. This is the reason why it often escapes our notice. For instance, the act of studying mechanics may seem to bear no relation to the two formulas already stated. On reflection, a true relation will be discovered between them. But as this act is highly complex, presupposing knowledge previously acquired, a certain mental aptitude, a special mental process, a certain professional or other aim— each of these secondary facts being itself highly complex—the moral element is, as it were, lost amid this great mass of elements, which are integrated in one single fact.

Hence the element which we have called invariable constitutes only a trifling part of our moral states and moral acts. The variable element consists of that sum of ideas, judgments, ratiocinations, recollections, passions, sentiments, habits, views often narrow and incomplete, prejudices and errors which vary from century to century, between nation and nation, and between individual and individual, according to the incessant evolution of the human mind.

By taking this point of view we see facts, apparently at total variance one with another, fall under one and the same moral formula, much as the ascent of balloons and the fall of bodies come under the one law of gravitation. If I take in a deserted child, if I care for and educate it, if I spare no pains to train it to good habits, and if thus I succeed in making it an accomplished man, assuredly every one will say that my conduct is worthy of praise. Now if in thought we go back two centuries, and imagine ourselves in Madrid or Seville at the instant when an auto-da-fé is about to take place, we see the court decked as for a holiday; crowds throng the streets, and there is procession of penitents and monks—the cruel pomp is revolting. Yet these two acts, unlike though they be, are reducible to one and the same moral idea—do good to others; but in the former instance this idea is applied only to true judgments, while in the latter case it is tangled in a web of false notions, such as an hypothetical belief accepted as certain, a right of coercion wrongfully exerted, etc., which eventually annihilate the moral idea.

It may be said that this is to assign a very small part to the moral element properly so called. But the fact is that this invariable basis is necessarily very restricted, as we have shown. What perfects it—and what varies—is the ideas and judgments that come into association with it. Hence we conclude that there is a great deal of truth in the much disputed adage—*Omnis peccans est ignorans.*

This brings us back to our subject, which we seemed to have forgotten. If it be admitted that the moral act comprises a great number of ideas, judgments and sentiments, as has been already shown by the influence of heredity on the development of sensibility and intelligence, then heredity must also exert a great influence on the formation of habits and of moral ideas—moral heredity is only a form of psychical heredity. It will suffice, then, to show briefly how heredity has contributed to insure the moral conditions of the evolution of society.

It is generally admitted that primitive societies must have passed through three phases—hunting, pastoral, and agricultural. It is only with the latter that civilization begins.

In the hunter stage, which is the condition of all existing savages, communities live by the chase, by fishing, and by war. This phase is characterized by the unlimited development of warlike instincts, bloodthirsty appetites, and a wandering, reckless life. Savages, like children, are prone to follow their sensual and turbulent passions. Communities that have been unable to rise out of this state, have either perished or drag out a miserable existence until some superior race shall exterminate them. Such as have been able to submit to the yoke of rude laws, imposed upon them by their sages, have in time acquired less brutal manners and less furious appetites. It is very likely that in this case heredity has acted by accumulation. The earlier generations submitted only with great repugnance to laws which galled them sorely, by restraining their most natural tendencies. Yet they in this way acquired somewhat gentler habits, and these habits, transmitted by heredity, made succeeding generations more ready to obey the law. And thus, amid many exceptions and frequent reversions to primitive appetites (phenomena of atavism), new steps in advance were ever possible, and savage instincts continually diminished.

The same is to be said of nomad peoples: for instance, the Tartars and the Mongols. Their manners are less fierce, and their habits more sociable than those of the hunter tribes, but yet their taste for an adventurous life detains them in a low form of civilization. Civilization must be attached to the soil; it requires a sedentary life, cities, roads, individual property—in short, those fixed elements which are its conditions of existence. The Turks and the Mant chus have succeeded, under the influence of laws and of heredity, in losing the nomad instincts of their races, and in adopting the civilization of the peoples they conquered. Others, the Mongols for instance, have shown themselves incapable of this, after their hour of glory under Gengis Khan and Tamerlane.

Nations destined for social life have early possessed the art of agriculture, together with all that it implies : division of property, agricultural arts and implements, and care for the future. Here would begin the really difficult and delicate part of our task, and this, for lack of a scientific genesis of moral ideas, we cannot attempt. It would be requisite to show how each progressive step of civilization presupposes new conditions of existence ; how to those very simple conditions of existence which, as we have said, are the groundwork of morals, succeed conditions of existence more and more complex, which have rendered possible every fresh stage in civilization. Then we should have to show the part played by heredity in the adaptation of successive generations to these new conditions. But we can here merely observe that, the primitive state of mankind being characterized by a lawless individualism, the development of sympathetic tendencies—those called 'altruistic' by the positivist school—becomes more and more necessary in proportion as civilization increases. These tendencies certainly exist, whatever may have been said of them by those who would reduce all our acts to egoism. They are natural, as is proved by psychological analysis. The attempt has even been ingeniously made to demonstrate this physically, by showing that in the lowest grade of the biological scale, where the sexes are not distinct, the individual is restricted to egoistic tendencies alone ; whereas, so soon as the difference of sex appears, it necessarily brings with itself tendencies of a different nature, which go beyond the individual. These gross sympathetic instincts of the lower organisms are developed in proportion with the growth of intelligence.

There is no doubt that there exist in man natural sympathetic tendencies, which are the germs of those ulterior complex sentiments which we call patriotism, philanthropy, devotion to a society or an idea. From what has been said in the preceding chapter as to the genesis of these complex ideas and sentiments, we can form some notion of the part played by heredity in the formation of moral habits, the evolution of morals being really but the evolution of intelligence.

Heredity, however, has a reverse side. If by accumulation it aids progress, it at the same time preserves or recalls, in the midst of civilization, sentiments and tendencies that are by no means related to such an environment. We have already given instances of this. It is perfectly natural to recognize facts of atavism in those sanguinary instincts, those savage tastes, that insane and objectless passion for wild pursuits, that insatiable desire for adventure, which we find in certain men who are, as it would seem, highly civilized. No doubt there is in these vices such a groundwork of power and greatness that the utter suppression of them would be a weakening of the living forces of humanity; and it is therefore the office of civilization to regulate these instincts, not to destroy them. It utilizes this troubled activity by directing it into wild lands, against unexplored regions. There, beyond the limits of civilization, these men work for civilization. Those of them who remain within her pale, but have the power of adapting themselves to it, are but a curse to society, for in them primitive humanity reappears, though its natural environment has vanished.

Then science verifies what many religions have discerned indistinctly, and expressed after their own fashion. It is a belief common to them that man is a fallen creature, and that he bears the stain of an original transgression, which is transmitted by heredity. Science interprets this vague hypothesis. Without inquiring what was the original state of humanity, we may confidently hold it to have been lowly enough. Primitive man, ignorant and idealess, the slave of his appetites and instincts, which were simply the forces of nature freely acting in him, rose but very gradually to the conception of the ideal. Art, poetry, science, morality, all those highest manifestations of the human soul, are like some frail and precious plant which has come late into being and been enriched by the long toil of generations. It is as impossible to govern life without the ideal as it is to steer a ship without compass or stars; still the ideal was not revealed to man all at once, but only little by little. Each people has had its own ideal; each generation has enabled the succeeding generation to aspire towards a more perfect ideal, as, in ascending some lofty mountain, we take in a wider horizon as we climb. And during this gradual conquest, in which humanity endeavours to strip off all that is low and base, primitive instincts, which are indeed an original stain, reappear every moment—indelible, though weakened—to remind us, not of a fall, but of the low estate from which we have risen.

CHAPTER IV.

SOCIAL CONSEQUENCES OF HEREDITY

It would be beside our subject and beyond the measure of our powers to examine here in detail the social consequences of heredity. To trace them through the manners, the legislation, the civil and political institutions, and the modes of government of various peoples, would require a separate work. Heredity presents itself to us under two forms, one natural, the other institutional. We have studied the former only, even so restricting ourselves to only one of its aspects, its psychological side; we have but incidentally touched on the ground of physiology, in order to confirm our positions. It will therefore suffice, in order to conclude this work, to show how the institutional heredity derives from natural heredity, and thus to refer the effects to their cause.

Every nation possesses at least a vague belief in hereditary transmission. Facts compel it : and indeed it may even be maintained that in primitive times this belief is stronger than it is under civilization. From this belief springs institutional heredity. It is certain that social and political considerations, or even prejudices, must have contributed to develop and strengthen it, but it were absurd to suppose that it has been invented. The characters which we have already often recognized in heredity —necessity, conservatism, and stability—are logically found in the institutions which spring from it. This a rapid examination of the subject will show. In exhibiting the part of heredity in the institution of the family, of castes, of nobility, of sovereignty, it will be our special study to throw light upon a point which, in our eyes, is of great philosophical importance—namely, the conflict of heredity and free-will.

I.

The family is a natural fact. Numerous works both in France and abroad show this, and have related the history of the family, described its various forms, and arranged the moral relations which subsist between its members. But with this we have here no concern.

From the stand-point of heredity—too generally overlooked by moralists—it may be said that all forms of the family are reducible to two principal and opposite types, around which oscillate a great number of intermediate forms. The one allows a very large part to heredity, and a very small part to individual free-will. The other allows a very large part to individual free-will, but regards hereditary transmission as the exception, not the law. The former is the rule of strict conservatism; the latter the rule of testamentary liberty.

If we examine the first of these types, we find it under various forms in all primitive civilizations, and it rests on a very firm faith in heredity. The child is regarded as the direct continuation of the parents; and indeed, properly speaking, between father and son, between mother and daughter, there is no distinction of persons—there is only one person under a two-fold appearance. If this idea be applied to the entire series of generations, we find the case to be thus:—in the first place is a family chief, a mysterious and revered being, usually ranked with the gods; then a succession of generations, each represented by the first-born son, who is the visible incarnation of the first father, and whose part is essentially conservative. He collects together the religious beliefs, the traditions and the possessions of the family, and transmits them in turn. He may not alienate anything or destroy anything. He can alter nothing in the invariable order of succession which wraps him round in its fatality. Under such a régime, individual free-will counts for little, while heredity is supreme. This is a pantheistic organization of the family; heredity being the invariable and indestructible ground whereon the ephemeral shadow of the individuals is thrown, and over which it flits.

In all primitive civilizations, the family came more or less near to this type wherein heredity is everything and free-will nothing.[1] Among the Hindus, Greeks, Romans, and Aryan peoples in general, the family was a natural community, having not only the same possessions, the same interests, the same traditions, but the same gods and the same rites. Religion was domestic, and hence Plato defines relationship to be 'a community of domestic gods.' These gods were of course worshipped by their own family, in their own sanctuary, and on an altar whereon the sacred fire was ever burning. No stranger could offer sacrifice to them without sacrilege.

To this necessary heredity of rites, which it was of obligation to maintain, was added the heredity of property. Originally among the Hindus, property was inalienable. In many Greek cities ancient laws forbad the citizen to sell his plot of land.[2] In Greece and in India succession was from male to male in order of primogeniture, and only at a late period in history was any share allowed to the younger sons, or to the daughters. It is probable that primitive Rome in like manner accepted the law of primogeniture.

It is equally instructive to notice that testaments were introduced at a late period, at the time when the state and the family had broken away from the immobility of inheritance, in order to give freer play to individual action. Thus, according to Fustel de Coulanges, ancient Hindu law knew nothing of testaments. The same is to be said of Athenian law prior to Solon. At Sparta testaments do not appear till after the Peloponnesian war; and at Rome they do not seem to have been in use before the law of the Twelve Tables. This allows to them the force of law: *Uti egassit (pater familias) super pecunia tutelave suæ rei, ita jus esto.*

The rule which subordinates the individual to heredity, by making the conservation of property obligatory, exists in a more or less perfect form in the great families of Sweden, Norway, Denmark, and Scotland; also over a large portion of Germany,

---

[1] On this subject see Fustel de Coulanges, *Le Cité Antique*, and *Le Play*, *La Réforme Sociale*, ch. ii.

[2] Aristotle, *Politics*, ii. 4.

particularly in Hanover, Brunswick, Mecklenburg, and Bavaria. In Russia, among the nomad tribes of the Ural, the Caspian, the lower Volga, and the Don, with the exception of personal pro-perty—limited to clothing—everything is possessed by the com-munity, and the heads of families cannot alienate anything.

At the other extremity we find the opposite type of testamen-tary liberty, where the individual, instead of being the slave of heredity, is its absolute master, and may at will establish, restrict, suspend, or do away with it. Here the freest play is accorded to free-will, and heredity, in place of being the rule, becomes the exception. Thus it is not surprising that this rule, unknown to primitive peoples, is propagated and extended in proportion as we depart from nature and her fatalistic laws. It is found in its most perfect form in the United States of America, and under a restricted form in England, in various German States, and in Italy. As we have seen, it made its appearance at an early period in ancient Rome.

We need not here inquire whether testamentary discretion has drawbacks. It is certain that if in France legislation is adverse to it, the reason is lest it should be abused ; and when we observe the evident tendency of those who demand it to go back to the *ancien régime*, we can but believe that it would there be attended by disastrous consequences. It is with testamentary as with all other liberty—in order to possess it a man must be worthy, and know how to use it.

It will be observed that the two opposite rules of which we have spoken imply two different views of property ; the one in which property exists completely, the other in which it hardly exists at all. Under the rule of testamentary discretion, owner-ship is absolute and without limit ; property forms part of the individual, who disposes of it as of himself.

Under the rule of obligatory conservation, ownership is reduced to usufruct. And since under the first arrangement heredity has no place in right, since it emanates wholly from free-will, and as under the second it always exists in right and in fact, being the law, we are again face to face with the same antinomy; and we may conclude that in the organization of the family there has ever existed an inverse proportion between the power of heredity and that of free-will.

II.

The family is the molecule of the social world. So soon as it is constituted society may take its rise. Families unite, associate together, amalgamate, and are perpetuated by thus commingling: the body social is the result of this fusion. After it has passed out of its embryonic phase—the hunter and the nomad states—and when the first forms of civilized life are beginning to be produced, then heredity appears as a social and political element in the institution of caste.

Caste is the result of various causes—difference of race, conquest, religious creeds—but everywhere its groundwork is the belief in heredity. Caste is exclusive : there is no entrance into it except by birth ; no art, no merit, no violence avail to burst open the doors of caste ; it reigns supreme over the destinies of the individual. Here we find heredity invested with its constant characteristics, viz., conservatism and stability. Nothing is more stagnant than nations that have accepted caste.

In India we find the ideal of this arrangement, for nowhere else is it more firmly grounded, more compactly constituted, or more minutely regulated. Moral heredity, its natural basis, is explicitly recognized in the sacred laws of Manu.

'A woman always brings into the world a son gifted with the same qualities as he who begat him.'

'We may know by his acts the man that belongs to a low class, or who is born of a disreputable mother.'

'A man of low birth has the evil dispositions of his father, or of his mother, or of both—he never can hide his descent.' [1]

Hindu law, as all are aware, admits four original castes : the Brahman, born from the mouth of Brahma; the Kshatriya, sprung from his arm ; the Vaishya, from his thigh, and Sudr from his feet. 'The priestly, the military, and the commercial castes are all regenerate ; the fourth, or servile caste, has only one birth.[2] There is no fifth caste.'

---

[1] *Manava Darma Shástra*, book x.

[2] *Ibid.* book x. ch. iv. According to the Hindu creed, to attain to supreme felicity (Nirvana), one must be born again successively into the noble castes, including that of the Brahmans. The latter complacently tell of a devout king

The Brahman has for his inheritance science, contemplation, the meditation of the mysteries, the care for divine worship, and the reading of the sacred books. He is recognized by his staff, by the cord he wears over his shoulder, by the girdle around his loins, but still more by his complexion, which differs from that of the other castes; for as travellers tell us, a Brahman who is a somewhat black, and a Pariah a somewhat white, are regarded as monstrosities, and in no other caste are there handsomer women or prettier children.

The Kshatriya is destined for active life, he is soldier or king; but he owes submission to the lord of all castes, the Brahman, a duty which he has not always discharged.

The Vaishyas practise the manual arts, agriculture and commerce; they support the priest and the noble, who pray for them or fight for them.

In the lowest grade, the only virtue of the Sudr is resignation. Devoted to servile labour, and treated with contumely, he knows no life but that of privations, but he has a faint glimpse of salvation in the distant future.

Thus each has his place, his environment, to which he is imprisoned by his birth. He may not aspire higher, neither may he marry outside his own caste. The time, however, had to come when these four primitive. divisions would no longer suffice. Though the law proscribes and anathematizes extra-caste marriage, still passion and the chances of life were necessarily stronger than the law; hence, besides the four pure castes, others have arisen, and these the laws of Manu, while pronouncing them impure, still condescends to regulate. It would be tedious to enumerate these hybrid classes; for as was to be expected, the development of institutions and the progress of civilization have produced an endless variety of crossings. Thus, half a century ago there were no less than four classes, subdivided into twenty others—and this simply among the Brahmans of the south. Among the Sudr there are about a hundred and twenty, which may be reduced to eighteen

who aspired to the Nirvana, but who, like any other person, had to obey his law, and to give up the practice of the austerities by means of which he was striving to obtain the miracle of a transformation impossible in the case of a Kshatriya.

principal classes. But, as Prosper Lucas observes, 'these non-race classes—all alike excluded from the sacrifices, and destined to exercise the vilest functions—have no more value in the eyes of Hindus than horses, cattle or dogs without pedigree would have in the eyes of an Arab, a farmer, or a huntsman.'

In all these subdivisions the only point which interests us is the part assigned to psychological heredity. It is very considerable indeed. According to Hindu belief, the father's influence preponderates in the procreation of the children; hence a marriage beyond caste on the part of the mothers is looked on as far more criminal than that of the fathers. When a Brahman woman marries a Sudr, the *chandal* (or cross-breed) born of their union 'is the most infamous of men.'

It is curious to observe that the law rests on heredity in assigning appropriate occupations to the impure castes. While admitting the preponderance of the father over the mother, it looks on the cross-breed as deriving from both. Thus, a child born of a Brahman and a Vaishya woman will practise medicine, a profession the practice of which is in one respect a liberal pursuit, while in another respect it approaches the manual arts. The son of a Kshatriya and a Brahman woman, will be at the same time a horseman, in reference to the warrior habits of his father, and a bard or singer like the Brahmans. The sons of a Kshatriya and a Sudr woman, will be hunters like their fathers, but their game will be serpents and animals that dwell in caves.

It is plain that this legislation has been skilfully elaborated and deduced from a single principle—heredity. Nowhere else is the institution of caste so firmly grounded or so complete. It is, however, found in a less perfect form under all primitive civilizations —among the Assyrians, the Persians, and the Egyptians, who reckoned seven classes according to Herodotus, five according to Diodorus Siculus. It was found by the Spaniards in Peru; in grades above the commonalty were the Curucas and the Incas. The latter, whose skulls, according to Morton *(Crania Americana)*, 'give evidence of a decided intellectual pre-eminence over the other races of the country,' constituted the high nobility.

We may even say that universally, in all nations who have risen above barbarism, we find, if not castes, at least classes, which constitute the mitigated form of caste. The class is not as exclusive as the caste. Though birth and heredity are its groundwork, and though it is natural to a privileged order that it should close its ranks against the new-comer, entrance is still possible; merit, energy, sometimes even chance, are strong enough to break down the barriers. History, moreover shows that class assumes every possible form, being sometimes inviolable, like caste, anon reduced to very slight differences for the sake of distinction.

The political institution of classes is found among the Greeks, the Romans, and Germanic nations. Perhaps even we may discover in the beginnings of their history some vestiges of caste. In Rome, at least, the distinction between patrician and plebeian was very sharply drawn at first, and among the Germans between the freeman and the slave. Indeed the institution of slavery, which was universal in ancient times, formed among all peoples at least two classes, based on heredity, and brought about the fact that all ancient communities, even the so-called democracies, were in reality aristocracies.

We may compare with castes and classes hereditary professions, which are but the same thing under another form. It is even probable, as Lucas says, ' that the heredity of professions is the primitive type, the elementary form of all institutions based on the heredity of the moral nature. Capacities are at first distributed naturally ; man follows his instincts, no less than the animal, the family no less than the species. Practice produces habit, habit produces art, and acquaintance with an art gives an interest in it: nature and education concentrate more and more a given art in a certain family, the common belief regards the art as belonging to that family; in course of time come institutions, religions, conquests, which, in the place of a fact, traditional but free, substitute an obligation, and in place of the spontaneous will of the father, or the instinctive dispositions of the child, set up the will of the law, the conqueror, or the priest.'

Here no doubt we must assign a large measure of influence to education, to external agencies—heredity is not all, yet it is much. If any one doubt this, let him remark how in ancient times certain professions of a purely moral nature, which necessarily presuppose definite psychological conditions, were hereditary, and he will see that this heredity cannot be altogether explained by external causes, by family traditions, or by secrets kept and transmitted.

Thus in Grecian antiquity medicine was originally cultivated by a few families. The Asclepiadæ, or family of Æsculapius, called themselves the descendants of that god. They practised their art in the Asclepia, and founded the schools of Cnidos, of Rhodes, and of Cos—Hippocrates was the seventeenth physician in his family.

The art of divination, the gift of prophecy, that high favour of the gods, was by the Greeks supposed to descend generally from father to son. This belief prevailed in Homeric times : Calchas was descended from a family of soothsayers.

The heredity of priesthood is found among many peoples who have not known caste distinctions. It is seen in Mexico, in Judæa, where the tribe of Judah alone supplied the priests, and even in Greece. In the latter country, where the religion was essentially local, and each city had its own gods, we find in most of the towns some sacerdotal family—at Delphi, the Deucalionidæ and Branchidæ; at Athens, the Eumolpidæ, and so on.

The conclusion to be drawn from all this is plain, that heredity is a law of nature from which a people frees itself in proportion as it grows in civilization. If we take one after another all the primitive civilizations, India, Persia, Egypt, Assyria, Judæa, Peru, Mexico, Greece and Rome, we shall often find in their earliest period the institution of caste, and of hereditary professions, and always that of classes. If, on the other hand, we notice how among very highly civilized nations—that is to say, those as far removed as possible from nature—the institution of caste and of hereditary professions is quite impracticable, and how even classes have disappeared; if we observe the advance toward liberty more and more marked through the transformation of castes into classes, and the abolition of classes, as also by the change from the heredity of professions to corporations and to freedom of occupation; if, furthermore, we remark how the influence of heredity is at first held to be absolute (caste), then relative (class), finally, though perhaps wrongly, as somewhat weak (the present period), we cannot but admit that these facts disclose to us a curious antagonism between heredity and free-will.

Heredity is a law of living nature, a biological law of destiny and necessity, like physical laws—a principle of conservatism and stability. Hence it is that so soon as civilizations have attained any growth, in accordance with the law of progress, of which variation is the essence, there arises a struggle between these two principles, and then either progress must overthrow caste, as in Greece, or caste hinder progress, as in India.

From this antagonism between heredity and free-will flow some weighty consequences. We will state these in the conclusion of this work, when we shall be able to generalize the facts more fully. We will now examine the relations between heredity and nobility.

III.

Nobility, whether we accept or reject it, has its natural causes. It is the result of the original inequality of talents and characters. History shows that though it has assumed various shapes, in different countries and at different periods, it has always and everywhere rested on a conscious and intentional selection, consolidated in an institution; this, at least, is what it has wished to be. With the exception of China, where nobility is conferred on principles the very reverse of those prevailing elsewhere,[1] we find this distinction always based on heredity. In the ancient east (India, Persia, Egypt, Assyria, etc.) where the rule of castes prevailed, we do not find nobility in the modern sense of the word—for though nobility is often called a caste, the two things are in reality incompatible. Nobility is impossible either in a community so simple as to be included in three or four divisions, or in a very mixed, very active community, such as that of the United States. But the social state of the east resembled the symbolic ladder of the worship of Mithra, each of the seven degrees of which was of a particular metal and answered to a special initiation into the infinite mysteries of the universe. Each man was born in his own degree, of iron or silver, lead or gold, as the case might be, and

---

[1] In China, when the sovereign confers a title of nobility on a subject, that title ennobles the ascendants, while the descendants remain commoners. This anomaly is explained by the great importance attached by the Chinaman to the cultus of his ancestors ; indeed, he scarcely knows any other religion than this.

there he must remain: the caste absorbed the individual. The westerns lengthened out this over-short ladder, and increased the number of degrees, and we might even say that in many countries this process has neutralized itself. Between these two extremes— the seven-stepped ladder on the one hand, and on the other the almost inappreciable gradient of modern times—stands the true period of nobility, Rome and mediæval Germany.

The great families which were to be perpetuated for centuries by heredity arose in many ways, of which history alone can give the full details. Some conquering race, inferior in numbers, superior in force, often formed a privileged class, and held the vanquished down—such were the Normans in England, the Incas in Peru, the Franks in Gaul. The latter were the only nation that possessed the 'terre salique,' 'alleu' or 'franc-alleu'—hereditary domain, which became later the fief. They were ennobled by the very fact of conquest. Oftener, nobility was conferred by the prince, in recompense for some brilliant action. There were also certain charges and functions that gave nobility, and even some kinds of commerce. Nobility was either transmissible or intransmissible, personal or territorial, of the gown or of the sword; in short, there were so many denominations, varieties, distinctions, and categories, that an author in the last century who tries to classify them reckons more than sixty.

But whatever its origin, nobility was always hereditary. This is its first law. It must perpetuate itself from its own resources; it must have a past history, and must preserve its memories and its traditions. In the state it represents stability. This character of continuousness and permanence, which is the essence of heredity, is also the essence of nobility. It has therefore always been careful to keep itself pure; this is its first duty. 'Nobility,' says the Comte de Boulainvilliers, 'is a natural privilege, incommunicable by any way other than that of birth.' There is no greater stain on character than to act in a manner derogatory to birth. To derogate from nobility is to deny ancestry and to ruin descendants; it is to break the golden chain and to let them fall down below the commonalty, into a category apart—to make them outcasts, for whom society has neither name nor place. Hence those genealogical trees, so carefully drawn and blazoned, extending backwards through the ages. Hence anxiety about alliances, always an important matter, not only for the German baron, who required in his wife six quarterings of nobility, but also of the Inca, who married his sister in order to perpetuate the race of the Sun.

'Nobility,' says Dr. Lucas, 'in the primitive vigour of its institution, made it a point of honour not to mingle its blood with the blood of other classes. In its minor alliances it scrutinized as minutely the purity of pedigree as the Arabs in Africa, or the members of jockey clubs in our day, with their eyes on the French or English stud books, scrutinize the pedigree of their horses.'

To us it appears clear and unquestionable that nobility is everywhere founded on the idea of heredity. The first step towards its institution is the hypothesis, distinctly expressed by some, indistinctly perceived by others, that all kinds of worth are transmissible; that a man inherits from his ancestors courage, regard for honour, loyalty, no less than lofty stature, robust health, and strong arms. *Bon sang ne peut mentir*—Blood must tell. Our old feudal poems delight to represent cowards and felons as bastards, unworthy scions of a great race that have soiled their blood. The brave spring from the brave, and love to proclaim their genealogy.[1]

Hence an illustrious writer of our day attributes to the belief in heredity a far too unimportant part when he says : 'The true idea of nobility is that it originates in merit, and as it is clear that merit is not hereditary, it is easily shown that hereditary nobility is an absurdity. But this is the universal French mistake of a distributive justice, with the state holding the balance. The social reason of nobility, regarded as an institution of public utility, was not to recompense merit, but to call forth, and render possible and even easy, certain kinds of merit.'[2] The author's stand-point is no doubt somewhat different from our own, since he considers more particularly the utility of nobility as an institution, not its legitimacy as a consequence; but we still hold that belief in the heredity of merit is the groundwork of nobility, and that, like every belief that is living and unshakable, it has survived all the attacks, criticisms, and reverses it has sustained from experience. In our view

---

[1] See Homer's poems, which have so much analogy with our feudal world.

[2] Renan, *La Monarchie Constitutionelle en France*, p. 25.

nobility is the result of two factors—the idea, whether true or false, of a certain merit above the common, and the opinion that this merit is transmissible. Undoubtedly, from the altogether ideal point of view, the institution of nobility may be considered an excellent one. To choose only the best; to keep intact the selections made, and from the cradle to fashion them by tradition, precept, and example; to care for them as we care for a choice and rare hot-house plant embedded in rich mould—to do this would be to prac-tise strict selection, with education added. But this is only a dream, as may be easily shown.

First, as regards its origin; nobility, while assuming to be a select class, has never been any such thing, save in a very restricted sense—that it fostered the warlike virtues. It had everywhere its rise in that period of the youth of nations when the imagination had no other ideal than the hero, no other cult than hero-worship, where the only virtue is honour, the only trade, war. Later, in more advanced ages, it was seen that the pacific virtues have also a nobility of their own—that an artist, a man of science, an in-ventor, belong also to the chosen class; but, apart from the nobility of the law, that aristocracy which it was attempted to establish under the title of 'literary nobility,' or 'spiritual nobility,' was never in any way to be compared with the warrior aristocracy —perhaps because it was soon perceived that genius is not so easily transmitted as courage. Hence, the selection which served as a basis for nobility was both very incomplete in principle and often very unsuccessful in fact. The only aristocracy that has practised this selection on a very liberal scale, while it has, in the words of Macaulay, become 'the most democratic aristocracy in the world,' is at the same time the only one in the world that has continued to be both powerful and respected.[1]

If selection is open to question, the dogma of hereditary trans-mission is no more stable. We have seen that heredity is a law of animated nature; that under purely ideal conditions it would lead to the continuous repetition of the same types, the same forms, the same properties, the same faculties; but in that most

---

[1] In the House of Lords, of the four hundred and twenty-seven lay peerages only forty-one are of date prior to the seventeenth century.

complex elaboration whence results the living being, so many laws are superimposed on one another, intersect one another, strengthen and neutralize one another; so many accidental facts intervene, often so as to confuse and destroy the whole, that the resemblance of children to parents is never more than approximative. Experience alone can decide whether this is sufficient or insufficient, whether the law has been stronger than the exceptions, or the exceptions than the law. But to submit nobility to the control of experience and to discuss its title at each accession by birth, would amount in fact to its suppression. But even if we admit that the law is stronger than the exceptions, and that the physical and moral qualities of the ancestors are transmitted to the descendants, there remains nevertheless another shoal on which the institution of nobility must wreck itself—the enfeeblement produced by heredity.

'The citizens of the ancient republics,' says Littré, 'were never able to maintain themselves by reproduction. The nine thousand Spartans of Lycurgus's time were reduced to nineteen hundred in the time of Aristotle. The people of Athens were often compelled to recruit their numbers by the admission of foreigners. Nor has the course of things been different in modern times. All aristocracies, all close corporations that fill up their ranks solely from among themselves, have suffered gradual losses which would have caused a certain reduction were it not for the additions made from time to time. There is not in Europe a single national nobility the majority of which dates from considerable antiquity.'[1]

Benoiston de Châteauneuf, in a curious *Mémoire statistique sur la durée des familles nobles en France*, shows that the average duration is not more than three hundred years. He finds the causes of this in primogeniture, consanguineous marriages, and, above all, war and duelling. We must, however, believe that the fact is regulated by more general causes, for the same author admits that his researches into the extinction of mercantile families and those of the lower classes have led to the same results. Of four hundred and eighty-seven families admitted into the citizenship of Berne between the years 1583 and 1654,

---

[1] *De la Philosophie Positive,* 1845.

less than half (two hundred and seven) remained at the end of a century, and in 1783 there remained only one hundred and sixty-eight, or one-third. Of the hundred and twelve families constituting the federal council of the canton of Berne in 1653, there remained, in the year 1796, only fifty-eight.[1]

'The degeneration of the race in noble families,' says Moreau of Tours, 'has been noted by sundry writers. Pope remarked that the noble air which the English aristocracy ought to have worn was the one thing they did not at all possess; that it was a saying in Spain that when a grandee was announced in a drawing-room you must expect to see a sort of abortion; finally, in France, any one who saw the men that constituted the higher ranks might suppose that he was in presence of a company of invalids. The Marquis de Mirabeau himself, in his *Ami des Hommes*, speaks of them as pygmies, or withered and starved plants.' We have already endeavoured to determine the causes of this physical and mental degeneration, by showing that heredity is a force ever contending against opposite forces, that it has its own struggle for life, and that in each generation, even when victorious, it comes out of the contest much weakened by its losses.

We have now seen the difficulties which criticism based on experience might bring against nobility considered as a natural fact. We need not here inquire into its value as an institution. It is certain that its influence has not been always evil, and that it has indeed 'called forth certain kinds of merit.' But such is the condition of human affairs that we must overlook much evil where a little good is done. Man is so small, that in order to become great he must cease to be himself—he must be blotted out, sacrificed in the interest of an idea, a caste, a corporation, a country, a lineage which he shall represent. Thrown into the infinity of time, like a waif on the boundless ocean, he seeks some stay for a longer, less ephemeral, and yet perishable life. This is presented to him by nobility. Who can tell how many vulgar souls have been upheld and uplifted by the thought of their ancestry! Many a man, as he has contemplated in some vast and silent hall the portraits of his forefathers, unimpassioned witnesses of his

---

[1] *Mémoire de l'Académie des Sciences Morales*, vol. v.

deeds, must have felt the heroic breath of those distant ages, whose extinct thoughts become conscious in him; he has been possessed with the instincts of his race, and, strengthened beyond the measure of his own lowliness, he has been uplifted to their height.

Those communities which have accepted the heredity of virtues and of merit, and who have seen fit to consecrate this belief by the official institution of nobility must of course have also accepted the heredity of vices and of criminal tendencies. Hence we have races that · are accursed, unclean castes, proscribed families, and the crimes of the father visited on the children and the grandchildren. History teaches that the further we go back into antiquity the more widespread is this belief, and the more numerous are the institutions and laws that give expression to it.

In China,[1] when a man has committed a capital crime, a minute inquiry is first made into his physical condition, his temperament, his mental complexion, his prior acts; nor does the investigation stop at the individual—it is concerned with the most inconsiderable antecedents of the members of his family, and is even carried back to his ancestry. This is in our view to do full justice to heredity. But in the case of high treason, or when a prince is assassinated, this same people, establishing an unfair solidarity between father and children, prescribe 'that the culprit shall be cut up into ten thousand pieces, and that his sons and grandsons shall be put to death.' The Japanese laws, it is said, include in the punishment the parents of the culprit.

The infliction on the children of the punishment due to the parents is very common under the Mosaic law. The whole human race inherit Adam's guilt, and suffer the penalty of the original sin.

In the Middle Ages the Jews, an object of loathing, restricted within their Ghetti, feared and at the same time despised by all, paid the penalty of their forefathers' guilt—the unheard of, the unique crime of having killed a god. This is the most striking instance afforded by history of a brand of reprobation and infamy hereditarily transmitted. The barbarous codes that sprung from

---

[1] *Gazette des Tribunaux,* 31 Décembre, 1844.

17

Germanic customs likewise accepted the heredity of guilt and punishment, and decreed a general proscription.

It is astonishing to find this doctrine clearly expounded and reasoned out by a respectable and judicious Greek writer, born in very enlightened times. Plutarch, in his essay on the *Delays of Divine Justice,* after a very strong argument showing that the family and the state form a true organism, declares that ' the fact that divine vengeance falls upon a state or a city long after the death of the guilty, has nothing in it that is contrary to reason.

' But if this is the case with the state, it must also hold good of a family sprung from a common stock, from which it derives a certain hidden force, a sort of communion of species and of qualities, that extends to all the individuals in the line of descent.

'Beings produced by generation are not like the products of art. What is generated comes from the very substance of the being that gendered it, so that it derives from the latter something that is most justly rewarded or punished on his account, inasmuch as this something is his very self.

' The children of vicious and wicked men are derived from the very essence of their fathers. That which was fundamental in the latter, which lived and was nurtured, which thought and spake, is precisely what they have given to their sons. It must not, therefore, seem strange or difficult to believe that there exists between the being which begets and the being begotten a sort of occult identity, capable of justly subjecting the second to all the consequences attending on the acts of the first.'

If we put in practice these conclusions of Plutarch we arrive at frightful consequences.

To sum up, we have found a perfect correspondence existing between effect and cause. Nobility is, like heredity, a conservative, permanent force that tends to immobility. But both are restricted within limits determinable only by experience. The institutions of modern nations appear more and more to accept this result, and to disregard all heredity save that which verifies itself. Bentham, we think, expressed a growing opinion when he said to the Americans : ' Beware of an hereditary nobility. The patrimony of merit soon comes to be one of birth. Bestow honour, erect statues, confer titles; but let these distinctions be personal. Preserve all the force and all the purity of honours in the state, and never part with this precious capital in favour of any proud class that would quickly turn their advantages against you.'

IV.

There still remain a few words to be said on the relations of natural and institutional heredity, with regard to sovereignty. Here again we find the same contrast between heredity and liberty, and between the belief of ancient times and the opinion of the modern world.

Originally, sovereignty concentrated in the hands of one man, the king, was absolute. Being supreme head, he was regarded as of a nature high above all other men, and as the peer of the gods.

' The earliest traditions represent rulers as gods or demigods. By their subjects, primitive kings were regarded as superhuman in origin, and superhuman in power. They possessed divine titles, received obeisances like those made before the altars of deities, and were in some cases actually worshipped. If there needs proof that the divine and half-divine characters originally ascribed to monarchs were ascribed literally, we have it in the fact that there are still existing savage races among whom it is held that the chiefs and their kindred are of celestial origin, or, as elsewhere, that only the chiefs have souls.'[1] At a later period it was deemed sufficient to regard kings as of divine race, descended from gods. Such were the Incas of Peru. This opinion still holds in the east, and notably in China.

It is easy to see that so long as this belief existed, heredity must have been the ground on which the sovereign power rested. Sovereignty being divine in its origin could only be transmitted by birth. Hence the important part played by hereditary transmission in the history of royal houses, traces of which are still found in the theory of divine right.

Modern ideas of the principle of sovereignty are the very opposite of this doctrine. The dogma of the national will having displaced the dogma of the royal will, the idea of a necessary transmission of the sovereignty by way of primogeniture is now

---

[1] Herbert Spencer, *First Principles*, § 2.

thought mere nonsense. The consequence is that all civilized
peoples either have abolished hereditary power—as is the case in
republics ; or only admit it as a part of the machinery of government—as is the case in parliamentary monarchies. And in this
latter case the thing accepted is not the permanence of inheritance, but the usefulness of machinery.

The question of heredity as a political institution has been fully
discussed. Its partisans and its opponents have never been able to
agree, for the simple reason that they have never looked at it from
the same side. It is very easy to attack heredity as a natural fact,
and it is very easy to defend heredity as an institution.

Facts prove, say its opponents, that neither genius, nor talent,
nor even uprightness and rectitude are hereditary; why then allow
power to fall into unworthy hands ? Besides, this sovereignty by
right of birth tends to make princes proud, indolent, ignorant, and
incapable. They might have added that, as we have seen, it is
proved by facts that even among the most highly-gifted races
heredity tends to enfeeblement, and that in the struggle for life,
and while battling with difficulties, it crumbles away, so to speak,
in its course. We must also bear in mind what has already been
said concerning the extinction of noble and royal families, their
ascending movement towards their apogee, and their subsequent
inevitable decay.

Its partisans make answer : Though mind may not be transmitted, traditions are, and this is a sufficient social result. The
object of heredity is to introduce into the state an element of
conservatism and stability. Without it, talents, time, and strength
are wasted, simply in winning place ; with the aid of institutional
heredity, a man is placed at once in the rank he deserves. Take
the case of the Earl of Chatham, a simple cornet in a regiment,
and the son of a widow who had but a very scanty income : he
attained to power only at the age of forty-eight. But his son, the
illustrious Pitt, had the advantage of a very careful education, and
was considered a prodigy at the age of twelve. He entered Parliament as early as the law allowed, when he spoke gained the
ear of the house, and at twenty-three became Prime Minister.
This is the history of every great family, and this perpetuation of
honours is of advantage as well to the state as to the individual.

Without discussing these opinions, we may say that in fact heredity, considered as a political institution, is tending to disappear. The idea of a right of sovereignty transmitted by birth finds but few adherents now, and it is commonly maintained only on the ground of utility. The same is to be said of that conservative body found in nearly every state under various names—such as House of Lords, of Seigneurs, or of Peers, Senate, etc. Inheritance, which was its original groundwork, has been abolished nearly everywhere. The English House of Lords, which is justly held to be utterly at variance in this respect with modern tendencies, does nevertheless admit elective members. Thus Scotland is represented by sixteen elective peers, and Ireland by twenty-eight.

In proportion, then, as we recede from primitive times, the political importance of heredity grows less. And if we hold, with the majority of thinkers, that the ideal towards which society must tend is the establishment of a political rule wherein the individual shall possess the largest possible liberty, and the government the least possible measure of power; where the liberty of each shall be limited only by a like measure accorded to all—the only duty of government being to enforce respect for this limitation—in such a government the heredity of power would have no meaning, the sovereignty being reduced to police duty. Here again we encounter the same antinomy—the maximum of free-will coinciding with the maximum of heredity.

We will close with a few remarks on the whole question of the consequences of heredity.

All progress, or, to speak more precisely, all development, presupposes evolution and heredity. Without the former there is no change; without the latter there is no fixity. But the action of heredity has its limits. As we have seen in the physiological introduction, deviations tend to disappear, and after a few generations the reversion to the primitive type is complete. In the moral order there are facts of the same nature—as, reversion to the savage life and to nomadic instincts, and the descent of certain highly-gifted families to the average level.

The opposition between these two kinds of facts, and the contradiction in saying on the one hand that heredity produces departure from the original type, and on the other hand it leads back to it, is only apparent. Reversion takes place when the race is left to itself. It does not occur in a race which, by the long-continued action of natural or artificial instrumentalities, has been adapted to its new surroundings. For every being, physical or moral, the condition of existence is a harmony between itself and its moral or physical surroundings. For every being the essential characteristics are those which are entirely in accord with its circumstances; accidental characteristics are those which are more or less so. Consequently the former are stable, as being sustained from within and from without; the latter are unstable, because, though sustained from within, they are opposed, or at least not sustained, from without. Reversion to the physical or mental type is therefore the result of natural laws, and by no means of a mysterious power or occult influence.

But if the natural or artificial surroundings favour the fixity of the acquired character, and make it a habit—for heredity is only a specific habit—it then becomes a second nature, which is so firmly grounded in the original nature that it cannot be distinguished from it. Heredity, which seemed divided against itself, comes into agreement with itself, and two cases apparently contradictory fall under one law. Other characteristics, however, cannot be fixed, and they appear but for a moment.

If this be understood, it is interesting to see how a contemporary philosopher infers from the two laws of heredity and of evolution the future progress of the human race. At the conclusion of his *Principles of Biology*, Mr. Herbert Spencer ingeniously shows that, in virtue of natural laws, civilization, the cause of which has been an excess of population, must result in a diminution of population. These considerations are so closely bound up with the consequences of psychological heredity that we shall be pardoned if we state them here in detail.

As the perfectness of a being consists in its more and more complete adaptation to its environment, it is logical to infer that all the progress of humanity will consist in an adjustment of this kind. But by what means, and by the development of what faculties?

'Will it be by the development of physical strength? Probably not to any considerable degree. Mechanical appliances are fast supplanting brute force, and the progress of social life has but little influence on bodily vigour.

'Will it be by the development of swiftness or agility? Probably not. In the savages they are important elements of the ability to maintain life; but in the civilized man they aid self-preservation in quite a minor degree, and there seems no circumstance likely to necessitate an increase of them.

'Will it be by development of mechanical skill? Most likely in some degree. Awkwardness is continually entailing injuries and deaths. Moreover, the complicated tools which civilization brings into use are constantly requiring greater delicacy of manipulation. All the arts, industrial and æsthetic, as they develop, imply a corresponding development of perceptive and executive faculties in men—the two necessarily act and react.

'Will it be by development of intelligence? Largely no doubt. There is ample room for advance in this direction, and ample demand for it. Our lives are universally shortened by our ignorance. In attaining complete knowledge of our own natures, and of the natures of surrounding things, we shall better understand the conditions of existence to which we must conform.

'Will it be by the development of morality, by a greater power of self-regulation? Largely so: perhaps most largely. Right conduct is usually come short of more from defect of will than defect of knowledge. To the due co-ordination of those complex actions which constitute human life in its civilized form, there goes not only the pre-requisite—recognition of the proper course; but the further pre-requisite—a due impulse to pursue that course. A further development of those feelings which civilization is developing in us must be acquired before the crimes, excesses, diseases, improvidences, dishonesties, and cruelties, that now so greatly diminish the duration of life, can cease.

'No more in the case of man than in the case of any other being, can we presume that evolution has taken place, or will hereafter take place, spontaneously. In the past, at present, and in the future, all modifications, functional and organic, have been, are, and must be immediately or remotely consequent on surrounding conditions. What, then, are those changes in the environment to which, by direct or indirect equilibration, the human organism has been adjusting itself, is adjusting itself now, and will continue to adjust itself? And how do they necessitate a higher evolution of the organism?

'Civilization, everywhere having for its antecedent the increase of population, and everywhere having for one of its consequences a decrease of certain race-destroying forces, has for a further consequence an increase of certain other race-destroying forces. Danger of death from predatory animals lessens as men grow more numerous. Though, as they spread over the earth and divide into tribes, men become wild beasts to one another, yet the danger of death from this cause also diminishes as tribes coalesce into nations. But the danger of death which does not diminish, is that produced by augmentation of numbers itself—the danger from deficiency of food. Manifestly, the wants of their redundant numbers constitute the only stimulus mankind have to obtain more necessaries of life; were not the demand beyond the supply, there would be no motive to increase the supply. . . . .

' This constant increase of people beyond the means of subsistence causes, then, a never-ceasing requirement for skill, intelligence, and self-control—involves, therefore, a constant exercise of these and gradual growth of them. Every industrial improvement is at once the product of a higher form of humanity, and demands that higher form of humanity to carry it into practice. The application of science to the arts is the bringing to bear greater intelligence for satisfying our wants; and implies continued progress of their intelligence. To get more produce from the acre, the farmer must study chemistry, must adopt new mechanical appliances, and must, by the multiplication of processes, cultivate both his own powers and the powers of his labourers. To meet the requirements of the market, the manufacturer is perpetually improving his old machines and inventing new ones; and by the premium of high wages incites artisans to acquire greater skill. The daily-widening ramifications of commerce entail on the merchant a need for more knowledge and more complex calculations; while the lessening profits of the ship-owner force him to build more scientifically, to get captains of higher intelligence, and better crews. In all cases, pressure of population is the original cause. Were it not for the competition this entails, more thought and energy would not daily be spent on the business of life, and growth of mental life would not take place. Difficulty in getting a living is alike the incentive to a higher education of childæn, and to a more intense and long-continued application in adults. In the mother it induces foresight, economy, and skilful house-keeping; in the father, laborious days and constant self-denial. Nothing but necessity could make men submit to this discipline; and nothing but this discipline could produce a continued progression.

'In this case, as in many others, nature secures each step in advance by a succession of trials, which are perpetually repeated, and cannot fail to be repeated, until success is achieved. . . .

'The proposition at which we have thus arrived is, then, that excess of fertility, through the changes it is ever working in man's environment, is itself the cause of man's further evolution; and the obvious corollary here to be drawn is, that man's further evolution, so brought about, itself necessitates a decline in his fertility.

'That future progress of civilization, which the never-ceasing pressure of population must produce, will be accompanied by an enhanced cost of individuation, both in structure and function, and more especially in nervous structure and function. The peaceful struggle for existence in societies ever growing more crowded and more complicated, must have for its concomitant an increase of the great nervous centres in mass, in complexity, in activity. The larger body of emotion needed as a fountain of energy for men who have to hold their places, and rear their families under the intensifying competition of social life, is, other things equal, the correlative of larger brain. Those higher feelings pre-supposed by the better self-regulation which, in a better society, can alone enable the individual to leave a persistent posterity, are, other things equal, the correlatives of a more complex brain; as are also those more numerous, more varied, more general, and more abstract ideas, which must also become increasingly requisite for successful life as society advances. And the genesis of this larger quantity of feeling and thought, in a brain thus augmented in size and developed in structure, is, other things equal, the correlative of a greater wear of nervous tissue and greater consumption of materials to repair it. So that, both in original cost of construction and in subsequent cost of working, the nervous system must become a heavier task on the organism. Already the brain of the civilized man is larger by nearly thirty per cent. than the brain of the savage. Already, too, it presents an increased heterogeneity, especially in the distribution of its convolutions. And further changes like these which have taken place under the discipline of life we infer will continue to take place.

'But, everywhere and always, evolution is antagonistic to procreative dissolution. . . . And we have seen reason to believe that this antagonism between individuation and genesis becomes unusually marked where the nervous system is concerned, because of the costliness of nervous structure and function. In another place was pointed out the apparent connection between high cerebral development and prolonged decay of sexual maturity, the evidence going to show that where exceptional fertility exists there is sluggishness of mind, and that where there has been during education excessive expenditure in mental action, there frequently follows a complete or partial infertility.[1] Hence, the particular kind of further evolution which man is hereafter to undergo is one which, more than any other, may be expected to cause a decline in his power of reproduction. . . .

'The necessary antagonism between individuation and genesis not only, then, fulfils with precision the *à priori* law of maintenance of race, from the monad up to man, but ensures final attainment of the highest form of this maintenance—a form in which the amount of life shall be the greatest possible, and the births and deaths the fewest possible. This antagonism could not fail to work out the results we see it working out. The excess of fertility has itself rendered the process of civilization inevitable; and the process of civilization must inevitably diminish fertility, and at last destroy its excess. From the beginning, pressure of population has been the proximate cause of progress. It produced the original diffusion of the race. It compelled men to abandon predatory habits and take to agriculture. It led to the clearing of the earth's surface. It forced men into the social state; made social organization inevitable, and has developed the social sentiments. It has stimulated to progressive improvements

---

[1] For details see Spencer's *Biology*, §§ 346, 366, and 367.

in production, and to increased skill and intelligence. It is daily thrusting us into closer contacts and more mutually-dependent relationships. And after having caused, as it ultimately must, the due peopling of the globe, and the raising of all its habitable parts into the highest state of culture; after having brought all processes for the satisfaction of human wants to perfection ; after having, at the same time, developed the intellect into complete competency for its work, and the feelings into complete fitness for social life—after having done all this, the pressure of population, as it gradually finishes its work, must gradually bring itself to an end.' [1]

CONCLUSION.

WE now sum up all that has been said, in order to get a general view of our subject. There are two ways of reaching a conclusion : either we may restrict ourselves to the facts, or we may strive to attach them to some probable hypothesis ; we may limit ourselves to experience ; or, starting from experience, we may endeavour to reach beyond it. In the first case, heredity is regarded as a law of life, of which the cause is the partial identity of the constituent elements of the organism in parent and in child. In the second case, it appears to us as a fragment of a far broader law, a law of the universe, and its cause is to be sought for in universal mechanism. We will examine the question according to both of these methods.

I.

Let us first look at it simply from the stand-point of experience. To this end we need but review what has already been said in the course of this work.

As regards specific characteristics, heredity comes before us with the evidence of an axiom, for it is without exception. In the physical, as in the moral order, every animal necessarily inherits the characteristics of its species. An animal which, *per impossibile*,

---

[1] Spencer's *Biology*, §§ 372—376.

should possess with the organism of its own species the instincts
of another, would be a monster in the psychological order.   The
spider can neither have the sensations nor perform the actions of
the bee, nor the beaver those of the wolf.   Just so in one and the
same species, whether animal or human, the races preserve their
psychical, precisely as they do their physiological characteristics.
Finally, as regards man, there is not one—even of those varieties
of the same race which we call peoples—that does not present
permanent moral characters, when we consider the sum of the
individuals.

Under the specific form, then, mental heredity is unquestionable,
and the only doubt possible would have reference to individual
characteristics.   We have shown from an enormous mass of facts,
which we might easily have made larger, that the cases of individual heredity are too numerous to be the result of mere chance,
as some have held them to be.   We have shown that all forms of
mental activity are transmissible—instincts, perceptive faculties,
imagination, aptitude for the fine arts, reason, aptitude for science
and abstract studies, sentiments, passions, force of character.   Nor
are the morbid forms less transmissible than the normal, as we
have seen in the case of insanity, hallucination, and idiocy.

Having got at the facts, the next thing was to interpret them, by
ascertaining their laws.   Here, in the inextricable tangle of conflicting causes, we reach only a theoretic determination of the law.
In practice, however, we can establish a few empiric formulas
which enable us to class the facts tolerably well.   Thus, heredity
is either direct or indirect ; now it passes from parent to child,
now again it must be referred to some remote ancestor.   We have
endeavoured to show how the phenomena of atavism, or of reversional heredity, may, not inaptly, be compared to alternate generations in lower species ; and how, at all events, those phenomena
may serve to give us a correct idea of heredity and of the stubborn
tenacity of its laws.

Passing from the laws to the causes, we have carefully avoided
all researches into ultimate reasons, and the only hypothesis we
have judged admissible with regard to the immediate cause of
heredity is this : psychological heredity has its cause in physiological heredity, and this in turn has its cause in the partial identity

of the materials constituting the organism of both parent and child, and in the division of this substance at reproduction. Heredity is really, therefore, partial identity. Thus we have been enabled, precisely—topographically, as it were—to define the position of our subject with reference to all other psychological studies. Heredity belongs to the science of the relations between the physical and the moral; it is one form of the influence of the physical over the moral; it is therefore a fraction of one great branch of that science.

The study of consequences led us to practical questions. Heredity transmits, preserves, accumulates. Is the result of this to create intellectual and moral habits—that all progress prepares further progress, all decadence further decadence? Two solutions occurred to us with regard to the general consequences of heredity, the one radical and hypothetical, and the other positive. The first, which attributes to heredity a creative part, explains thereby the very genesis of our faculties; the second, which attributes to it the conservative part, explains thereby the development of our faculties. We accepted the first, as any bolder solution seemed premature.

The question of the consequences appeared to us to be really dominated by this general law, which is verified by experience—the transmission of any acquired modification. When the fact of mental heredity shall be better known; when our vague intuitions of this matter have become evident truths—then its social importance, as yet hardly suspected, will be better understood; and many a question which it were now idle to discuss will perhaps arise and furnish their own solution. Yet it is hardly possible for even the most inattentive observer not to ask whether, if the laws of psychological heredity were known, man might not employ them for his own intellectual and moral improvement, thus bending to his own purposes, here as elsewhere, the forces of nature. It is now some forty years since Spurzheim and others put the question, whether one day we might not be able to foresee the intellectual character of children, the psychological constitution of their parents being known, and whether 'we could not easily create races of able men, by employing the means adopted for the production of different species of animals.'

A categorical answer is impossible at present. Hitherto man has thought more of perfecting other races than his own, probably from ignorance of natural laws. Yet we may affirm, on the strength of an incontestable calculation of probabilities, that parents of superior mental ability are likely to produce intellectual children, and that, however numerous the deviations and anomalies (and we have seen that numerous they must be), still—since among facts of the same order, depending in part on constant, and in part on variable causes, law must at last carry the day—a conscious selection, carried on for a long time, would have good results. But the race so formed could never be left to itself, for, not to speak of atavism, which would bring back abruptly mental forms apparently extinct, we know that heredity always tends to revert to the primitive type, or, to speak without metaphor, what was acquired but recently possesses little stability; perhaps, too, these selected constitutions resemble those very unstable compounds which it is very difficult to fix.

We do not know what man was originally, nor can we tell what he yet will be. But compare for a moment the state of nature with that of the highest civilization. Compare the almost naked savage, his brain filled with images and void of ideas, with his rude speech and his fetiches—a man associated with nature, living her life, and forming one with her—with the man that is very remote from nature, highly civilized, highly refined—initiated into all the niceties of art, literature, and science, all the elegancies and all the complexities of social life, and practising that maxim of Goethe, Strive to understand thyself and to understand all things beside. The distance between these two extremes appears infinite, and yet it has been travelled over step by step. No doubt this evolution—the result of the complex play of numerous causes—is not due exclusively to heredity; but we have succeeded ill with our task if the reader does not now see that it has contributed largely to bringing it about.

II.

Quitting now experience, though not forgetting it, we will endeavour to trace back the law of heredity to some more general law which shall explain it. Whatever may be thought of the theoretic considerations which follow, it must be borne in mind that they are independent of our investigations of the facts: they give completeness to the facts, but they do not alter them. We have nowhere confounded proof with hypothesis.

If we except cut-and-dry solutions and certain narrow partisan views, we may say that contemporary investigation in England, France, and Germany, manifests one common tendency—conscious in some writers, unconscious in others—to hold that, whatever we know, and consequently whatever exists for us, whether in the physical or in the moral order, is reducible under one or other head of this antithesis : mechanism and spontaneity ; determinism and free-will.

In the view of one school, mechanism explains, or will one day explain, everything, and any other hypothesis does but mask our ignorance. For another school, universal mechanism is only the empty form of existence, the totality of its conditions, not existence itself—the appearance of things, not the reality. They cannot conceive of a mechanism without a *primum movens* to give it impulse and vitality. The absolute determinism of phenomena is incontestable; the end of all science is to study it; the office of all science is to ascertain it; the progress of the human mind to detect it where all seems fortuitous and lawless. Every science must accept determinism—at least, so far as regards its empiric conditions —its constitution as a science depends on this. Even those sciences which most resist it will be compelled to accept it. We have applied this principle to psychological phenomena under a peculiar aspect, that of hereditary transmission—for heredity is one form of determinism. Mental activity is subject to divers laws, which are but divers forms of determinism, of which the most general is the law of association or of habit. With this subject we did not concern ourselves. From the complicated laws, each one of which performs its part in binding on us the yoke of necessity, we have selected one. It now remains for us to show that it is in fact a form of mechanism.

In the order of physico-chemical phenomena it is universally admitted that everything may be explained by emotion and its transformations, and that consequently the most absolute determinism reigns in the inorganic world.

With regard to vital phenomena there is no such uniformity of opinion. Many hold that the harmony of the functions which support life in plants and animals cannot be merely the result of the general laws of motion, and that it necessitates the hypothesis of some principle distinct from the organism and subject to different laws. It cannot, however, be denied that all these vitalist explanations have a provisional character, that they yield daily to mechanical explanations, and that it looks as though eventually their only stay would be our ignorance. Furthermore, inasmuch as the quantity of motion in the universe is invariable, the hypothesis of a force possessed of the power of creating motion, of suspending it, and varying it, is full of difficulties and contradictions. Hence the conclusion which meets us at the end of all our scientific researches is that 'we are warranted in bringing life under the laws of inorganic matter, though there are some special processes peculiar to life.' (Claude Bernard.)

There is still less disposition to admit determinism in the order of psychological phenomena. Yet whatever progress has been made by experimental psychology during the past forty years—real progress, though as yet but little known—consists in the investigation of laws—that is to say, of invariable simultaneousness and succession—in other words of determinism. So recent is this study, so little has been done, compared with what remains to do, that psychological determinism necessarily finds many opponents and few adherents. Yet it is contrary to all logic to hold that this category of phenomena is not subject to determinism. In the first place, perception, which is the necessary starting-point of all conscious mental activity, is subject to physical and physiological laws with which we are partially acquainted ; and we have seen that every sensation is resolved by analysis into slight motions. In the next place, intellectual activity (judgment, reason, memory, imagination) is governed by the great law of association or of habit, which is evidently only a form of determinism. Finally, as regards even the voluntary act, we have seen that, besides being subject to the law of habit, which reduces it to automatism, since it is always determined by motives, it always enters, as far as regards its empirical conditions, into the web of universal mechanism.

It would still remain for us to show that social and historical phenomena are not exempt from determinism; but it is impossible to do this here in a satisfactory manner. We may simply observe that it is the necessary consequence of all that has been said. History results from the action of nature on man, and of man on nature; but if nature is subject to determinism, and man no less so, the resultant historical and social development cannot escape.

Thus we find necessity everywhere—at the beginning, in the middle, and at the end of all things. It is almost superfluous to show that heredity is only a form of it. If vital actions, in their production and in their evolution are subject to determinism, and if physiological heredity is bound up with organic heredity, is it not plain that hereditary transmission is one of the causes that introduce mechanism into mental activity, and which introduce nature into the domain of free-will? We have seen that in practice —that is, in the moral, the social, and the political order, free-will loses what heredity gains. The totality of the motions which, according to mechanical laws, determine an organism to be, and to be in such a manner rather than in another, determine indirectly the mental constitution, which, as regards its empiric conditions, is bound up with that organism.

Heredity, therefore, is a form of determinism; but what distinguishes this from all other forms is, that it is a specific determinism,—the habit of a family, a race, or a species. 'The disposition possessed by the living economy to follow the directions previously impressed upon it—that tendency to repetition whence often results the apparently spontaneous reproduction of certain phenomena— is inherent in the organization; it is by it that animals are led to imitate themselves, that is, to repeat what they have previously done; and this, too, leads them to imitate their ancestors.' (Dutrochet.) In other words, nothing that ever has been can cease to be; hence, in the individual, habit; in the species, heredity. This it is which fixes us in the indestructible series of causes and effects, and by this our poor personality is connected with the ultimate origin of things, through an infinite concatenation of necessities. Heredity is but one form of that ultimate law which by physicists is called the conservation of energy, and by metaphysicians universal casuality.

But it is difficult to admit that everything is reducible to mechanism. To us it seems impossible to see in mechanism anything else than the sum of the bare conditions and purely logical possibilities of existence: so that to accept mechanism is to accept the form instead of the reality. We firmly believe that wherever there are facts, of whatever kind, there is determinism; that wherever there is determinism there is science; and that science can neither go beyond determinism nor fall short of it. But is there not beyond science a something that does not come under its law, high above all that science can know, by processes peculiar to it. To do away with it would be a contradiction, to explain it would be only to offer an hypothesis. It is impossible alike to deny and to determine it, for it comes to us at once as necessary and as unknowable. At most we can only say that this unknown is the reality that lies concealed beneath psychological determinism —the end towards which the vital processes tend in every being, and the obscure tendency which is manifested even in the absolute determinism of inorganic matter.

This supreme antithesis between free-will and mechanism, which underlies the antithesis of science and art, of the individual and the general, is insoluble to us.

At times we are inclined to believe that all reality is in the person, that perfection consists in the most complete individuation, and that the general is but an ephemeral form of existence, produced by what is common to the individuals; that beneath the veil of universal mechanism there exists in nature, as it were, a dispersed thought, which is unconscious of itself in inorganic matter, seeks itself in the animal, and finds itself in man.

At another time we are inclined to the belief that individuality is but the transitory product of the interaction of eternal laws; that, lost in a little nook in the universe, the best thing for us is to regard personality as an illusion, and to look with disdain on our griefs, which are so vain, and on our pleasures, which are so brief, to enter into communion with nature, and share in the imperturbable serenity of her laws.

At times, too, we are disposed to think that this supreme antithesis might be resolved without sacrificing either free-will to mechanism, or mechanism to free-will; that, were we to occupy a higher stand-point, we should see that what is given us from without as science, under the form of mechanism, is given us from within as æsthetics or morals, under the form of free-will.

In our opinion, the progress of the present and of future sciences will enable us better and better to state this antinomy; it were rash to hope for its solution.

THE END.

A LIBRARY

OF THE MOST IMPORTANT

STANDARD WORKS ON EVOLUTION.

I.

Origin of Species by Means of Natural Selection, or the Preservation of Favored Races in the Struggle for Life. By CHARLES DARWIN, LL. D., F. R. S. New and revised edition, with Additions. 12mo. Cloth, $2.00.

"Personally and practically exercised in zoölogy, in minute anatomy, in geology, a student of geographical distribution, not in maps and in museums, but by long voyages and laborious collection; having largely advanced each of these branches of science, and having spent many years in gathering and sifting materials for his present work, the store of accurately-registered facts upon which the author of the 'Origin of Species' is able to draw at will is prodigious."—*Professor T. H. Huxley.*

II.

Variation of Animals and Plants under Domestication. By CHARLES DARWIN, LL. D., F. R. S. With Illustrations. Revised edition. 2 vols., 12mo. Cloth, $5.00.

"We shall learn something of the laws of inheritance, of the effects of crossing different breeds, and on that sterility which often supervenes when organic beings are removed from their natural conditions of life, and likewise when they are too closely interbred."—*From the Introduction.*

III.

Descent of Man, and Selection in Relation to Sex. By CHARLES DARWIN, LL. D., F. R. S. With many Illustrations. A new edition. 12mo. Cloth, $3.00.

"In these volumes Mr. Darwin has brought forward all the facts and arguments which science has to offer in favor of the doctrine that man has arisen by gradual development from the lowest point of animal life. Aside from the logical purpose which Mr. Darwin had in view, his work is an original and fascinating contribution to the most interesting portion of natural history."

IV.

On the Origin of Species; or, The Causes of the Phenomena of Organic Nature. By Professor T. H. HUXLEY, F. R. S. 12mo. Cloth, $1.00.

"Those who disencumber Darwinism of its difficulties, simplify its statements, relieve it of technicalities, and bring it so distinctly within the horizon of ordinary apprehension that persons of common sense may judge for themselves, perform an invaluable service. Such is the character of the present volume."—*From the Preface to the American edition.*

V.

Darwiniana. Essays and Reviews pertaining to Darwinism. By ASA GRAY, Fisher Professor of Natural History (Botany) in Harvard University. 12mo. Cloth, $2.00.

"Although Professor Gray is widely known in the world of science for his botanical researches, but few are aware that he is a pronounced and unflinching Darwinian. His contributions to the discussion are varied and valuable, and as collected in the present volume they will be seen to establish a claim upon the thinking world, which will be extensively felt and cordially acknowledged. These papers not only illustrate the history of the controversy, and the progress of the discussion, but they form perhaps the fullest and most trustworthy exposition of what is to be properly understood by 'Darwinism' that is to be found in our language. To all those timid souls who are worried about the progress of science, and the danger that it will subvert the foundations of their faith, we recommend the dispassionate perusal of this volume."—*The Popular Science Monthly.*

VI.

Heredity: A Psychological Study of its Phenomena, Laws, Causes, and Consequences. From the French of TH. RIBOT. 12mo. Cloth, $2.00.

"Heredity is that biological law by which all beings endowed with life tend to repeat themselves in their descendants: it is for the species what personal identity is for the individual. The physiological side of this subject has been diligently studied, but not so its psychological side. We propose to supply this deficiency in the present work."—*From the Introduction.*

VII.

Hereditary Genius: An Inquiry into its Laws and Consequences. By FRANCIS GALTON, F. R. S., etc. New and revised edition, with an American Preface. 12mo. Cloth, $2.00.

"The following pages embody the result of the first vigorous and methodical effort to treat the question in the true scientific spirit, and place it upon the proper inductive basis. Mr. Galton proves, by overwhelming evidence, that genius, talent, or whatever we term great mental capacity, follows the law of organic transmission—runs in families, and is an affair of blood and breed; and that a sphere of phenomena hitherto deemed capricious and defiant of rule is, nevertheless, within the operation of ascertainable law."—*From the American Preface.*

VIII.

The Evolution of Man. A Popular Exposition of the Principal Points of Human Ontogeny and Phylogeny. From the German of ERNST HAECKEL, Professor in the University of Jena. With numerous Illustrations. 2 vols., 12mo. Cloth, $5.00.

"In this excellent translation of Professor Haeckel's work, the English reader has access to the latest doctrines of the Continental school of evolution, in its application to the history of man."

IX.

The History of Creation; or, the Development of the Earth and its Inhabitants by the Action of Natural Causes. A Popular Exposition of the Doctrine of Evolution in General, and of that of Darwin, Goethe, and Lamarck in Particular. By ERNST HAECKEL, Professor in the University of Jena. The translation revised by Professor E. RAY LANKESTER. Illustrated with Lithographic Plates. 2 vols., 12mo. Cloth, $5.00.

"The book has been translated into several languages. I hope that it may also find sympathy in the fatherland of Darwin, the more so since it contains special morphological evidence in favor of many of the most important doctrines with which this greatest naturalist of our century has enriched science."—*From the Preface.*

A STANDARD EVOLUTION LIBRARY.

X.

Religion and Science. A Series of Sunday Lectures on the Rlatione of Natural and Revealed Religion, or the Truths revealed in Nature and Scripture. By JOSEPH LE CONTE, LL. D. 12mo. Cloth, $1.50.

XI.

Prehistoric Times, as illustrated by Ancient Remains and the Manners and Customs of Modern Savages. By Sir JOHN LUBBOCK, Bart. Illustrated. Entirely new revised edition. 8vo. Cloth, $5.00.

The book ranks among the noblest works of the interesting and important class to which it belongs. As a *résumé* of our present knowledge of prehistoric man, it leaves nothing to be desired. It is not only a good book of reference, but the best on the subject.

XII.

Winners in Life's Race; or, The Great Backboned Family. By ANABELLA B. BUCKLEY, author of "The Fairy-Land of Science" and "Life and her Children." With numerous Illustrations. 12mo. Cloth, gilt side and back, $1.50.

XIII.

Physics and Politics; or, Thoughts on the Application of the Principles of "Natural Selection" and "Inheritance" to Political Society. By WALTER BAGEHOT. 12mo. Cloth, $1.50.

XIV.

The Theory of Descent and Darwinism. By Professor OSCAR SCHMIDT. With 26 Woodcuts. 12mo. $1.50.

"The facts upon which the Darwinian theory is based are presented in an effective manner, conclusions are ably defended, and the question is treated in more compact and available style than in any other work on the same topic that has yet appeared. It is a valuable addition to the 'International Scientific Series.'"—*Boston Post.*

XV.

Outline of the Evolution Philosophy. By Dr. M. E. CAZELLES. Translated from the French, by the Rev. O. B. FROTHINGHAM; with an Appendix, by E. L. YOUMANS, M. D. 12mo. Cloth, $1.00.

"This unpretentious little work will, no doubt, be used by thousands to whom the publications of Mr. Herbert Spencer are inaccessible and those of Auguste Comte repellent, by reason of their prolixity and vagueness. In a short space Dr. Cazelles has managed to compress the whole outline and scope of Mr. Spencer's system, with his views of the doctrine of progress and law of evolution, and a clear view of the principles of positivism."—*Nature (London).*

XVI.

Principles of Geology; or, The Modern Changes of the Earth and its Inhabitants, considered as illustrative of Geology. By Sir CHARLES LYELL, Bart. Illustrated with Maps, Plates, and Woodcuts. A new and entirely revised edition. 2 vols. Royal 8vo. Cloth, $8.00.

The "Principles of Geology" may be looked upon with pride, not only as a representative of English science, but as without a rival of its kind anywhere. Growing in fullness and accuracy with the growth of experience and observation in every region of the world, the work has incorporated with itself each established discovery, and has been modified by every hypothesis of value which has been brought to bear upon, or been evolved from, the most recent body of facts.

XVII.

Elements of Geology. A Text-Book for Colleges and for the General Reader. By Joseph Le Conte, LL. D., Professor of Geology and Natural History in the University of California. Revised and enlarged edition. 12mo. With upward of 900 Illustrations. Cloth, $4.00.

XVIII.

Evolution and its Relation to Religious Thought. By Joseph Le Conte, LL. D. Illustrated. 12mo. Cloth, $1.50.

XIX.

The Origin of the Fittest: Essays on Evolution. By Professor E. D. Cope, Member of the National Academy of Sciences. Illustrated. 8vo. Cloth, $3.00.

XX.

Animal Life, as affected by the Natural Conditions of Existence. By Karl Semper, Professor of the University of Würzburg. With Maps and 100 Woodcuts. 12mo. Cloth, $2.00.

XXI.

Anthropology: An Introduction to the Study of Man and Civilization. By Edward B. Tylor, F. R. S. Illustrated. 12mo. Cloth, $2.00.

XXII.

First Principles. By Herbert Spencer. Part I. The Unknowable. Part II. The Knowable. 1 vol., 12mo. $2.00.

XXIII.

The Principles of Biology. By Herbert Spencer. 2 vols., 12mo. $4.00.

XXIV.

The Principles of Psychology. By Herbert Spencer. 2 vols., 12mo. $4.00.

XXV.

The Principles of Sociology. By Herbert Spencer. 12mo. 2 vols. $4.00.

XXVI.

The Data of Ethics. By Herbert Spencer. Being Part I, Vol. I, of "The Principles of Morality." 12mo. Cloth, $1.25.

XXVII.

Illustrations of Universal Progress. By Herbert Spencer. 12mo. Cloth, $2.00.

New York: D. APPLETON & CO., 1, 3, & 5 Bond Street.

www.ingramcontent.com/pod-product-compliance
Lightning Source LLC
Chambersburg PA
CBHW031350290326
41932CB00044B/861